D1708431

Nephrology and Fluid/Electrolyte Physiology: Neonatology Questions and Controversies

Nephrology and Fluid/Electrolyte Physiology

Neonatology Questions and Controversies

Series Editor
Richard A. Polin, MD
Professor of Pediatrics
College of Physicians and Surgeons
Columbia University
Director, Division of Neonatology
Morgan Stanley Children's Hospital of New York-Presbyterian
Columbia University Medical Center
New York, New York

Other Volumes in the Neonatology Questions and Controversies Series
Cardiology
Gastroenterology and Nutrition
Hematology, Immunology and Infectious Disease
Neurology
The Newborn Lung

Nephrology and Fluid/ Electrolyte Physiology

Neonatology Questions and Controversies

William Oh, MD
Professor of Pediatrics
Warren Alpert Medical School of Brown University
Attending Neonatologist
Women and Infants' Hospital of Rhode Island
Providence, Rhode Island

Jean-Pierre Guignard, MD
Honorary Professor of Pediatrics
Lausanne University Medical School
Centre Hospitalier Universitaire Vaudois
Lausanne, Switzerland

Stephen Baumgart, MD
Professor of Pediatrics
School of Medicine & Health Sciences
George Washington University
Department of Neonatology
The Children's National Medical Center
Washington, District of Columbia

Consulting Editor
Richard A. Polin, MD
Professor of Pediatrics
College of Physicians and Surgeons
Columbia University
Director, Division of Neonatology
Morgan Stanley Children's Hospital of New York-Presbyterian
Columbia University Medical Center
New York, New York

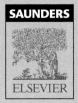

SAUNDERS

ELSEVIER

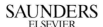

SAUNDERS
ELSEVIER

1600 John F. Kennedy Blvd.
Suite 1800
Philadelphia, PA 19103-2899

NEPHROLOGY AND FLUID/ELECTROLYTE PHYSIOLOGY: Neonatology Questions and Controversies
ISBN: 978-1-4160-3163-5

Copyright © 2008 by Saunders, an imprint of Elsevier Inc.

All rights reserved. No part of this publication may be reproduced or transmitted in any form or by any means, electronic or mechanical, including photocopying, recording, or any information storage and retrieval system, without permission in writing from the publisher. Permissions may be sought directly from Elsevier's Rights Department: phone: (+1) 215 239 3804 (US) or (+44) 1865 843830 (UK); fax: (+44) 1865 853333; e-mail: healthpermissions@elsevier.com. You may also complete your request on-line via the Elsevier website at http://www.elsevier.com/permissions.

Notice

Knowledge and best practice in this field are constantly changing. As new research and experience broaden our knowledge, changes in practice, treatment and drug therapy may become necessary or appropriate. Readers are advised to check the most current information provided (i) on procedures featured or (ii) by the manufacturer of each product to be administered, to verify the recommended dose or formula, the method and duration of administration, and contraindications. It is the responsibility of the practitioner, relying on their own experience and knowledge of the patient, to make diagnoses, to determine dosages and the best treatment for each individual patient, and to take all appropriate safety precautions. To the fullest extent of the law, neither the Publisher nor the Authors assumes any liability for any injury and/or damage to persons or property arising out of or related to any use of the material contained in this book.

The Publisher

Library of Congress Cataloging-in-Publication Data

Nephrology and Fluid/Electrolyte Physiology: neonatology questions and controversies/[edited by]
William Oh, Jean-Pierre Guignard, Stephen Baumgart; consulting editor, Richard A. Polin.—1st ed.
    p.; cm
  Includes bibliographical references
  ISBN: 978-1-4160-3163-5
  1. Pediatric nephrology. 2. Newborn infants—Diseases. I. Guignard, J.-P (Jean-Pierre) II. Oh, William.
III. Baumgart, Stephen. IV. Polin, Richard A. (Richard Alan), 1945-
  [DNLM: 1. Infant, Newborn, Diseases. 2. Kidney Diseases. 3. Infant, Newborn. 4. Water-Electrolyte Imbalance. WS 320 N4395 2008]

RJ278.N47 2008
618.92′61—dc22

2007044396

Publishing Director: Judith Fletcher
Developmental Editor: Lisa Barnes
Associate Development Editor: Bernard Buckholtz
Senior Project Manager: David Saltzberg
Design Direction: Karen O'Keefe-Owens

Working together to grow libraries in developing countries

www.elsevier.com | www.bookaid.org | www.sabre.org

ELSEVIER | **BOOK AID International** | **Sabre Foundation**

Printed in China

Last digit is the print number 9 8 7 6 5 4 3 2

Contents

Section IV
SPECIAL PATHOLOGY, 147

[†]Deceased. The Editors dedicate this volume to Professor Bauer, a brilliant neonatologist/scientist and a friend.

Contributors

Sharon P. Andreoli, MD

Byron P. and Frances D. Hollet Professor of Pediatrics
Director of Pediatric Nephrology
James Whitcomb Riley Hospital for Children
Indiana University Medical Center
Indianapolis, Indiana
Renal Failure in the Neonate

Karl Bauer, MD[†]

Professor of Neonatology
Head, Division of Neonatology
Neonatology, Department of Pediatrics
Johann Wolfgang von Goethe University
Frankfurt, Germany
Body Fluid Compartments in the Fetus and Newborn Infant with Growth Aberration

Stephen Baumgart, MD

Professor of Pediatrics
School of Medicine & Health Sciences
George Washington University
Department of Neonatology
The Children's National Medical Center
Washington, District of Columbia
Acute Problems of Prematurity: Balancing Fluid Volume and Electrolyte Replacements in Very Low Birth Weight (VLBW) and Extremely Low Birth Weight (ELBW) Neonates

Marie H. Beall, MD

Professor of Obstetrics and Gynecology
David Geffen School of Medicine at UCLA
Harbor-UCLA Medical Center
Torrance, California
Water Flux and Amniotic Fluid Volume: Understanding Fetal Water Flow

Richard D. Bland, MD

Professor of Pediatrics
Stanford University School of Medicine
Stanford, California
Lung Fluid Balance in Developing Lungs and its Role in Neonatal Transition

---

[†]Deceased.

Farid Boubred, MD

Division of Neonatology
Hôpital de la Conception
Assistance Publique-Hôpitaux de Marseille, France
Faculté de Médecine
Université de la Méditerranée
Marseille, France
The Developing Kidney and the Fetal Origins of Adult Cardiovascular Disease

Caroline D. Boyd, MD

Fellow in Critical Care Pediatrics
Thomas Jefferson University–Jefferson Medical College
Philadelphia, Pennsylvania
Pediatric Intensivist in Critical Care
Department of Anesthesiology & Critical Care Medicine
Alfred I. DuPont Hospital for Children
Wilmington, Delaware
Edema

Christophe Buffat, PharmD

Assistant Hospitalo-Universitaire
Laboratory of Biochemistry and Molecular Biology
Hôpital de la Conception
Assistance Publique–Hopitaux de Marseille, France
University School of Medicine
Marseille, France
The Developing Kidney and the Fetal Origins of Adult Cardiovascular Disease

Robert L. Chevalier, MD

Professor and Chair
Department of Pediatrics
The University of Virginia
Charlottesville, Virginia
Obstructive Uropathy: Assessment of Renal Function in the Fetus

Andrew T. Costarino, MD

Professor of Anesthesiology and Pediatrics
The Thomas Jefferson University–Jefferson Medical College
Philadelphia, Pennsylvania
Chairman, Department of Anesthesiology &
  Critical Care Medicine
Alfred I. DuPont Hospital for Children
Wilmington, Delaware
Edema

Francesco Emma, MD
Head, Division of Nephrology and Dialysis
Bambino Gesù Children's Hospital and Research Institute
Rome, Italy
Renal Modulation: Arginine Vasopressin and Atrial Natriuretic Peptide

Jean-Bernard Gouyon, MD
Professor of Pediatrics
Dijon Children's Hospital
Dijon, France
Glomerular Filtration Rate in Neonates

Jean-Pierre Guignard, MD
Honorary Professor of Pediatrics
Lausanne University Medical School
Centre Hospitalier Universitaire Vaudois
Lausanne, Switzerland
Glomerular Filtration Rate in Neonates

Lucky Jain, MD
Professor of Pediatrics
Division of Neonatal and Developmental Medicine
Emory University School of Medicine
Atlanta, Georgia
Lung Fluid Balance in Developing Lungs and its Role in Neonatal Transition

Pedro A. Jose, MD, PhD
Professor of Pediatrics and Physiology and Biophysics
Georgetown University Medical Center
Washington, District of Columbia
Renal Modulation: The Renin-Angiotensin-Aldosterone System (RAAS)

John M. Lorenz, MD
Professor of Clinical Pediatrics
College of Physicians and Surgeons
Columbia University
Morgan Stanley Children's Hospital of New York-Presbyterian
New York, New York
Potassium Metabolism

Aruna Natarajan, MD, DCh
Assistant Professor
Department of Pediatrics
Division of Critical Care
Georgetown University Hospital
Washington, District of Columbia
Renal Modulation: The Renin-Angiotensin-Aldosterone System (RAAS)

Maria Antonietta Procaccino, MD

Pediatrician, Division of Nephrology and Dialysis
Bambino Gesù Children's Hospital and Research Institute
Rome, Italy
Renal Modulation: Arginine Vasopressin and Atrial Natriuretic Peptide

Michael G. Ross, MD, MPH

Professor of Obstetrics and Gynecology and Public Health
David Geffen School of Medicine at UCLA
Chairman of Obstetrics and Gynecology
Harbor-UCLA Medical Center
Torrance, California
Water Flux and Amniotic Fluid Volume: Understanding Fetal Water Flow

Istvan Seri, MD, PhD

Professor of Pediatrics
Keck School of Medicine
University of Southern California
Director, Center for Fetal and Neonatal Medicine
CHLA-Director, Institute for Fetal-Maternal Health
Head, USC Division of Neonatal Medicine
Children's Hospital Los Angeles
Los Angeles, California
Acid-base Homeostasis in the Fetus and Newborn

Umberto Simeoni, MD

Professor of Pediatrics
Université de la Méditerranée
Marseille, France
The Developing Kidney and the Fetal Origins of Adult Cardiovascular Disease

Gilda Stringini, MD

Physician, Division of Nephrology and Dialysis
Bambino Gesù Children's Hospital and Research Institute
Rome, Italy
Renal Modulation: Arginine Vasopressin and Atrial Natriuretic Peptide

Endre Sulyok, MD, PhD, DSc

Professor of Pediatrics
Faculty of Health Sciences
Institute of Health Promotion and Family Care
University of Pécs
Director of Center for Child Health
Country Teaching Hospital
Pécs, Hungary
Renal Aspects of Sodium Metabolism in the Fetus and Neonate

Daniel Vaiman, PhD

Department of Genetics and Development
Cochin Institute and Faculty of Medicine
René Descartes
Paris V University
Paris, France

The Developing Kidney and the Fetal Origins of Adult Cardiovascular Disease

Jeroen van den Wijngaard, PhD

Postdoctoral Fellow
Department of Medical Physics
Academic Medical Center
University of Amsterdam
Amsterdam, The Netherlands

Water Flux and Amniotic Fluid Volume: Understanding Fetal Water Flow

Martin van Gemert, PhD

Professor of Clinical Applications of Laser Physics
Director, The Laser Center
Academic Medical Center
University of Amsterdam
Amsterdam, The Netherlands

Water Flux and Amniotic Fluid Volume: Understanding Fetal Water Flow

Marco Zaffanello, MD, PhD

Department of Mother-Child and Biology-Genetics
University of Verona
Verona, Italy

Renal Modulation: Arginine Vasopressin and Atrial Natriuretic Peptide

Foreword

Interest in the care of the premature baby developed more than 100 years ago. Nevertheless, newborn babies had to wait until the 1940s for investigators to focus on their immature kidneys. Jean Oliver, Edith Louise Potter, George Fetterman and Robert Vernier were among the first to study and describe the structures of the immature kidney. Most of the basic knowledge on the function of the neonatal kidney was also developed between the early 1940s and the early 1970s. While Homer Smith at New York University College of Medicine was in the process of establishing the basic concepts of mature renal physiology, two investigators explored the function of the immature kidney and founded the scientific basis of modern perinatal nephrology: Henry Barnett at Albert Einstein College of Medicine in New York and Reginald McCance at the University of Cambridge in the UK. Quantification of glomerular filtration rate was established, first in infants, then in term neonates and later on in tiny premature neonates. The ability of the immature kidney to modify the glomerular ultrafiltrate, to dilute or concentrate the urine, to get rid of an acid load, to produce and respond to various hormones, and to maintain constant the neonate's body fluid volume and composition, was subsequently investigated. When it became clear that dysfunction and dysgenesis of the kidney could have long lasting consequences, fetal developmental studies were conducted with the aim of understanding the pathogenesis of renal diseases and dysfunctions from the early days of gestation.

Studies on the key role played by the placenta in maintaining the homeostasis of the fetus, as well as research on the formation and function of the fetal and the postnatal kidney have grown exponentially in the last decades. A bewildering amount of results, sometimes contradictory, has been produced, clarifying many yet unsolved problems, but also raising new questions. The interpretation of published clinical or experimental data, as well as the establishment of practical guidelines most often based on poorly or ill-controlled clinical trials generated controversies that sometimes disconcerted the physician in charge of still-unborn or newly-born infants.

The purpose of this new series entitled *Neonatology Questions and Controversies* is to discuss precisely the scientific basis of perinatal medicine. It also aims to present a rational, critical analysis of current concepts in different fields related to fetuses and newborn infants. To cover the various topics presented in this *Nephrology and Fluid/Electrolyte Physiology* volume, such as placental and perinatal physiology, pathophysiology and pathology, the editors gathered a distinguished group of contributors who are all leading experts in their respective fields. It is our conviction that physicians and students will benefit from this authoritative source of critical knowledge to improve the fate of fetuses and neonates under their care.

We thank all our contributors for their dedication and generous cooperation.

Jean-Pierre Guignard, MD

Series Foreword

"Learn from yesterday, live for today, hope for tomorrow. The important thing is not to stop questioning."

ALBERT EINSTEIN

"The art and science of asking questions is the source of all knowledge."

THOMAS BERGER

In the mid-1960s W.B. Saunders began publishing a series of books focused on the care of newborn infants. The series was entitled *Major Problems in Clinical Pediatrics.* The original series (1964–1979) consisted of ten titles dealing with problems of the newborn infant (*The Lung and its Disorders in the Newborn Infant* edited by Mary Ellen Avery, *Disorders of Carbohydrate Metabolism in Infancy* edited by Marvin Cornblath and Robert Schwartz, *Hematologic Problems in the Newborn* edited by Frank A. Oski and J. Lawrence Naiman, *The Neonate with Congenital Heart Disease* edited by Richard D. Rowe and Ali Mehrizi, *Recognizable Patterns of Human Malformation* edited by David W. Smith, *Neonatal Dermatology* edited by Lawrence M. Solomon and Nancy B. Esterly, *Amino Acid Metabolism and its Disorders* edited by Charles L. Scriver and Leon E. Rosenberg, *The High Risk Infant* edited by Lula O. Lubchenco, *Gastrointestinal Problems in the Infant* edited by Joyce Gryboski and *Viral Diseases of the Fetus and Newborn* edited by James B. Hanshaw and John A. Dudgeon. Dr. Alexander J. Schaffer was asked to be the consulting editor for the entire series. Dr. Schaffer coined the term "neonatology" and edited the first clinical textbook of neonatology entitled *Diseases of the Newborn.* For those of us training in the 1970s, this series and Dr. Schaffer's textbook of neonatology provided exciting, up-to-date information that attracted many of us into the subspecialty. Dr. Schaffer's role as "consulting editor" allowed him to select leading scientists and practitioners to serve as editors for each individual volume. As the "consulting editor" *for Neonatology Questions and Controversies*, I had the challenge of identifying the topics and editors for each volume in this series. The six volumes encompass the major issues encountered in the neonatal intensive care unit (newborn lung, fluid and electrolytes, neonatal cardiology and hemodynamics, hematology, immunology and infectious disease, gastroenterology, and neurology). The editors for each volume were challenged to combine discussions of fetal and neonatal physiology with disease pathophysiology and selected controversial topics in clinical care. It is my hope that this series (like *Major Problems in Clinical Pediatrics*) will excite a new generation of trainees to question existing dogma (from my own generation) and seek new information through scientific investigation. I wish to congratulate and thank each of the volume editors (Drs. Bancalari, Oh, Guignard, Baumgart, Kleinman, Seri, Ohls, Yoder, Neu and Perlman) for their extraordinary effort and finished products. I also wish to acknowledge Judy Fletcher at Elsevier who conceived the idea for the series and who has been my "editor and friend" throughout my academic career.

Richard A. Polin, MD

Preface

During the past decades, scientific advances in several fields of perinatal medicine have contributed significantly in the increase in the number of neonatal survivors. One of these fields is the management of infants with fluid, electrolyte and renal disorders. To discuss recent advances in this topic and the controversies that are often generated by new discoveries, the editors have assembled a group of well-respected perinatologists, neonatologists, pediatric nephrologists and their colleagues. They have contributed their expertise in discussing different aspects of normal and abnormal development and functions of the kidney and urinary tract, as well as normal and abnormal fluid and electrolyte homeostasis.

The volume is divided into four sections. Section I deals with the role of the placenta in the regulation of fetal water metabolism and amniotic fluid volume and composition. The role of the aquaporin water channels in this regulation is also discussed. Section II presents the normal regulation of sodium, potassium and acid-base balance along with a discussion of management when imbalance occurs. Section III deals with the exogenous and endogenous factors that affect the maturation of glomerular functions. We also discuss the late consequences of impaired or incomplete nephrogenesis observed in growth-restricted neonates or very premature infants. The key role played by various hormones such as angiotensin II, aldosterone, arginine vasopressin and the atrial natriuretic peptide in regulating renal development and function is also discussed. Section IV consists of six chapters discussing various aspects of fluid and electrolyte balance including (1) The disturbances in fluid balance observed in small or large for gestational age infants, and the methods available for measuring body fluid compartments; (2) The controversial issue of high versus low fluid intake in very low birth weight infants with respect to the development of patent ductus arteriosus and chronic lung disease; (3) The physiology and pathophysiology of water balance in the developing lung, the formation and clearance of lung fluid and the importance of secreted liquid for normal lung growth before birth; (4) The importance of lymphatic drainage, and the pathogenesis and management of edema; (5) Etiology, pathogenesis and management of acute renal failure; (6) The current management of obstructive uropathy.

The goal of this volume is to summarize recent advances in various aspects of fetal and neonatal fluid balance, and major clinical problems in neonatal nephrology for physicians involved in the care of the fetus and newborn infant. The information will serve as the foundation for the diagnosis and management of renal and fluid and electrolyte disorders resulting from clinical illness or iatrogenic factors. We trust that the contributions of our experts will achieve this goal, and enhance the clinicians' abilities to provide optimal care to high-risk newborn infants.

William Oh, MD
Jean-Pierre Guignard, MD
Stephen Baumgart, MD

Section I

Placental and Fetal Water Flux

Chapter 1

Water Flux and Amniotic Fluid Volume: Understanding Fetal Water Flow

Marie H. Beall, MD • Jeroen van den Wijngaard, PhD • Martin van Gemert, PhD • Michael G. Ross, MD, MPH

Clinical Scenarios
Fetal Water
Mechanisms of Water Flow
Aquaporins
Conclusion

In a term human gestation, the amount of water in the fetal compartments, including fetus, placenta and amniotic fluid (AF) may exceed 5 L; in pathologic states the amount may be much more, due to excessive amniotic fluid and/or fetal hydrops. Water largely flows from the maternal circulation to the fetus via the placenta, and the rate of fetal water acquisition is dependent on placental water permeability characteristics. Once in the gestational compartment, water is circulated between the fetus and AF. In the latter part of pregnancy, an important facet of this circulation is water flux from the AF to the fetal circulation across the amnion. Normal AF water dynamics are critical, as insufficient (oligohydramnios) or excessive (polyhydramnios) amounts of amniotic fluid are associated with impaired fetal outcome, even in the absence of structural fetal abnormalities. This chapter aims to review data regarding the placental transfer of water and to examine the circulation of water within the gestation, specifically the water flux across the amnion, as factors influencing AF volume. Finally, some controversies regarding the mechanics of these events will be discussed.

CLINICAL SCENARIOS

Water flux in the placenta and chorioamnion is a matter of more than theoretical interest. Clinical experience in humans suggests that altered placental water flow occurs, and can cause deleterious fetal effects in association with excessive or reduced AF volume.

Maternal Dehydration

Maternal dehydration has been associated with reduced fetal compartment water and oligohydramnios. As an example, the following case has been reported: A 14-year-old girl was admitted at 33 weeks' gestation with cramping and vaginal spotting. A sonogram indicated oligohydramnios and an amniotic fluid index (AFI) of 2.6, with normal fetal kidneys and bladder. On hospital day 2, the AFI was 0. Recorded maternal fluid balance was 8 L in and 13.6 L out. Serum sodium was 153 mEq/L. Diabetes insipidus was diagnosed and treated with intranasal desmopressin acetate. The oligohydramnios resolved rapidly, and the patient delivered a healthy 2700-g male infant at 38 weeks (1).

Reduced Maternal Plasma Oncotic Pressure

Maternal malnutrition may predispose a patient to increased fetal water transfer and polyhydramnios. We recently encountered a patient who illustrated this condition: A 35-year-old gravida 4, para 3 presented at 32–33 weeks of gestation complaining of premature labor. On admission, the maternal hematocrit was 18.9% and hemoglobin was 5.6 g/dL with a mean corpuscular volume of 57.9. Blood chemistries were normal, except that the patient's serum albumin was 1.9 g/dL (normal 3.3–4.9 g/dL). A diagnosis of maternal malnutrition was made. On ultrasound examination, the AFI was 24.5 cm and the fetal bladder was noted to be significantly enlarged consistent with increased urine output. Subsequently, the patient delivered a 1784 g male infant with Apgar scores of 3 at 1 minute and 7 at 5 minutes. The infant was transferred to the neonatal intensive care unit (NICU) for significant respiratory distress.

As described below, although the forces driving normal maternal to fetal water flux are uncertain, changes in the osmotic/oncotic difference between the maternal and fetal sera can affect the volume of water flowing from the mother to the fetus. In the first case, presumably due to an environment of increased maternal osmolality, less water crossed the placenta to the fetus. Similarly, maternal dehydration due to water restriction (in a sheep model) (2) or due to hot weather (in the human) (3) have been associated with reduced AF volumes. Conversely, reduced maternal oncotic pressure likely contributed to increased maternal to fetal water transfer in the second patient. Fetal homeostatic mechanisms then led to increased fetal urine output and increased AF volume. Similarly, studies with DDAVP in both humans (4) and sheep (5) have demonstrated that a pharmacologic reduction in maternal serum osmolality can lead to an increase in AF. As these examples illustrate, fetal water flow is a carefully balanced system that can be perturbed with clinically significant effect. The material presented below will detail the mechanisms regulating fetal-maternal-AF fluid homeostasis.

FETAL WATER

Placental Water Flux

Net water flux across the placenta is relatively small. In sheep, a water flow to the fetus of 0.5 mL/min (6) is sufficient for fetal needs at term. By contrast, tracer studies suggest that the total water exchanged (i.e. diffusionary flow) between the fetus and the mother is much larger, up to 70 mL/min (7). Most of this flow is bi-directional, resulting in no net accumulation of water. Although the mechanisms regulating the maternal–fetal flux of water are speculative, the permeability of the placenta to water changes with gestation (8), suggesting that placental water permeability may be a factor in regulating the water available to the fetus.

Although fetal water may derive from sources other than transplacental flux, these other sources appear to be of minor importance. Water could, theoretically, pass from the maternal circulation to the amniotic fluid across the fetal membranes (i.e., transmembrane flow), though this effect is thought to be small (9), in part because the amniotic fluid is hypotonic compared to maternal serum. The driving force resulting from osmotic and oncotic gradients between hypotonic, low protein amniotic fluid and isotonic maternal serum is far greater than that induced by maternal vascular versus amniotic fluid hydrostatic pressure. Any direct water flux between maternal serum and amniotic fluid should therefore be from fetus to mother. In addition, a small amount of water is produced as a byproduct of fetal metabolic processes. As these alternative routes contribute only a minor proportion of the fetal water, it is apparent that the fetus is dependent on placental flux for the bulk of water requirements.

Fetal Water Compartments

In the gestation, water is partitioned between the fetus, placenta and membranes, and the amniotic fluid. Although term human fetuses may vary considerably in size, an average fetus contains 3000 mL of water, of which about 350 mL are in the vascular compartment. In addition, the placenta contains another 500 mL of water. More precisely, the volume of fetal and placental water is proportionate to the fetal weight. Amniotic fluid volume is less correlated with fetal weight, and there is a significant variation in volume between individuals. In normal human gestations at term, the AF volume may vary from 500 mL to more than 1200 mL (10). In pathologic states, the AF volume may vary more widely. Below we present what is known regarding the formation of AF, the circulation of AF water, and the mechanisms controlling this circulation.

AF Volume and Composition

During the first trimester, AF is isotonic with maternal plasma (11) but contains minimal protein. It is thought that the fluid arises either from a transudate of fetal plasma through nonkeratinized fetal skin, or maternal plasma across the uterine decidua and/or placenta surface (12). With advancing gestation, AF osmolality and sodium concentration decrease, a result of the mixture of dilute fetal urine and isotonic fetal lung liquid production. In comparison with the first half of pregnancy, AF osmolality decreases by 20–30 mOsm/kg H_2O with advancing gestation to levels approximately 85–90% of maternal serum osmolality (13) in the human, although there was no osmolality decrease in the AF near term in the rat (14). AF urea, creatinine and uric acid increase during the second half of pregnancy resulting in AF concentrations of the urinary byproducts two to three times higher than fetal plasma (13).

Concordant with the changes in AF content, AF volume changes dramatically during human pregnancy (Fig. 1-1). Average AF volume increases progressively from 20 mL at 10 weeks to 630 mL at 22 weeks and to 770 mL at 28 weeks' gestation (15). Between 29 and 37 weeks, there is little change in volume. Beyond 39 weeks, AF volume decreases sharply, averaging 515 ml at 41 weeks. Once the patient becomes post-date, there is a 33% decline in AF volume per week (16–18), consistent with the increased incidence of oligohydramnios in post-term gestations.

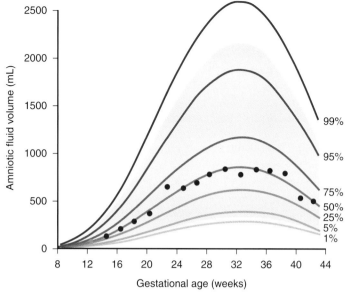

Figure 1-1 Normal range of amniotic fluid (AF) volume in human gestation.

Fetal Water Circulation

Amniotic fluid is produced and resorbed in a dynamic process with large volumes of water circulated between the AF and fetal compartments (Fig. 1-2). During the latter half of gestation, the primary sources of AF include fetal urine excretion and fluid secreted by the fetal lung. The primary pathways for water exit from the AF include removal by fetal swallowing and intramembranous absorption into fetal blood. Although some data on these processes in the human fetus is available, the bulk of the information about fetal AF circulation derives from animal models, especially the sheep.

Urine production

In humans, fetal urine production changes with increasing gestation. The amount of urine produced by the human fetus has been estimated by the use of ultrasound

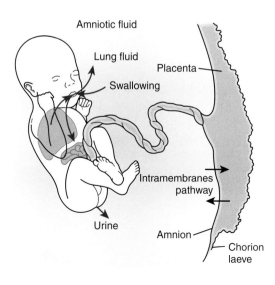

Figure 1-2 Water circulation between the fetus and amniotic fluid (AF). The major sources of AF water are fetal urine and lung liquid, the routes of absorption are through fetal swallowing and intramembranous flow (see text).

assessment of fetal bladder volume (19), although the accuracy of these measurements has been called into question. Exact human fetal urine production rates across gestation are not established but appear to be in the range of 25% of body weight per day or nearly 1000 mL/day near term (20,19).

In the near term ovine fetus, 500 to 1200 mL/day of urine are distributed to the AF and allantoic cavities (21–23). During the last third of gestation, the fetal glomerular filtration rate (GFR) increases in parallel to fetal weight, with a similar though variable increase in reabsorption of sodium, chloride and free water (24). Fetal urine output can be modulated, as numerous endocrine factors, including arginine vasopressin, atrial natriuretic factor, aldosterone and prostaglandins, have been demonstrated to alter fetal renal blood flow, glomerular filtration rate, or urine flow rates (25,26). Importantly, physiologic increases in fetal plasma arginine vasopressin significantly increase fetal urine osmolality and reduce urine flow rates (27,28).

Lung Fluid Production

It appears that all mammalian fetuses normally secrete fluid from their lungs. The absolute rate of fluid production by human fetal lungs has not been estimated; the fluid production rate has been extensively studied in the ovine fetus only. During the last third of gestation, the fetal lamb secretes an average of 100 mL/day per kg fetal weight. Under physiological conditions, half of the fluid exiting the lungs enters the AF and half is swallowed (29), therefore an average of approximately 165 mL/day of lung liquid enters the AF near term. Fetal lung fluid production is affected by physiologic and endocrine factors, but nearly all stimuli have been demonstrated to reduce fetal lung liquid production, with no evidence of stimulated production and nominal changes in fluid composition. Increased arginine vasopressin (30), catecholamines (31) and cortisol (32), even acute intravascular volume expansion (33), decrease lung fluid production. Given this lack of evidence of bi-directional regulation, it appears that, unlike the kidney, the fetal lung may not play an important role in the maintenance of AF volume homeostasis. Current opinion is that fetal lung fluid secretion is likely most important in providing pulmonary expansion, which promotes airway and alveolar development.

Fetal Swallowing

Studies of near term pregnancies suggest that the human fetus swallows an average of 210–760 mL/day (34), which is considerably less than the volume of urine produced each day. However, fetal swallowing may be reduced beginning a few days before delivery (35), so the rate of human fetal swallowing is probably underestimated. Little other data on human fetal swallowed volumes is available. In fetal sheep there is a steady increase in the volume of fluid swallowed over the last third of gestation. In contrast to a relatively constant daily urine production/kg body weight, the daily volume swallowed increases from approximately 130 mL/kg per day at 0.75 term to over 400 mL/kg per day near-term (36). A series of studies have measured ovine fetal swallowing activity with esophageal electromyograms and swallowed volume using a flow probe placed around the fetal esophagus (37). These studies demonstrate that fetal swallowing increases in response to dipsogenic (e.g., central or systemic hypertonicity (38) or central angiotensin II (39) or orexigenic (central neuropeptide Y (40)) stimulation, and decreases with acute arterial hypotension (41) or hypoxia (29,42). Thus, near term fetal swallowed volume is subject to periodic increases as mechanisms for 'thirst' and 'appetite' develop functionality, although decreases in swallowed volume appear to be more reflective of deteriorating fetal condition.

Intramembranous (IM) Flow

The amount of fluid swallowed by the fetus does not equal the amount of fluid produced by both the kidneys and the lungs in either human or ovine gestation.

As the volume of amniotic fluid does not greatly increase during the last half of pregnancy, another route of fluid absorption is needed. This route is the intramembranous (IM) pathway.

The IM pathway refers to the route of absorption between the fetal circulation and the amniotic cavity directly across the amnion. Although the contribution of the IM pathway to the overall regulation and maintenance of AF volume and composition has yet to be completely understood, results from in vivo and in vitro studies of ovine membrane permeability suggest that the permeability of the fetal chorioamnion is important for determining AF composition and volume (43–45). This IM flow, recirculating AF water to the fetal compartment, is thought to be driven by the significant osmotic gradient between the hypotonic AF and isotonic fetal plasma (46). In addition, electrolytes (e.g., Na^+) may diffuse down a concentration gradient from fetal plasma into the AF while intraamniotic peptides (e.g., arginine vasopressin (47,48)) and other electrolytes (e.g., Cl^-) may be recirculated to the fetal plasma.

Although it has never been directly measured in humans, indirect evidence supports the presence of IM flow. Studies of intraamniotic ^{51}Cr injection demonstrated the appearance of the tracer in the circulation of fetuses with impaired swallowing (49). Additionally, alterations in IM flow may contribute to AF clinical abnormalities, as membrane ultrastructure changes are noted with polyhydramnios or oligohydramnios (50).

Experimental estimates of the net IM flow averages 200–250 mL/day in fetal sheep and likely balances the flow of urine and lung liquid with fetal swallowing under homeostatic conditions. Filtration coefficients have been calculated (51), though IM flow rates under control conditions have not been directly measured. Mathematical models of human AF dynamics also suggest significant IM water and electrolyte fluxes (52,53), whereas *trans*membranous flow (AF to maternal) is extremely small in comparison to IM flow (54,55).

This detailed understanding of fetal fluid production and resorption, provides little explanation as to how AF volume homeostasis is maintained throughout gestation, and does not account for gestational alterations in AF volume, or post-term or acute-onset oligohydramnios. As an example, the acute reduction in fetal swallowing in response to hypotension or hypoxia seen in the ovine model would not produce the reduced amniotic fluid volume noted in stressed human fetuses. For this reason, recent research has addressed the regulation of water flow in the placenta and fetal membranes. We will discuss the possible mechanisms for the regulation of fetal water flow, beginning with a review of the general principles of membrane water flow.

MECHANISMS OF WATER FLOW

Biologic membranes exist (in part) to regulate water flux. Flow may occur through the cell (i.e., transcellular) or between cells (i.e., paracellular), and the type of flow affects the composition of the fluid crossing the membrane. In addition, transcellular flow may occur across the lipid bilayer, or through membrane channels or pores (i.e., aquaporins); the latter route is more efficient as the water permeability of the lipid membrane is low. As the aquaporins allow the passage of water only (and sometimes other small non-polar molecules), transcellular flow is predominantly free water. Paracellular flow occurs through relatively wide spaces between cells, and consists of both water and solutes in the proportions present in the extracellular space; large molecules may be excluded. Although water molecules can randomly cross the membrane by diffusion without net water flow, net flow occurs only in response to concentration (osmotic) or pressure (hydrostatic) differences.

Osmotic and hydrostatic forces are created when there is a difference in osmotic or hydrostatic pressure on either side of the membrane. Osmotic differences arise when there is a difference in solute concentration across the membrane. In order for this difference to be maintained, membrane permeability of the solute must be low (i.e., a high reflection coefficient). Commonly, osmotic differences are maintained by charged ions such as sodium, or large molecules such as proteins (also called oncotic pressure). These solutes do not cross the cell membrane readily. Osmotic differences can be *created* locally by the active transport of sodium across the membrane, with water following due to the osmotic force created by the sodium imbalance. It should be noted that, although the transport of sodium is active, water flux is always a passive, non-energy-dependent process. Hydrostatic differences occur when the pressure of fluid is greater on one side of the membrane. The most obvious example is the difference between the inside of a blood vessel and the interstitial space. Hydrostatic differences may also be created locally by controlling the relative direction of two flows. Even with equal initial pressures, a hydrostatic difference will exist if venous outflow is matched with arterial inflow (countercurrent flow). The actual movement of water in response to these gradients may be more complex as a result of additional physical properties, including unstirred layer effects and solvent drag.

Net membrane water flux is a function of the membrane properties, and the osmotic and hydrostatic forces. Formally, this is expressed as the Starling equation:

$$J_v = LpS(\Delta P - \sigma RT(c_1 - c_2))$$

where J_v is the volume flux, LpS is a description of membrane properties (hydraulic conductance times the surface area for diffusion), ΔP is the hydrostatic pressure difference and $-\sigma RT(c_1 - c_2)$ is the osmotic pressure difference, with T being the temperature in degrees Kelvin, R the gas constant in Nm/Kmol, σ the reflection coefficient (a measure of the permeability of the membrane to the solute) and c_1 and c_2 the solute concentrations on the two sides of the membrane. Experimental studies most often report the membrane water permeability (a characteristic of the individual membrane). Permeability is proportionate to flux (amount of flow per second per cm^2 of membrane) divided by the concentration difference on different sides of the membrane (amount per cubic cm). Membrane water permeabilities are reported as the permeability associated with flux of water in a given direction, and under a given type of force, or as the diffusional permeability. As one membrane may have different osmotic versus hydrostatic versus diffusional permeabilities (56), an understanding of the forces driving membrane water flow is critical for understanding flow regulatory mechanisms. This area remains controversial, however the anatomy of placenta and membranes suggests possible mechanisms for promoting water flux in one direction.

Mechanism of Placental Water Flow

Placental Anatomy (57,58)

The placenta is a complex organ, and the anatomic variation in the placentas of various species is substantial. Rodents have often been used for the study of placental water flux, as primates and rodents share a hemochorial placental structure. In hemochorial placentas, the maternal blood is contained in sinuses in direct contact with one or more layers of fetal epithelium. In the human, this epithelium is the syncytiotrophoblast, a layer of contiguous cells with few or no intercellular spaces. Beneath the syncytium, there are layers of connective tissue, and fetal blood vessel endothelium. (In early pregnancy, human placentas have a layer of cytotrophoblast underlying the syncytium, however, by the third trimester this layer is not continuous, and is therefore not a limiting factor for placental permeability.) The human placenta is therefore monochorial. The guinea pig placenta is also monochorial; the fetal vessels are covered with connective tissue that is, in turn, covered with a single layer of syncytium (59). In the mouse, the layer immediately apposed to the maternal blood is a cytotrophoblast layer, covering two layers of syncytium. Due to the presence of three layers in much of the placenta, the mouse placenta is labeled trichorial. Similar to the human, the mouse cytotrophoblast does not appear to be continuous, suggesting that the cytotrophoblast layer does not limit membrane permeability. The rat placenta is similar to the mouse.

The syncytium is, therefore, a common structure in all of these placental forms, and a likely site of regulation of membrane permeability. In support of this hypothesis, membrane vesicles derived from human syncytial brush border were used to evaluate the permeability of the placenta. At 37°C, the osmotic permeability of apical vesicles was $1.9 +/- 0.06 \times 10^{-3}$ cm/s, whereas the permeability of basal membrane (maternal side) vesicles was higher at $3.1 +/- 0.20 \times 10^{-3}$ cm/s (60). The difference between basal and apical sides of the syncytiotrophoblasts was taken to indicate that the apical (fetal) side of the trophoblast was the rate-limiting structure for water flow through the placenta. In all placentas, the fetal blood is contained in vessels, suggesting that fetal capillary endothelium may also serve as a barrier to flow between maternal and fetal circulations. Experimental evidence suggests, however, that the capillary endothelium is a less significant barrier to small polar molecules than the syncytium (58).

Although the sheep has been extensively used in studies of fetal physiology and placental permeability, it has a placenta that differs from that of the human in important respects. The sheep placenta is classified as epitheliochorial, meaning that the maternal and fetal circulations are contained within blood vessels, with maternal and fetal epithelial layers interposed between them. In general, as compared to the hemochorial placenta, the epithelialchorial placenta would be expected to demonstrate decreased water permeability based on the increase in membrane layers. In addition, the forces driving water permeability may differ between the two placental types, as the presence of maternal vessels in the sheep placenta increase the likelihood that a hydrostatic pressure difference could be maintained favoring water flux from maternal to fetal circulations.

In all of the rodent placentas, fetal and maternal blood circulate in opposite directions (countercurrent flow), potentially increasing the opportunity for exchange between circulations based on local differences. The direction of maternal blood circulation in human placentas is from the inside to the outside of the placental lobule, and therefore at cross-current to the fetal blood flow (61) (Fig. 1-3). Unlike the mouse and rat, investigation has not revealed countercurrent blood flow in the ovine placenta (62).

The forgoing is not intended to imply that there are not important differences between human and rodent placentas. The human placenta is organized into cotyledons, each with a central fetal vessel. Fetal–maternal exchange in the mouse and rat placenta occurs in the placental labyrinth. In addition, the rat and mouse have an 'inverted yolk sac placenta,' a structure with no analogy in the primate placenta. The reader is referred to Faber and Thornberg (57) and Benirschke (63) for additional details.

Controversies in Placental Flow

In the placenta the flux of water may be driven by either hydrostatic or osmotic forces. Hydrostatic forces can be developed in the placenta by alterations in the flow in maternal and fetal circulations. Osmotic forces may be generated locally, due to

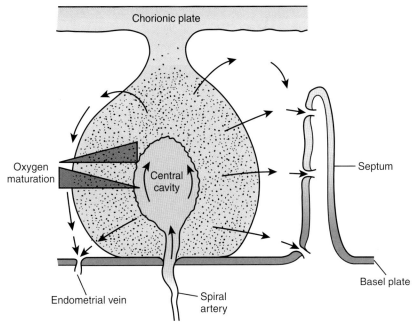

Figure 1-3 Maternal blood flow in the human placenta. Blood flow proceeds from the spiral artery to the center of the placental lobule. Blood then crosses the lobule laterally, exiting through the endometrial vein. This creates a gradient in oxygen content from the inside to the outside of the lobule due to the changing oxygen content of the maternal blood.

active transport of solutes such as sodium or due to depletion of solute from the local perimembrane environment (due to the so-called 'unstirred layer' effect). The relative direction of maternal and fetal blood flows can be concurrent, counter-current, crosscurrent, or in part combinations of these flows (64), and differences in the direction of blood flow may be important in establishing either osmotic or hydrostatic gradients within the placenta. It has not been possible to directly study possible local pressure or osmotic differences at the level of the syncytium, therefore theories regarding the driving forces for placental water flux are inferences from available data.

Water may be transferred from mother to fetus driven osmotically by the active transport of solutes such as sodium (65). In the rat, inert solutes such as mannitol and inulin are transferred *to* the maternal circulation from the fetus more readily than *from* mother to fetus (66), and, conversely, sodium is actively transported to the fetus in excess of fetal needs. This was taken to indicate that water was being driven to the fetal side by a local osmotic effect created by the sodium flux. Water, with dissolved solutes, then differentially crossed from fetus to mother, probably by a paracellular route. Perfusion of the guinea pig placenta with dextran-containing solution demonstrates that the flow of water can also be influenced by colloid osmotic pressure (67). In the sheep, intact gestations have yielded estimates of osmotic placental water flow of 0.062 mL/kg min per mOsm/kg H_2O (68). The importance of osmotically-driven water flow in the sheep is uncertain, as the same authors found that the maternal plasma was consistently hyperosmolar to the fetal plasma. Theoretical considerations have been used, however, to argue that known electrolyte active transport, and a modest hydrostatic pressure gradient, could maintain maternal-to-fetal water flow against this osmotic gradient (69).

Others have argued that the motive force for water flux in the placenta is hydrostatic. In perfused placenta of the guinea pig, reversal of the direction of the fetal flow reduced the rate of water transfer (70), and increasing the fetal-side perfusion pressure increased the fetal-to-maternal water flow in both the perfused guinea pig placenta (71) and in an intact sheep model (72). Both findings suggest that water transfer is flow-dependent.

As a whole, the available data suggests that either osmotic or hydrostatic forces *can* promote placental water flux. The actual motive force in normal pregnancy is uncertain, and may vary with the species and/or the pregnancy stage. Whatever the driving force, at least some part of placental water flux involves the flow of solute-free water transcellularly, suggesting the involvement of membrane water channels in the process.

Mechanism of IM Flow

Membrane Anatomy

In sheep, an extensive network of microscopic blood vessels is located between the outer surface of the amnion and the chorion (73), providing an extensive surface area available for IM flow. In primates including humans, IM fluxes likely occur across the fetal surface of the placenta as the amnion and chorion are not vascularized per se. The close proximity of fetal blood vessels to the placental surface provides accessibility to the fetal circulation, explaining the absorption of AF technetium (46) and arginine vasopressin (48) in subhuman fetal primates with esophageal ligation. The potential for the membranes overlying the placenta to serve as a selective barrier of exchange is further supported by in vitro experiments of isolated layers of human amnion and chorion (74).

Studies in the ovine model suggest that the IM pathway can be regulated to restore homeostasis. Since fetal swallowing is a major route of AF fluid resorption, esophageal ligation would be expected to increase AF volume significantly. Although AF volume increased significantly 3 days after ovine fetal esophageal occlusion (75), longer periods (9 days) of esophageal ligation reduced AF volume in preterm sheep (76). Similarly, esophageal ligation of fetal sheep over a period of one month did not increase AF volume (77). In the absence of swallowing, normalized AF volume suggests an increase in IM flow. In addition, IM flow markedly increased following the infusion of exogenous fluid to the AF cavity (78). Collectively, these studies suggest that AF resorption pathways and likely IM flow are under dynamic feedback regulation. That is, AF volume expansion increases IM resorption, ultimately resulting in a normalization of AF volume. Importantly, factors downregulating IM flow are less studied, and there is no evidence of reduced IM resorption as an adaptive response to oligohydramnios. Studies have revealed that prolactin reduced the upregulation of IM flow due to osmotic challenge in the sheep model (79), and reduced diffusional permeability to water in human amnion (80) and guinea pig (81) amnion.

Controversies Regarding IM Flow

The specific mechanism and regulation of IM flow is key to AF homeostasis. A number of theories have been put forward to account for the observed results. Esophageal ligation of fetal sheep resulted in the upregulation of fetal chorioamnion vascular endothelial growth factor (VEGF) gene expression (82). It was proposed that VEGF-induced neovascularization potentiates AF water resorption. These authors also speculated that fetal urine and/or lung fluid may contain factors that upregulate VEGF. Their further studies demonstrated an increased water flow despite a constant membrane diffusional permeability (to technetium) in animals in whom the fetal urine output had been increased by an intravenous volume load, and a concurrent flow of water and solutes against a concentration gradient by the IM route (83,84). Finally, artificial regulation of the osmolality and oncotic pressure of the AF revealed that the major force promoting IM flow in the sheep was osmotic, however there was an additional flow of about 24 mL/h, which was not osmotic-dependent. As protein was also transferred to the fetal circulation, this flow was felt to be similar to fluid flow in the lymph system (85).

These findings, in aggregate, have been interpreted to require active bulk fluid flow across the amnion; Brace et al (83) have proposed that this fluid transport occurs via membrane vesicles (bulk vesicular flow), as evidenced by the high prevalence of amnion intracellular vesicles seen in electron microscopy (86). This theory is poorly accepted, as vesicle water flow has not been demonstrated in any other tissue and is highly energy dependent. Most others believe that IM flow occurs through conventional para- and trans-cellular channels, driven by osmotic and hydrostatic forces. Mathematical modeling indicates that relatively small IM sodium fluxes could be associated with significant changes in AF volume, suggesting that sodium flux may be a regulator of IM flow (53), although the observation that IM flow was independent of AF composition suggests that other forces (such as hydrostatic forces) may also drive IM flow (87).

Importantly, upregulation of VEGF or sodium transfer alone cannot explain AF composition changes following fetal esophageal ligation as AF electrolyte composition indicates that water flow increases disproportionately to solute flow (76). The passage of free water across a biological membrane without solutes is a characteristic of transcellular flow, a process mediated by water channels in the cell membrane. Although water flow through these channels is passive, the expression and location of the channels can be modulated in order to regulate water flux. We will review the characteristics of aquaporin water channels, and then comment on the evidence that aquaporins may be involved in regulating gestational water flow.

AQUAPORINS

Aquaporins (AQPs) are cell membrane proteins approximately 30 kD in size (26–34 kD). Similarities in amino acid sequence suggest that the 3-dimensional structure of all AQPs is similar. AQP proteins organize in the cell membrane as tetramers, however each monomer forms a hydrophilic pore in its center and functions independently as a water channel (88) (Fig. 1-4). Although all AQPs function as water channels, some AQPs also allow the passage of glycerol, urea and other small, non polar molecules. These have also been called aquaglyceroporins. Multiple AQPs have been identified (up to 13, depending on the mammalian species). Some are widely expressed throughout the body, others appear to be more tissue-specific.

AQP function is dependent upon cellular location. In the kidney, several AQPs are expressed in specific areas of the collecting duct: AQP3 and AQP4 are both present in the basolateral membrane of the collecting duct principal cells while AQP2 is present in the apical portion of the membrane of these same cells (89). The presence of these different AQPs on opposite membrane sides of the same cell is important for the regulation of water transfer across the cell, as altered AQP properties or AQP expression may differentially regulate water entry from the collecting duct lumen and water exit to the interstitial fluid compartment. Absence of the various renal AQPs leads to renal concentrating defects; in particular the absence of AQP2 in the human is responsible for nephrogenic diabetes insipidus.

AQP function is also dependent upon the cellular milieu. This regulation may occur through the insertion or removal of AQP into the membrane from the intracellular compartment. For example, in the renal tubule, AQP2 is transferred from cytoplasm vesicles to the apical cell membrane in response to arginine vasopressin (90) or forskolin (91). AQP8 is similarly transferred from hepatocyte vesicles to the cell membrane in response to dibutyryl cAMP and glucagon (92).

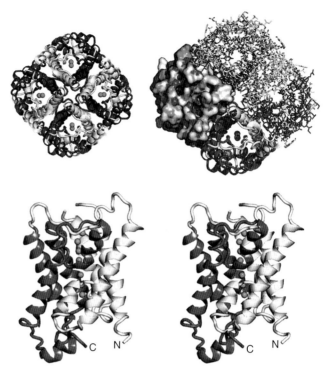

Figure 1-4 Structure of aquaporin (bovine AQP0). Upper left shows the structure from the extracellular side of the membrane. Upper right shows each monomer in a different format. Lower figure shows a side view of an AQP monomer, extracellular side upper. Two figures to be viewed in crossed eye stereo.

In longer time frames, the expression of various AQPs may be induced by external conditions. For example, AQP3 expression in cultured keratinocytes is increased when the cell culture medium is made hypertonic (93). In summary, AQPs are important in the regulation of water flow across biological membranes, and their expression and activity can be regulated according to the hydration status of the organism.

AQPs in Placenta and Membranes

Four AQPs (i.e., AQP 1, 3, 8 and 9) have been found in the placenta and fetal membranes of a variety of species. AQP1 mRNA has been demonstrated in ovine placenta, and it appears to be associated with the placental vessels (94). Ovine placental AQP1 expression levels are highest early in pregnancy, with a decline thereafter, although there is a rise in expression near term (95). AQP1 protein expression has been demonstrated in the fetal chorioamnion at term in human gestations (96), though the cellular location of the protein has not been studied. AQP3 message has also been demonstrated in the placenta and fetal chorioamnion of humans (96,97), in sheep placenta (94,95) and in rat placenta (98), while protein expression has been demonstrated in ovine and human placentas. In the human, AQP3 protein is expressed on the apical membranes of the syncytiotrophoblast (97). Less is known about the remaining two AQPs: AQP8 mRNA has been detected in mouse placenta (99), sheep placenta (95) and human placenta, and in human fetal chorioamnion (100). (AQP8 protein expression has not been studied in these tissues.) AQP9 protein and mRNA have been demonstrated in human placenta (97).

Indirect evidence suggests that AQPs may be involved in the regulation of placental water flow. Some experimental data (8) suggests that the permeability of the placenta changes (increases, then decreases) with advancing gestation in the human. Interestingly, this pattern of increase and decrease is also seen in the placental expression of membrane AQPs in both the sheep (95) and mouse (101), suggesting that AQPs may be involved in regulating placental permeability changes. In particular, in our studies AQP3 followed this pattern in the mouse. This data, together with the location of AQP3 on the apical membrane of the syncytiotrophoblasts, makes it a candidate regulator of placental water flow.

AQP and IM Water Flow

IM flow may also be regulated by AQPs and there is evidence that AQP1 is necessary for normal AF homeostasis. Mice lacking the AQP1 gene have significantly increased AF volume (102). Furthermore, AQP1 expression is altered in conditions with pathologic AF volume. AQP1 expression was increased in human amnion derived from patients with increased AF volumes (103); this upregulation was postulated to be a response to, rather than a cause of, polyhydramnios. AQP 1 protein increased in sheep fetal chorioallantoic membranes in response to fetal hypoxia, suggesting increased IM flow as a mechanism for the oligohydramnios associated with fetal compromise (104). In addition, AQP expression in the chorioamnion is subject to hormonal regulation. In work done in our laboratory, AQP3, AQP8 and AQP9 expression is up-regulated in cultured human amnion cells following incubation with cyclic AMP (cAMP) or forskolin, a cAMP-elevating agent (105,106). These data together support the hypothesis that AQPs, and specifically AQP1, are important mediators of water flow out of the gestational sac across the amnion.

In summary, we would propose the following model for human fetal water flow. Water crosses from the maternal to fetal circulation in the placenta, perhaps under the influence of local osmotic differences created by the active transport of sodium. Transplacental water flow, at least in the maternal to fetal direction, is through AQP water channels. Membrane permeability in the placenta is therefore subject to regulation by up- or down-regulating the number of AQP channels in the membrane. There is no evidence of acute changes in placental water permeability, but changes in permeability have been described over time; these could be due to changes in the expression of AQPs with advancing gestation. AQP3 is expressed on the apical membrane of the syncytiotrophoblasts; the membrane barrier thought to be rate-limiting for placental water flux, and its expression increases with gestation. AQP3 is therefore a candidate for the regulation of placental water flow.

Once in the gestational compartment, water circulates between the fetus and the AF. The available evidence suggests that the IM component of this flow is likely mediated by AQP1. IM flow can be altered over gestation, and also in response to acute events (e.g., increased AF volume). These alterations in IM flow are likely affected by alterations in the membrane expression of AQP1. Normally, AQP1 expression in the amnion decreases with gestation, associated with increasing AF volume, but expression can be increased by various humeral factors, by polyhydramnios or by fetal acidosis.

CONCLUSION

The circulation of water between mother and fetus, and within the fetal compartment, is complex, and the mechanisms regulating water flow remain poorly understood. Water flow across the placenta must increase with increasing fetal water needs, and must be relatively insensitive to transient changes in maternal status. Water circulation within the gestation must sustain fetal growth and plasma volume, while also allowing for appropriate amounts of amniotic fluid for fetal growth and development.

Experimental data suggests that placental water flow is affected by both hydrostatic and osmotic forces, and that both transcellular and paracellular water flow occurs. IM water flow is more likely to be osmotically driven, although there are other contributing forces as well. The observation that water crosses the membrane in excess of solutes suggests a role for aquaporin water channels in placental and IM water flow. Experimental data has confirmed the expression of AQPs in the placenta and fetal membranes, as well as modulation of this expression by a variety of factors. AQP3 is an exciting prospect for the regulation of placental water flow given its cellular location and gestational pattern of expression. AQP1 has been implicated in the mechanism of IM flow using a variety of experimental models. The availability of agents known to regulate the expression of AQPs suggests the possibility of treatments for AF volume abnormalities based on the stimulation or suppression of the appropriate water channel.

REFERENCES

1. Hanson RS, Powrie RO, Larson L. Diabetes insipidus in pregnancy: a treatable cause of oligohydramnios. Obstet Gynecol 89:816, 1997.
2. Schreyer P, Sherman DJ, Ervin MG, Day L, Ross MG. Maternal dehydration: impact on ovine amniotic fluid volume and composition. J Dev Physiol 13:283, 1990.
3. Sciscione AC, Costigan KA, Johnson TR. Increase in ambient temperature may explain decrease in amniotic fluid index. Am J Perinatol 14:249, 1997.
4. Ross MG, Cedars L, Nijland MJ, Ogundipe A. Treatment of oligohydramnios with maternal 1-deamino-[8-D-arginine] vasopressin-induced plasma hypoosmolality. Am J Obstet Gynecol 174:1608, 1996.
5. Ross MG, Nijland MJ, Kullama LK. 1-Deamino-[8-D-arginine] vasopressin-induced maternal plasma hypoosmolality increases ovine amniotic fluid volume. Am J Obstet Gynecol 174:1118, 1996.
6. Lumbers ER, Smith FG, Stevens AD. Measurement of net transplacental transfer of fluid to the fetal sheep. J Physiol 364:289, 1985.
7. Faichney GJ, Fawcett AA, Boston RC. Water exchange between the pregnant ewe, the foetus and its amniotic and allantoic fluids. J Comp Physiol [B] 174:503, 2004.
8. Jansson T, Powell TL, Illsley NP. Gestational development of water and non-electrolyte permeability of human syncytiotrophoblast plasma membranes. Placenta 20:155, 1999.
9. Brace RA. Progress toward understanding the regulation of amniotic fluid volume: water and solute fluxes in and through the fetal membranes. Placenta 16:1, 1995.
10. Goodwin, JW, Godden JO, Chance GW. Perinatal medicine: the basic science underlying clinical practice. Baltimore, MD: Williams & Wilkins, 1976.
11. Campbell J, Wathen N, Macintosh M, Cass P, Chard T, Mainwaring BR. Biochemical composition of amniotic fluid and extraembryonic coelomic fluid in the first trimester of pregnancy. Br J Obstet Gynaecol 99:563, 1992.
12. Faber JJ, Gault CF, Green TJ, Long LR, Thornburg KL. Chloride and the generation of amniotic fluid in the early embryo. J Exp Zool 183:343, 1973.
13. Gillibrand PN. Changes in the electrolytes, urea and osmolality of the amniotic fluid with advancing pregnancy. J Obstet Gynaecol Br Commonw 76:898, 1969.
14. Desai M, Ladella S, Ross MG. Reversal of pregnancy-mediated plasma hypotonicity in the near-term rat. J Matern Fetal Neonatal Med 13:197, 2003.
15. Brace RA, Wolf EJ. Normal amniotic fluid volume changes throughout pregnancy. Am J Obstet Gynecol 161:382, 1989.
16. Gadd RL. The volume of the liquor amnii in normal and abnormal pregnancies. J Obstet Gynaecol Br Commonw 73:11, 1966.
17. Beischer NA, Brown JB, Townsend L. Studies in prolonged pregnancy. 3. Amniocentesis in prolonged pregnancy. Am J Obstet Gynecol 103:496, 1969.
18. Queenan JT, Thompson W, Whitfield CR, Shah SI. Amniotic fluid volumes in normal pregnancies. Am J Obstet Gynecol 114:34, 1972.
19. Rabinowitz R, Peters MT, Vyas S, Campbell S, Nicolaides KH. Measurement of fetal urine production in normal pregnancy by real-time ultrasonography. Am J Obstet Gynecol 161:1264, 1989.
20. Fagerquist M, Fagerquist U, Oden A, Blomberg SG. Fetal urine production and accuracy when estimating fetal urinary bladder volume. Ultrasound Obstet Gynecol 17:132, 2001.
21. Ross MG, Ervin MG, Rappaport VJ, Youssef A, Leake RD, Fisher DA. Ovine fetal urine contribution to amniotic and allantoic compartments. Biol Neonate 53:98, 1988.
22. Wlodek ME, Challis JR, Patrick J. Urethral and urachal urine output to the amniotic and allantoic sacs in fetal sheep. J Dev Physiol 10:309, 1988.
23. Gresham EL, Rankin JH, Makowski EL, Meschia G, Battaglia FC. An evaluation of fetal renal function in a chronic sheep preparation. J Clin Invest 51:149, 1972.

24. Robillard JE, Matson JR, Sessions C, Smith FG, Jr. Developmental aspects of renal tubular reabsorption of water in the lamb fetus. Pediatr Res 13:1172, 1979.
25. Robillard JE, Weitzman RE. Developmental aspects of the fetal renal response to exogenous arginine vasopressin. Am J Physiol 238:F407, 1980.
26. Lingwood B, Hardy KJ, Coghlan JP, Wintour EM. Effect of aldosterone on urine composition in the chronically cannulated ovine foetus. J Endocrinol 76:553, 1978.
27. Lingwood B, Hardy KJ, Horacek I, McPhee ML, Scoggins BA, Wintour EM. The effects of antidiuretic hormone on urine flow and composition in the chronically-cannulated ovine fetus. Q J Exp Physiol Cogn Med Sci 63:315, 1978.
28. Ervin MG, Ross MG, Leake RD, Fisher DA. V1- and V2-receptor contributions to ovine fetal renal and cardiovascular responses to vasopressin. Am J Physiol 262:R636, 1992.
29. Brace RA, Wlodek ME, Cock ML, Harding R. Swallowing of lung liquid and amniotic fluid by the ovine fetus under normoxic and hypoxic conditions. Am J Obstet Gynecol 171:764, 1994.
30. Ross MG, Ervin G, Leake RD, Fu P, Fisher DA. Fetal lung liquid regulation by neuropeptides. Am J Obstet Gynecol 150:421, 1984.
31. Lawson EE, Brown ER, Torday JS, Madansky DL, Taeusch HW, Jr. The effect of epinephrine on tracheal fluid flow and surfactant efflux in fetal sheep. Am Rev Respir Dis 118:1023, 1978.
32. Dodic M, Wintour EM. Effects of prolonged (48 h) infusion of cortisol on blood pressure, renal function and fetal fluids in the immature ovine fetus. Clin Exp Pharmacol Physiol 21:971, 1994.
33. Sherman DJ, Ross MG, Ervin MG, Castro R, Hobel CJ, Fisher DA. Ovine fetal lung fluid response to intravenous saline solution infusion: fetal atrial natriuretic factor effect. Am J Obstet Gynecol 159:1347, 1988.
34. Pritchard JA. Fetal swallowing and amniotic fluid volume. Obstet Gynecol 28:606, 1966.
35. Bradley RM, Mistretta CM. Swallowing in fetal sheep. Science 179:1016, 1973.
36. Nijland MJ, Day L, Ross MG. Ovine fetal swallowing: expression of preterm neurobehavioral rhythms. J Matern Fetal Med 10:251, 2001.
37. Sherman DJ, Ross MG, Day L, Ervin MG. Fetal swallowing: correlation of electromyography and esophageal fluid flow. Am J Physiol 258:R1386, 1990.
38. Xu Z, Nijland MJ, Ross MG. Plasma osmolality dipsogenic thresholds and c-fos expression in the near-term ovine fetus. Pediatr Res 49:678, 2001.
39. El-Haddad MA, Ismail Y, Gayle D, Ross MG. Central angiotensin II AT1 receptors mediate fetal swallowing and pressor responses in the near term ovine fetus. Am J Physiol Regul Integr Comp Physiol 288:R1014–20, 2004.
40. El-Haddad MA, Ismail Y, Guerra C, Day L, Ross MG. Neuropeptide Y administered into cerebral ventricles stimulates sucrose ingestion in the near-term ovine fetus. Am J Obstet Gynecol 189:949, 2003.
41. El-Haddad MA, Ismail Y, Guerra C, Day L, Ross MG. Effect of oral sucrose on ingestive behavior in the near-term ovine fetus. Am J Obstet Gynecol 187:898, 2002.
42. Sherman DJ, Ross MG, Day L, Humme J, Ervin MG. Fetal swallowing: response to graded maternal hypoxemia. J Appl Physiol 71:1856, 1991.
43. Lingwood BE, Wintour EM. Amniotic fluid volume and in vivo permeability of ovine fetal membranes. Obstet Gynecol 64:368, 1984.
44. Gilbert WM, Newman PS, Eby-Wilkens E, Brace RA. Technetium Tc 99m rapidly crosses the ovine placenta and intramembranous pathway. Am J Obstet Gynecol 175:1557, 1996.
45. Lingwood BE, Wintour EM. Permeability of ovine amnion and amniochorion to urea and water. Obstet Gynecol 61:227, 1983.
46. Gilbert WM, Brace RA. The missing link in amniotic fluid volume regulation: intramembranous absorption. Obstet Gynecol 74:748, 1989.
47. Ervin MG, Ross MG, Leake RD, Fisher DA. Fetal recirculation of amniotic fluid arginine vasopressin. Am J Physiol 250:E253, 1986.
48. Gilbert WM, Cheung CY, Brace RA. Rapid intramembranous absorption into the fetal circulation of arginine vasopressin injected intraamniotically. Am J Obstet Gynecol 164:1013, 1991.
49. Queenan JT, Allen FH, Jr, Fuchs F, Stakemann G, Freisleben E, Fogh J, Soelvsten S. Studies on the method of intrauterine transfusion. I. Question of erythrocyte absorption from amniotic fluid. Am J Obstet Gynecol 92:1009, 1965.
50. Hebertson RM, Hammond ME, Bryson MJ. Amniotic epithelial ultrastructure in normal, polyhydramnic, and oligohydramnic pregnancies. Obstet Gynecol 68:74, 1986.
51. Gilbert WM, Brace RA. Novel determination of filtration coefficient of ovine placenta and intramembranous pathway. Am J Physiol 259:R1281, 1990.
52. Mann SE, Nijland MJ, Ross MG. Mathematic modeling of human amniotic fluid dynamics. Am J Obstet Gynecol 175:937, 1996.
53. Curran MA, Nijland MJ, Mann SE, Ross MG. Human amniotic fluid mathematical model: determination and effect of intramembranous sodium flux. Am J Obstet Gynecol 178:484, 1998.
54. Anderson DF, Faber JJ, Parks CM. Extraplacental transfer of water in the sheep. J Physiol 406:75, 1988.
55. Anderson DF, Borst NJ, Boyd RD, Faber JJ. Filtration of water from mother to conceptus via paths independent of fetal placental circulation in sheep. J Physiol 431:1, 1990.
56. Capurro C, Escobar E, Ibarra C, Porta M, Parisi M. Water permeability in different epithelial barriers. Biol Cell 66:145, 1989.
57. Faber, JJ, Thornberg, KL. Placental physiology: structure and function of fetomaternal exchange. Philadelphia, PA: Lippincott Williams & Wilkins, 1983.

58. Stulc J. Placental transfer of inorganic ions and water. Physiol Rev 77:805, 1997.

59. Georgiades P, Ferguson-Smith AC, Burton GJ. Comparative developmental anatomy of the murine and human definitive placentae. Placenta 23:3, 2002.

60. Jansson T, Illsley NP. Osmotic water permeabilities of human placental microvillous and basal membranes. J Membr Biol 132:147, 1993.

61. Hempstock J, Bao YP, Bar-Issac M, Segaren N, Watson AL, Charnock-Jones DS, Jauniaux E, Burton GJ. Intralobular differences in antioxidant enzyme expression and activity reflect the pattern of maternal arterial bloodflow within the human placenta. Placenta 24:517, 2003.

62. Makowski EL, Meschia G, Droegemueller W, Battaglia FC. Distribution of uterine blood flow in the pregnant sheep. Am J Obstet Gynecol 101:409, 1968.

63. Benirschke K: Comparative placentation. Available: http://medicine ucsd edu/cpa/homefs html 2006.

64. Schroder HJ. Basics of placental structures and transfer functions. In Brace RA, Ross MG and Robillard JE (eds), Fetal and neonatal body fluids: the scientific basis for clinical practice (pp. 187–226). Ithaca, NY: Perinatology Press. 1989.

65. Stulc J, Stulcova B, Sibley CP. Evidence for active maternal-fetal transport of Na+ across the placenta of the anaesthetized rat. J Physiol 470:637, 1993.

66. Stulc J, Stulcova B. Asymmetrical transfer of inert hydrophilic solutes across rat placenta. Am J Physiol 265:R670, 1993.

67. Schroder H, Nelson P, Power G. Fluid shift across the placenta: I. The effect of dextran T 40 in the isolated guinea-pig placenta. Placenta 3:327, 1982.

68. Ervin MG, Amico JA, Leake RD, Ross MG, Robinson AG, Fisher DA. Arginine vasotocin-like immunoreactivity in plasma of pregnant women and newborns. West Soc Ped Res Clin Res 33:115A, 1985.

69. Conrad EE, Jr, Faber JJ. Water and electrolyte acquisition across the placenta of the sheep. Am J Physiol 233:H475, 1977.

70. Schroder H, Leichtweiss HP. Perfusion rates and the transfer of water across isolated guinea pig placenta. Am J Physiol 232:H666, 1977.

71. Leichtweiss HP, Schroder H. The effect of elevated outflow pressure on flow resistance and the transfer of THO, albumin and glucose in the isolated guinea pig placenta. Pflugers Arch 371:251, 1977.

72. Brace RA, Moore TR. Transplacental, amniotic, urinary, and fetal fluid dynamics during very-large-volume fetal intravenous infusions. Am J Obstet Gynecol 164:907, 1991.

73. Brace RA, Gilbert WM, Thornburg KL. Vascularization of the ovine amnion and chorion: a morphometric characterization of the surface area of the intramembranous pathway. Am J Obstet Gynecol 167:1747, 1992.

74. Battaglia FC, Hellegers AE, Meschia G, Barron DH. In vitro investigations of the human chorion as a membrane system. Nature 196:1061, 1962.

75. Fujino Y, Agnew CL, Schreyer P, Ervin MG, Sherman DJ, Ross MG. Amniotic fluid volume response to esophageal occlusion in fetal sheep. Am J Obstet Gynecol 165:1620, 1991.

76. Matsumoto LC, Cheung CY, Brace RA. Effect of esophageal ligation on amniotic fluid volume and urinary flow rate in fetal sheep. Am J Obstet Gynecol 182:699, 2000.

77. Wintour EM, Barnes A, Brown EH, Hardy KJ, Horacek I, McDougall JG, Scoggins BA. Regulation of amniotic fluid volume and composition in the ovine fetus. Obstet Gynecol 52:689, 1978.

78. Faber JJ, Anderson DF. Regulatory response of intramembranous absorption of amniotic fluid to infusion of exogenous fluid in sheep. Am J Physiol 277:R236, 1999.

79. Ross MG, Ervin MG, Leake RD, Oakes G, Hobel C, Fisher DA. Bulk flow of amniotic fluid water in response to maternal osmotic challenge. Am J Obstet Gynecol 147:697, 1983.

80. Leontic EA, Tyson JE. Prolactin and fetal osmoregulation: water transport across isolated human amnion. Am J Physiol 232:R124, 1977.

81. Holt WF, Perks AM. The effect of prolactin on water movement through the isolated amniotic membrane of the guinea pig. Gen Comp Endocrinol 26:153, 1975.

82. Matsumoto LC, Bogic L, Brace RA, Cheung CY. Fetal esophageal ligation induces expression of vascular endothelial growth factor messenger ribonucleic acid in fetal membranes. Am J Obstet Gynecol 184:175, 2001.

83. Daneshmand SS, Cheung CY, Brace RA. Regulation of amniotic fluid volume by intramembranous absorption in sheep: role of passive permeability and vascular endothelial growth factor. Am J Obstet Gynecol 188:786, 2003.

84. Brace RA, Vermin ML, Huijssoon E. Regulation of amniotic fluid volume: intramembranous solute and volume fluxes in late gestation fetal sheep. Am J Obstet Gynecol 191:837, 2004.

85. Faber JJ, Anderson DF. Absorption of amniotic fluid by amniochorion in sheep. Am J Physiol Heart Circ Physiol 282:H850, 2002.

86. Wynn RM, French GL. Comparative ultrastructure of the mammalian amnion. Obstet Gynecol 31:759, 1968.

87. Anderson D, Yang Q, Hohimer A, Faber J, Giraud G, Davis L. Intramembranous absorption rate is unaffected by changes in amniotic fluid composition. Am J Physiol Renal Physiol 288:F964, 2005.

88. Knepper MA, Wade JB, Terris J, Ecelbarger CA, Marples D, Mandon B, Chou CL, Kishore BK, Nielsen S. Renal aquaporins. Kidney Int 49:1712, 1996.

89. Nielsen S, Frokiaer J, Marples D, Kwon TH, Agre P, Knepper MA. Aquaporins in the kidney: from molecules to medicine. Physiol Rev 82:205, 2002.

90. Klussmann E, Maric K, Rosenthal W. The mechanisms of aquaporin control in the renal collecting duct. Rev Physiol Biochem Pharmacol 141:33, 2000.

91. Tajika Y, Matsuzaki T, Suzuki T, Aoki T, Hagiwara H, Kuwahara M, Sasaki S, Takata K. Aquaporin-2 is retrieved to the apical storage compartment via early endosomes and phosphatidylinositol 3-kinase-dependent pathway. Endocrinol 145:4375, 2004.
92. Gradilone SA, Garcia F, Huebert RC, Tietz PS, Larocca MC, Kierbel A, Carreras FI, LaRusso NF, Marinelli RA. Glucagon induces the plasma membrane insertion of functional aquaporin-8 water channels in isolated rat hepatocytes. Hepatology 37:1435, 2003.
93. Sugiyama Y, Ota Y, Hara M, Inoue S. Osmotic stress up-regulates aquaporin-3 gene expression in cultured human keratinocytes. Biochim Biophys Acta 1522:82, 2001.
94. Johnston H, Koukoulas I, Jeyaseelan K, Armugam A, Earnest L, Baird R, Dawson N, Ferraro T, Wintour EM. Ontogeny of aquaporins 1 and 3 in ovine placenta and fetal membranes. Placenta 21:88, 2000.
95. Liu H, Koukoulas I, Ross MC, Wang S, Wintour EM. Quantitative comparison of placental expression of three aquaporin genes. Placenta 25:475, 2004.
96. Mann SE, Ricke EA, Yang BA, Verkman AS, Taylor RN. Expression and localization of aquaporin 1 and 3 in human fetal membranes. Am J Obstet Gynecol 187:902, 2002.
97. Damiano A, Zotta E, Goldstein J, Reisin I, Ibarra C. Water channel proteins AQP3 and AQP9 are present in syncytiotrophoblast of human term placenta. Placenta 22:776, 2001.
98. Umenishi F, Verkman AS, Gropper MA. Quantitative analysis of aquaporin mRNA expression in rat tissues by RNase protection assay. DNA Cell Biol 15:475, 1996.
99. Ma T, Yang B, Verkman AS. Cloning of a novel water and urea-permeable aquaporin from mouse expressed strongly in colon, placenta, liver, and heart. Biochem Biophys Res Commun 240:324, 1997.
100. Wang S, Kallichanda N, Song W, Ramirez BA, Ross MG. Expression of aquaporin-8 in human placenta and chorioamniotic membranes: evidence of molecular mechanism for intramembranous amniotic fluid resorption. Am J Obstet Gynecol 185:1226, 2001.
101. Beall MH, Chaudhri N, Amidi F, Wang S, Yang B, Ross MG. Increased expression of aquaporins in placenta of the late gestation mouse fetus. J Soc Gynecol Invest 12:780, 2005.
102. Mann SE, Ricke EA, Torres EA, Taylor RN. A novel model of polyhydramnios: amniotic fluid volume is increased in aquaporin 1 knockout mice. Am J Obstet Gynecol 192:2041, 2005.
103. Mann S, Dvorak N, Taylor R. Changes in aquaporin 1 expression affect amniotic fluid volume. Am J Obstet Gyn 191:S132, 2004.
104. Bos HB, Nygard KL, Gratton RJ, Richardson BS. Expression of aquaporin 1 (AQP1) in chorioallantoic membranes of near term ovine fetuses with induced hypoxia. J Soc Gynecol Invest 12:333A, 2005.
105. Wang S, Chen J, Au KT, Ross MG. Expression of aquaporin 8 and its up-regulation by cyclic adenosine monophosphate in human WISH cells. Am J Obstet Gynecol 188:997, 2003.
106. Wang S, Amidi F, Beall MH, Ross MG. Differential regulation of aquaporin water channels in human amnion cell culture. J Soc Gynecol Invest 12:344A, 2005.

Section II

Electrolyte Balance During Normal Fetal and Neonatal Development

Chapter 2

Renal Aspects of Sodium Metabolism in the Fetus and Neonate*

Endre Sulyok, MD, PhD, DSc

Body Water Compartments
Body Water Compartments and Initial Weight Loss
Physical Water Compartments
Sodium Homeostasis
Disturbances in Plasma Sodium Concentrations
Sodium Homeostasis and Acid-Base Balance

Sodium and volume homeostasis in the fetus and neonates has been the subject of intensive research for decades. Several aspects of the developmental changes in renal sodium handling have been revealed. It is now apparent that in addition to the intrinsic limitations of tubular transport of sodium by the immature kidney, extra-renal factors play an important role in maintaining sodium balance. In this chapter an attempt has been made to summarize our current knowledge of the sodium homeostasis in the fetus and the neonate, and to present a revised concept of perinatal redistribution of body fluids. In the light of recent clinical, experimental and molecular biological research, our understanding of the developmental changes in salt and water metabolism is greatly improved, and consequently a more targeted approach can be applied to the clinical management of healthy and sick neonates.

BODY WATER COMPARTMENTS

Body water is distributed in well-defined compartments that undergo marked developmental changes. Total body water (TBW) and extracellular water (ECW) gradually decrease, whereas intracellular water (ICW) increases as the gestation advances. The decrease of ECW is mainly confined to the interstitial water (ISW); the plasma water remains relatively unaffected (1).

Individual estimates of body water compartments over this period vary greatly and are related to several factors, including intrauterine growth rate, gender, pregnancy pathology, mode of delivery, maternal fluid management during labor, neonatal renal function, and postnatal fluid intake. For example, growth-retarded neonates have significantly higher ECW (as a percentage of body weight) than their appropriate-for-gestational age matches (2). Infants born to mothers with

---

*To commemorate the 100th anniversary of the birth of my teacher Professor Edmund Kerpel-Fronius.

Table 2-1	**Body Composition of the Reference Fetus**								
		Per 100g fat-free weight							
Gestational age (weeks)	Body weight (g)	Water (g)	Protein (g)	Ca (mg)	P (mg)	Mg (g)	Na (mEq)	K (mEq)	Cl (mEq)
24	690	88.6	8.8	621	387	17.8	9.9	4.0	7.0
25	770	88.4	9.1	615	385	17.6	9.8	4.0	7.0
26	880	88.1	9.4	611	384	17.5	9.7	4.1	7.0
27	1010	87.8	9.7	609	383	17.4	9.5	4.1	6.9
28	1160	87.5	10.0	610	385	17.4	9.4	4.2	6.9
29	1318	87.2	10.3	613	387	17.4	9.3	4.2	6.8
30	1480	86.8	10.6	619	392	17.4	9.2	4.3	6.8
31	1650	86.5	10.9	628	398	17.6	9.1	4.3	6.7
32	1830	86.1	11.3	640	406	17.8	9.1	4.3	6.6
33	2020	85.8	11.6	656	416	18.0	9.0	4.4	6.5
34	2230	85.4	11.9	675	428	18.3	8.9	4.4	6.4
35	2450	85.0	12.2	699	443	18.6	8.9	4.5	6.3
36	2690	84.6	12.5	726	460	19.0	8.8	4.5	6.1
37	2940	84.3	12.8	758	479	19.5	8.8	4.5	6.0
38	3160	83.9	13.1	795	501	20.0	8.8	4.5	5.9
39	3330	83.6	13.3	836	525	20.5	8.7	4.6	5.8
40	3450	83.3	13.5	882	551	21.1	8.7	4.6	5.7

From Ziegler EE, O'Donnell AM, Nelson SE, Fomon SJ: Body composition of the reference fetus. Growth 40: 329-341, 1976.

toxemia and those delivered by elective caesarean section or after maternal fluid administration during labor have greater ECW (3). Infants of diabetic mothers have increased body fat. As a result, the TBW is reduced but the relationship between ECW and ICW and fat-free body mass is normal (4). Newborn infants with severe respiratory distress syndrome (RDS) who have impaired renal function are likely to have an expanded ECW when sodium and fluid intake is not restricted (5,6).

Body fat apposition is less than 1% in the fetus with gestational age below 26 weeks; it approximates 12% in full-term neonates and reaches about 30% of body weight in 3-month-old infants.

The perinatal redistribution of body fluid compartments is associated with changes in ionic composition of tissue water (Table 2-1). Accordingly, at the early stage of development the body has high sodium and low potassium contents that progress to the opposite with increasing maturation.

As shown by Ziegler et al (7), the sodium and chloride content per 100 g fat-free weight, the principal electrolytes of ECW, decrease, while protein, phosphorous, magnesium and potassium content, the major constituents of the ICW, increase. More specifically, body sodium decreased progressively from 9.9 mEq at 24 weeks' gestation to 8.7 mEq at term as opposed to the steady rise of body potassium from 4.0 mEq to 4.6 mEq during the same period of gestation.

When individual tissues of various species were analyzed separately there were variations in the rate of chemical development, possibly reflecting differences in their functional maturation. Interestingly, the developmental pattern of brain electrolytes in fetal sheep and guinea-pigs followed paraboloid relations with gestational age; brain sodium and chloride content reached its peak value in the second part of gestation, which was mirrored by the minimum value of brain potassium (8). This phenomenon may represent corresponding alterations in the volume of ECW and/or in the transport activity of the Na^+/K^+ exchanger. It is also of interest that when distinct brain areas representing various stages of phylogenetic development were investigated, brain water content and sodium concentration were found to vary from high for the youngest cortex to low for the oldest medulla, the respective values for other brain areas fell between these extremes (9).

Cell Volume Regulation

The volume and composition of body fluid compartments are strictly controlled. ECW is under neuroendocrine control and the final regulation is accomplished by the kidney through retaining or excreting solutes and fluids. By contrast, ICW volume is regulated by osmotically driven passive water flux across the cell membrane.

In this regard it is to be noted that cells of the brain and transporting epithelia respond to perturbations of ECW osmolality, not only with inducing the appropriate water flow in or out of cells, but also with gaining or losing cellular organic and anorganic osmolytes to limit osmotic water flux and to preserve cell volume. This volume regulatory response develops in the brain of ovine fetuses in a region-and age-related fashion. Namely in fetuses with 60% of gestation this volume regulatory response is impaired when compared with more mature animals and it starts operating in the younger cortex then in the phylogenetically older medulla (10). It is to be stressed that the elevated tissue sodium levels, and more importantly, the elevated sodium to potassium ratio in the developing brain indicates that the proccss of 'chemical maturation' has not been completed (11) and the immature brain is not capable of controlling its volume by ionic movements, but rather by the accumulation or extrusion of the predominant organic osmolyte, i.e., taurine (12).

In addition to the well-defined volume regulatory response by the cellular osmolytes the cell membrane itself is also involved in the adaptation of cells to osmotic challenges. Brain-specific water channel membrane protein, aquaporin-4 (AQP4), is widely distributed in cells at the blood/brain and brain/cerebrospinal fluid interfaces, where it facilitates water movement.

AQP4 protein is expressed abundantly in a highly polarized distribution in ependymal cells and astroglial membranes facing capillaries and forming the glia limitans (13).

A growing body of evidence suggests that complete lack, reduced expression, mislocalization, deficient membrane anchoring and dysfunction of brain AQP4 limits transmembrane water flux and provides first-line defense mechanisms to maintain cerebral water balance and to protect brain volume (14).

In support of this notion Manley et al (15) demonstrated that AQP4 deficiency protected the brain and reduced edema formation in mice exposed to acute water intoxication and focal ischemic stroke. When compared to their wild-type counterparts the AQP4 knockout mice had less brain water content, better neurological outcome and improved survival. Almost simultaneously our group, using a different experimental model, came essentially to the same conclusion. Namely, we found that in response to severe systemic hyponatremia, a rapid increase occurred in the immunoreactivity of astroglial AQP4 protein without significant changes in AQP4 mRNA levels or subcellular distribution of AQP4 protein. According to our interpretation the hypoosmotic stress-related post-transcriptional AQP4 protein changes may potentially be accounted for by enhanced phosphorylation and subsequent altered conformation and immunogenity of the channel protein (16). Phosphorylated AQP4 has been shown to reduce water conductivity (17). Furthermore, the dystrophin-associated protein (DAP) complex that connects extracellular matrix components to the cytoskeleton is closely related to AQP4. Neuronal dystrophin isoform and the related proteins are co-localized with brain AQP4 in the astrocyte endfeet and AQP4 is markedly reduced in dystrophin deficient states. Additionally, α-syntrophin, a member at the DAP family, has also been shown to be involved in polarized trafficking, regulated surface expression and membrane anchoring of AQP4. The complex interrelationship between dystrophin, α-syntrophin, AQP4 and brain water metabolism has been documented by demonstrating a marked reduction in the abundance of both AQP4 and α-syntrophin protein expression in the perivascular astrocyte endfeet of animals missing dystrophin. It is to be stressed that dystrophin-null mice subjected to water intoxication had delayed intracellular water accumulation and prolonged survival (18). These observations can be regarded as indicating that functioning AQP4 favors development of brain edema, while AQP4 deficiency protects against edemagenesis when animals are challenged by pathological conditions known to cause brain water accumulation.

Recent studies on the ontogeny of the expression of brain AQP4 protein and mRNA in four mammalian species, including humans, have revealed their very low levels at the early stage of gestation and their gradual increase as the gestation progressed to term (19). AQP4 protein expression levels in rat cerebellum during different stages of postnatal development have proved to be hardly detectable in the first week, increasing from 2% of adult levels on day 7 to 25% and 63% on days 14 and 28, respectively (20). These observations provide suggestive evidences that the low expression of AQP4 may limit transmembranous water flux and may contribute to maintaining water balance in the maturing brain, which has no fully developed osmolyte-related volume regulatory reaction.

Fetal Sodium Metabolism

The dynamic interactions between maternal and fetal circulation and amniotic fluid throughout gestation ensure fetal homeostasis and supply nutrients, solutes and water for growth. The placenta and fetal membranes play an essential role in regulating transport processes as they behave like a low-permeability barrier and/or contain specific transcellular transport mechanisms. In general, minerals that are contained in the plasma at low concentrations and are mainly intracellular or sequestered in bones (K^+, Mg, Ca, phosphate) are transported to the fetus actively, whereas the transfer of major extracellular ions (Na^+, Cl^-) has great interspecies variations and may occur through active or passive transport (21).

To accomplish normal fetal growth the accretion rate of sodium and potassium has been estimated to be 1.8 mMol/kg/day (22) and the volume of transplacental water flux is approximately 20 mL/kg/day in near-term human fetuses (23).

Fetal plasma sodium concentrations are stable in relation to gestational age of 18 to 40 weeks, and are not significantly different from maternal plasma sodium concentrations or they are slightly lower, which allows passive sodium flow to the fetus (24). It has been well-documented, however, that the placental syncytiotrophoblast is equipped with transport systems needed for transcellular sodium transfer. Sodium flux from mother to fetus is 10–100 times higher than the rate of sodium accretion by the fetus, indicating that most of the sodium transferred to the fetus returns to the mother by paracellular diffusion so the transplacental sodium flux is bidirectional and nearly symmetrical (25).

Amniotic Fluid Dynamics

Although there are fairly wide variations, the volume and composition of amniotic fluid undergo characteristic changes during gestation (26). Its volume increases from 40 mL at 11 weeks' gestation to approximately 700 mL at 25 weeks' gestation, then increases further to reach its maximum of about 920 mL at 35 weeks' gestation. Later in gestation it begins to decrease to about 720 mL at term, followed by a more marked reduction in post-term pregnancies. During the first trimester of gestation, osmolality and electrolyte composition of the amniotic fluid correspond to fetal plasma. When the fetus begins to void hypotonic urine at approximately 11 weeks of gestation, amniotic fluid osmolality decreases progressively with advancing gestational age to reach the value of 250–260 mOsm/L near term. Sodium concentration in fetal urine decreases accordingly, and contributes to the generation of hypotonic amniotic fluid. The low amniotic fluid osmolality provides an

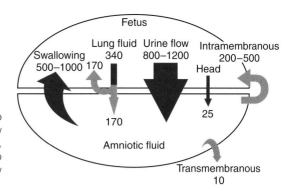

Figure 2-1 Schematic presentation of water flows into and out of the amniotic space in late gestation. Arrow size is proportional to flow rate. (From Gilbert WM, Brace RA: Amniotic fluid volume and normal flows to and from the amniotic cavity. Seminar of Perinatology 17:150-157, 1993, with permission.)

osmotic driving force for the outward water flow across the intra- and transmembranous pathways. The volume and composition of amniotic fluid during late gestation are therefore determined by fetal urine and lung fluid secretion as the two primary sources of amniotic fluid, and fetal swallowing and intramembranous absorption as the two primary routes of amniotic water clearance (Fig. 2-1). Quantitative estimates for the dynamic state of amniotic fluid sodium are presented in Table 2-2.

Mechanisms of Placental Sodium Transfer

Convincing evidences have been provided to indicate that in the rat and pig the maternal–fetal sodium flux is accomplished by active transcellular transport, which is saturable, highly dependent on temperature and can be inhibited by ouabain added to the fetal side (27). The presence of Na^+-K^+-ATPase in the trophoblast plasma membrane has been demonstrated (28). Moreover, in rat placenta the activity and expression of the α-subunit of Na^+-K^+-ATPase increase in parallel with the maternal–fetal sodium flux during the last trimester of pregnancy (29,30). These observations are in line with the conclusion that the sodium-pump enzyme serves as the major common pathway of sodium extrusion from the syncytiotrophoblast at the fetal side of the membrane. Attempts to explore the sites of sodium entry at the brush-border plasma membrane (maternal side facing) have identified several mechanisms. The Na^+/H^+ exchanger (NHE) family of transport proteins have been shown to be present in the placental microvillous plasma membrane. These transport proteins mediate the electroneutral exchange of extracellular Na^+ for intracellular H^+ and play a role in regulating intracellular pH, transepithelial Na transport and cell volume homeostasis.

Table 2-2   Sodium and Volume Metabolism in Human Amniotic Fluid

Gestational age (weeks)	Amniotic fluid Volume (ml)	Amniotic fluid Na (mEq/L)	Urine Volume (ml)	Urine Na (mEq/L)	Lung Volume (ml)	Lung Na (mEq/L)	Flow calculations IM_D (ml)	Flow calculations S_D (ml)
11	40	135	11	122	0	140	1	10
15	151	135	49	110	2	140	9	37
20	393	135	122	89	10	140	42	83
25	665	135	239	71	27	140	112	147
30	872	134	427	57	58	140	241	239
35	924	131	728	50	114	140	438	403
40	726	126	1211	50	169	140	701	686

From Curran MA, Nijland MJM, Mann SE, Ross MG: Human amniotic fluid mathematical model: Determination and effect of intramembranous sodium flux. American Journal of Obstetrics and Gynecology 178:484–490, 1998.

IM_D, dynamic intramembranous flow; S_D, dynamic swallowed volume.

Three isoforms of the NHE protein family have been detected in the microvillous membrane of syncytiotrophoblast (NHE1, NHE2 and NHE3). NHE1 proved to be the predominant isoform responsible for the amiloride-sensitive maternofetal sodium transfer (31). NHE activity increases over gestation and the amiloride-sensitive Na^+ uptake by the microvillous membrane is markedly elevated in term placenta as compared to the first trimester placenta (32). A similar gestational pattern was seen for the expression of NHE1 and NHE2 mRNA. NHE1 protein expression did not change over gestation, but NHE2 and NHE3 protein showed a marked increase in their expression between the second trimester and term (33). Interestingly, when placental NHE1 activity and expression were compared between normally grown and growth-retarded preterm and full-term infants both the expression and activity of NHE1 were lower in the growth-retarded group delivered preterm. It has been suggested that the limited Na^+/H^+ exchange may contribute to the development of fetal acidosis frequently seen in these infants without apparent birth asphyxia (34). Studies to reveal the control mechanisms of Na^+ transport by Na^+/H^+ exchanger in brush-border membrane vesicles, isolated from human placental villous tissue have shown that ethylisopropylamiloride, the specific inhibitor of the transporter, decreased Na uptake by 98%, whereas benzamil, the Na channel blocker, had no effect. Similarly, the activity of Na^+/H^+ exchanger remained unaffected by cAMP, phorbol ester, insulin, angiotensin II, or parathyroid hormone, all known to regulate Na^+/H^+ exchange by the isoform present in the renal brush border membrane (35).

In addition to the Na^+/H^+ antiporter, other transport mechanisms have been assumed to be involved in the passive entry of Na^+ into the trophoblast from the maternal side. Furosemide-sensitive Na-K-2Cl co-transporter and hydrochlorothiazide-sensitive Na-Cl co-transporter appear to be absent from placental brush-border membrane vesicles (27), although bumetanide-sensitive Na-K-2Cl co-transporter has been shown to be expressed in BeWo cells, a human trophoblastic cell line (36). The involvement of epithelial sodium channel (ENaC) in placental sodium transport has not been confirmed, however, there has been suggestive evidence for the presence and gestational increase of ENaC-α-subunit in the allantoic membrane and trophoblast of the porcine placenta (37). The substrate-specific (phosphate, amino acids) cotransporter-mediated Na uptake by the microvillous membrane of the syncytiotrophoblast has been widely accepted (35).

Fetal Homeostatic Reactions

Fetal sheep infused intravascularly with normal saline had a modest increase in amniotic fluid volume and a substantial rise in urine flow rate. These increases roughly equalled the intramembranous absorption that occurred in parallel with an increase in vascular endothelial growth factor gene expression in the amnion, chorion and placenta. Based on these findings it has been suggested that the increased intramembranous absorption induced by volume-loading diuresis may be mediated by vascular endothelial growth factor via stimulating active transport processes (38).

Persistent fetal diuresis can also be induced by maternal administration of DDAVP combined with oral water load. Water retention results in maternal hyponatremia followed by a slow decline in fetal plasma sodium and increased fetal urine flow. Fetal diuresis has been assumed to be due to fetal hyponatremia rather than to the reduction in maternal-to-fetal osmotic gradient. This notion appears to be supported by the close inverse relationship of fetal urine flow rate to fetal plasma sodium concentration and by the persistent diuresis despite placental osmotic equilibrium (39).

Furthermore, to maintain sodium homeostasis in the fetus of sodium-depleted, severely hyponatremic pregnant rats, net sodium transfer to the growing fetus increases markedly against a significant sodium concentration gradient between maternal and fetal plasma (40). By contrast, long-term hypertonic NaCl infusion into late-gestation fetal sheep caused a significant increase in fetal plasma sodium, chloride and osmolality but their values in the maternal plasma remained unaltered. Most of the infused sodium and chloride was excreted by the fetus in large volumes of hypotonic urine. There was a transient rise in amniotic fluid volume with unchanged osmolality and sodium concentration. Interestingly, as the infused NaCl was retained neither in the fetus nor in the amniotic fluid, it has been suggested that NaCl was lost from the fetal into the maternal compartment despite osmotic and concentration gradients favoring the opposite direction of transfer (41).

Fetal sheep undergoing continuous drainage of fetal fluids in late gestation attempt to maintain their salt-and water balance by a compensatory reduction in renal sodium excretion. The fall in fetal renal sodium excretion, however, accounted for only about 11% of total sodium conservation, the rest of the compensation was achieved by the mother (42).

All these observations can be regarded as strong evidence that the fetal sodium and volume homeostasis is effectively regulated and when challenged by depletion or loading feto-maternal control mechanisms comes into operation to restore volume and salt balance to normal. The control of fetal homeostatic mechanisms operating to limit or enhance salt and fluid flux across the kidney or fetal membrane barriers has not been clearly defined. However, there have been reports that in addition to the traditional volume regulatory hormones, prolactin plays an important role. Namely, fetal prolactin has been shown to be released in response to increasing cord serum sodium concentration and osmolality. Fetal prolactin in turn has a significant positive correlation with amniotic fluid sodium concentration and osmolality but an inverse relationship with amniotic fluid volume suggesting the suppression of hypotonic fetal urine excretion (43). The additional roles of maternal and amniotic fluid prolactin, derived from maternal decidua in fetal-amniotic fluid salt and water balance, have also been proposed (44). In good agreement with these findings we have demonstrated significantly elevated plasma prolactin levels in full-term newborn infants presenting with idiopathic edema (45) and an increase in plasma prolactin in sodium-depleted low-birth weight premature infants and its restoration to normal when supplemental sodium was given (46).

BODY WATER COMPARTMENTS AND INITIAL WEIGHT LOSS

Soon after birth, redistribution of body fluid compartments occurs, which is a subject of controversy. Most authors agree that early postnatal weight loss corresponds to the isotonic contraction of ECW and the disposal of excess sodium and water through the kidney (47,48). It is greater and lasts longer in infants with less advanced maturation (49). The weight loss and the contraction of ECW is a physiological adaptation to extrauterine life rather than dehydration or starvation, in as much as body solids increase and nitrogen balance is positive during the period of weight loss. Longitudinal studies to assess changes in body composition of preterm neonates with and without respiratory distress syndrome (RDS) during the immediate postnatal period support this notion. Providing adequate nutritional support, postnatal weight loss and loss of TBW is accompanied by a steady increase in the accretion of body solids. The rate of increase, however, proved to be greater in healthy preterm infants than in those with RDS (50). Contrasting reports have been published by others showing some evidence for tissue catabolism and for failure to gain solids (51–54).

In addition to renal excretion a fluid 'shift' from ECW to ICW has also been described, but this is more likely a result of ECW loss than growth in cell mass (55).

In low-birth weight premature infants, the initial weight loss of 15% or more is confined to the extravascular ECW. Plasma volume remains unchanged, and there are no clinical signs of dehydration or hypovolemic circulatory failure. Plasma protein levels that would reflect a shift in oncotic pressure differences favoring water loss from interstitium into the vascular space do not change (56).

Renal salt wasting and hyponatremia during the early postnatal weight loss in low-birth weight prematures is not compatible with isotonic contraction of ECW but rather it indicates that these infants are not capable of maintaining the volume of their ECW within the physiological limits.

Cheek has developed the concept that there was a significant decrease in cell water content rather than in ECW during the first days of life (57). MacLaurin (58), using thiocyanate as a marker for ECW, identified ICW as the source of neonatal water loss. In this study, ICW fell in parallel with TBW, while ECW rose slightly and plasma volume remained constant. He argued that ECW is more effectively maintained than ICW during adaptation to early extrauterine life. In good agreement with these observations Coulter and Avery (59) and Coulter (60) demonstrated a paradoxical reduction in hydration of fat-free (FF) body mass (mL water/100g FF body mass) in neonatal rabbit pups, which correlated with increasing weight gain during the first 72 h of life. The extent of relative reduction in tissue water varied considerably among individual tissues; the greatest losses were observed in the skin (24%) and skeletal muscle (5–8%). Whereas lean body mass and skin and skeletal muscle water related inversely to weight gain and fluid intake, the liver and brain related directly. Based on these findings, the authors concluded that there is an ICW reservoir located mainly in the skin and muscle from which water is released in a regulated manner according to the actual need. Thus when sufficient fluid intake is provided, the superfluous ICW is rapidly released and excreted. However, when fluid intake is restricted, the release is considerably slower and contributes to maintaining circulating plasma volume (59). It has been claimed that prolactin is involved in the regulation of these processes (60).

The mechanisms triggering and controlling the process of initial weight loss have not been clearly established. Recently it has been proposed that the postnatal fall in pulmonary vascular resistance and the subsequent increase of left atrial return result in the release of atrial natriuretic peptide (ANP), which induces sodium chloride and water diuresis (61,62). However, plasma ANP does not correlate with either urinary flow rate or urinary sodium excretion (6). Furthermore, the effective circulating blood volume in healthy term infants varies directly with the ECF volume.

PHYSICAL WATER COMPARTMENTS

To reconcile the apparently conflicting views on the source of neonatal water loss, a concept has been recently put forward implying that not only the compartmentalization but also the mobility of tissue water is of importance in neonatal body fluid redistribution. Accordingly, motionally distinct water fractions have been established; the free bulky water and the relatively constrained, slow-motion bound water. From this latter fraction water can be liberated in a regulated manner according to the actual need of volume regulation irrespective of its location in the cellular or extracellular phase (63).

The Principle of Physical Water Compartments

The term 'physical water compartments' designates the physical state of tissue water and implies interactions between dipole water molecules and tissue biopolymers including proteins and glycosaminoglycans. The interaction of the polar solid surface of intra-or extracellular macromolecules with water results in the formation of the dynamic structure of polarized water multilayer. The degree of water polarization depends on the number of exposed active, polar groups of the water polarizing macromolecules. The first oriented layer of water molecules on the surfaces can induce a second layer to orient, the second will likewise influence the third and so on. As a result, a picture of hydrophylic surfaces bounded by a coat of structured water emerges. The range of interactions generating the polarized water multilayer has been variously suggested extending from nanometers to several micrometers. With respect to the electrical polarization and spatial orientation of tissue water, intra-and extracellular macromolecules, therefore, create microcompartments with different size and stability. The extent of water polarization is assumed to be proportional to the limitation of tissue water mobility (64,65).

Determination of Motionally Distinct Water Fractions

H^1-NMR measurements have been applied to assess quantitative changes in tissue water mobility since it provides an estimate of the physical state of tissue water, including volume fraction, proton residence time and intrinsic magnetic relaxation rate within the compartments. The theoretical basis for this estimate is that the magnetic relaxation rates for ordered (bound) water protons are faster than those for non-ordered (free) water protons. For quantitative assessment of tissue water fractions with different mobility multicomponent analysis of the T_2 relaxation decay curves has been applied. The free induction decay of the proton relaxation process follows an exponential function. This function can be described by a multi-exponential equation, provided that in the tissues studied there are water compartments with different rates of relaxation and these compartments are not interdependent at the time of measurement. Biexponential analysis of the T_2 relaxation curves allows us to estimate the bound and free water fractions by determining the fast and the slow components of the curves. Using triexponential analysis, further partition of the T_2 curves is possible and a distinction can be made between the fast, middle and slow components corresponding to the tightly bound, the loosely bound, and the free water fractions (66).

Physical Water Compartments during the Early Postnatal Period

In a series of recent studies we attempted to quantitate the free and bound water fractions in the skin, skeletal muscle, brain, and liver of two groups of newborn rabbits during the first 3–4 days of life. Rabbit pups of one group were nursed conventionally by their mothers, suckling ad libitum while the other group included pups separated from their mothers and completely withheld from fluid intake (67,68).

Biexponential analysis of the T_2 relaxation curves revealed that the bound water fractions amounted to 42–47% in the skin, 50–57% in the muscle, and 34–40% in the liver, respectively, of the total tissue water. This pattern of distribution did not change either with age or fluid intake. By contrast, the percent contribution of bound water fraction in the brain fell progressively from 61% at birth to 3–4% at the age of 72–96 h. In response to complete fluid deprival the reduction of bound water fraction was accelerated to attain a value of as low as 4% already on the first day of life (Fig. 2-2).

Using triexponential analysis we found that most of the skin (48–64%) and muscle water (54–64%) is loosely bound followed by the free (skin: 26–45%, muscle: 25–32%) and tightly bound water fractions (skin: 6–14%, muscle: 10–16%). Postnatal age and fluid intake had no apparent influence on this pattern of partition. Interestingly, in the liver, more water was tightly bound than in the other tissues, this fraction increased from 14% at birth to 26–33% later on, mostly at the expense of loosely bound water fraction. The postnatal increase of the tightly bound fraction proved to be more pronounced in the starving pups. In the brain

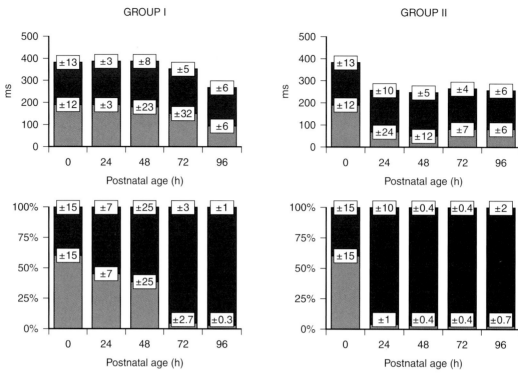

Figure 2-2 Relaxation times and partition of brain water fractions according to their mobility as derived from the biexponential analysis of T2 decay curves in newborn rabbits nursed conventionally (group I) and completely withheld from fluid intake (group II). Symbols □ = fast-bound, ■ = slow-free components. Upper panels represent absolute values; lower panels represent percent distribution of different water fractions. Data are given as mean ± SE. (From Berényi E, Repa I, Bogner P, Dóczi T, Sulyok E: Water content and proton magnetic resonance relaxation times of the brain in newborn rabbits. Pediatric Research 43:421–425, 1998, with permission.)

loosely bound water (48–94%) also predominated over the free (3–49%) and tightly bound water fraction (3–29%). Starving pups responded to fluid deprivation with a 3- to 6- fold decrease in the tightly bound water and with a simultaneous 4-fold increase in the free water fractions.

The postnatal increase of the free water fraction can be regarded as a supportive evidence for restructuring brain water in order to maintain brain volume.

The different water mobility in individual newborn rabbit tissues and its response pattern to complete withdrawal of fluid intake appear to be the result of the differences in water content, water-free chemical composition, qualitative or quantitative alterations in macromolecular compounds and metabolic activity of the tissues investigated.

Role of Hyaluronan (HA) in the Perinatal Lung and Brain Water Metabolism

Hyaluronan (HA), with its polyanionic nature and gel-like properties, has been claimed to be the major macromolecular compound controlling water mobility and water balance in the lung (69). During the fetal and neonatal periods HA concentration in the lung tissue is elevated and inversely proportional to the maturity of the neonate. Its role as a determinant of tissue water content during pulmonary adaptation has been established (70,71).

Recently, parameters of lung water metabolism and lung HA concentrations have been studied simultaneously in the late fetal and early postnatal periods. It has been demonstrated that the T_2-derived free water fraction increased, whereas the bound water fraction decreased progressively with advancing maturation. HA correlated positively with total lung water but not with the bound water fraction. The elimination of lung fluid, therefore, is associated with an increase in free water at the expense of bound water fraction.

The underlying mechanisms of the release of water molecules from macromolecular bindings remain to be established as HA does not appear to be directly involved in this process (72).

Parameters of brain water metabolism and brain HA concentration undergo similar developmental changes. With increasing maturation the motionally constrained bound water is restructured to freely moving water fraction and it proves to be independent of total brain water and tissue HA content (73).

On the basis of these observations one can conclude that in addition to the well-defined channel-mediated water transport and a reduction in ECW, the redistribution of the bound to free water fraction is an important but still unappreciated mechanism of the physiological dehydration of immature lung and brain.

Role of Hyaluronan in Neonatal Renal Concentration

The possible involvement of renal papillary HA in renal water handling has also been proposed. A large amount of HA is accumulated in the inner medulla and papilla that limits water flow by influencing interstitial hydrostatic pressure (74,75).

Inducing water diuresis by increased body hydration results in elevated HA content in renal papilla, whereas opposite changes are seen after water deprivation. As a result, renal papillary HA positively correlates with urine flow rate and there is an inverse relationship of papillary HA to urine osmolality. These findings support the notion that increased papillary interstitial HA can antagonize renal tubular water reabsorption (76).

In the light of these observations it is relevant to postulate that the impaired concentration performance of the immature kidney can be accounted for, not only by the decreased corticopapillary osmotic gradient and diminished renal tubular responsiveness to arginine vasopressin (AVP), but also by the markedly elevated HA content-related limited water flow in the neonatal renal papilla. This additional mechanism may be of great importance in neonatal adaptation when excess water needs to be excreted (77).

SODIUM HOMEOSTASIS

Sodium chloride balance is normally maintained by renal sodium conservation and excretion over a broad range of intakes. Newborn infants are limited in conserving sodium when challenged by sodium restriction and in excreting sodium when challenged by a sodium load.

Renal Sodium Excretion under Basal Conditions

In the first week of life, urinary sodium excretion and fractional sodium excretion, in particular, are high and are inversely proportional to the maturity of the neonate (78–82) (Fig. 2-3). Premature infants of less than 35 weeks' gestation have an obligatory sodium loss with subsequent negative sodium balance, which is believed to be a physiologic measure for adjustments to extrauterine existence. It is assumed to result from isotonic contraction of expanded ECW present at birth and the disposal of excess extracellular sodium through the kidney. This concept has been supported by the observation that the practice of giving a high fluid and sodium intake to replace water and sodium loss was associated with increased incidence

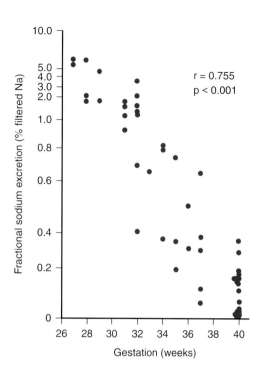

Figure 2-3 Scattergram showing the inverse correlation between fractional sodium excretion and gestational age. (From Siegel BR, Oh W: Renal function as a marker of human fetal maturation. Acta Paediatrica Scandinavica 65:481–485, 1976, with permission.)

of patent ductus arteriosus (PDA), cardiac failure, bronchopulmonary dysplasia (BPD), necrotizing enterocolitis (NEC), and intracranial hemorrhage (ICH), all conditions known to relate to fluid overload and protracted expansion of ECW.

Tang et al (50) have shown that loss of body water after birth occurs to the same extent in healthy preterm infant and in babies with RDS and is unrelated to the volume of fluid administered.

Bell and Acarregui (83) reviewed the results of randomized trials on water restriction and BPD, and concluded that although there is a trend for lower incidence of BPD in preterm infants who received restricted fluid intake during the first days of life, the difference is not statistically significant. Based on the result of this metaanalysis, the most prudent prescription for water intake to premature infants would seem to be careful restriction of water intake so that physiological needs are met without allowing significant dehydration.

Recently Oh et al (84) demonstrated that higher fluid intake and less weight loss during the first 10 days of life were associated with an increased risk of BPD.

Sodium, along with chloride concentration in plasma, often falls to low levels, and urinary sodium excretion remains high relative to plasma sodium. It has become apparent, therefore, that the redistribution of body fluid compartments alone does not account for the high rate of urinary sodium excretion, but rather may be caused by renal immaturity (85–87).

This contention is supported by the gestational age-related changes in sodium balance and in the activity of the renin-angiotensin-aldosterone system (RAAS) in one-week-old newborn infants with gestational ages of 31–41 weeks. It has been demonstrated that in response to renal salt wasting and to the subsequent negative sodium balance, premature infants augmented their plasma renin activity above values found for full-term infants. Plasma renin activity correlated positively with urinary sodium excretion, but negatively with sodium balance. Plasma aldosterone concentration did not change with gestational age; urinary aldosterone excretion, however, increased steadily as the gestation advanced. The clear dissociation between plasma renin activity and aldosterone status strongly suggests that the adrenals of premature infants do not respond adequately to stimulation in the

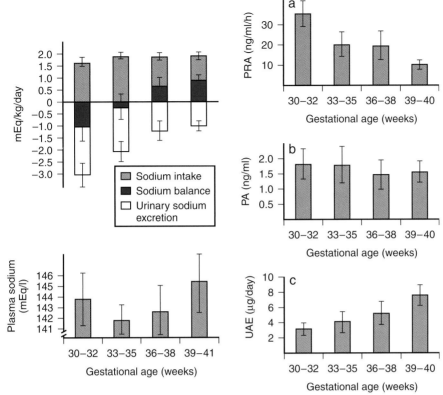

Figure 2-4 Sodium balance and the activity of the renin-angiotensin-aldosterone system in one-week-old newborn infants with gestational ages of 30–41 weeks. PRA = plasma renin activity, PA = plasma aldosterone concentration, UAE = urinary aldosterone excretion. (From Sulyok E, Németh M, Tényi J et al: Relationship between maturity, electrolyte balance and the function of the renin-angiotension-aldosterone system in newborn infants. Biology of the Neonate 35:60–65, 1979, with permission.)

first week of life. Urinary aldosterone excretion was found to relate inversely to renal sodium excretion, but directly to sodium balance (Fig. 2-4). These findings indicate that the improvement of renal sodium conservation and establishment of positive sodium balance with increasing maturation is causally related to aldosterone secretion and/or renal tubular aldosterone-reactivity (88).

Clinical and experimental studies, attempting to define the nephron segments responsible for urinary sodium loss, indicate that the higher fractional sodium excretion in premature infants is caused by deficient proximal and distal tubular reabsorption of sodium. With advancing gestational and postnatal ages, significant improvement occurs in renal sodium conservation (89,90).

Aldosterone-mediated distal reabsorption improves more rapidly to keep up with the sodium load presented to this nephron site (91,92). According to the concept of glomerulotubular imbalance, there is a morphologic and functional preponderance of glomeruli to proximal tubules in immature nephrons. Consequently, it is argued that a greater fraction of glomerular filtrate escapes proximal tubular reabsorption (93,94).

Indeed, in the neonatal kidney the volume of proximal tubules (the membrane area available for reabsorption), the net oncotic pressure favoring reabsorption and the capacity of transporters involved in active sodium reabsorption are reduced (95–97).

It is of note, however, that the distal nephron also exhibits immature sodium transport characteristics consisting of high passive permeability, low baseline active transport, and mineralocorticoid unresponsiveness with low density and activity of aplical Na^+ channels (98,99).

Molecular Basis of Proximal Tubular Sodium Reabsorption

The sodium transporting capacity of the proximal tubule undergoes maturational changes. Most of the luminal sodium uptake is mediated by the Na^+/H^+ exchanger (NHE) via electroneutral exchange of extracellular Na^+ for intracellular H^+. The NHEs are a widely distributed family of transport proteins containing six members (NHE 1–6). They have 10–12 transmembrane spanning domains with an intracellular C-terminal region. Their amino acid sequences show 45–65% homology. The six isoforms vary in terms of cellular location to the apical or basolateral membrane, amiloride sensitivity and mode of regulation (100).

NHE3, which predominantly mediates sodium-dependent apical proton secretion in the proximal tubules, is stimulated by the low intracellular sodium generated and maintained by basolateral Na^+-K^+-ATPase. Membrane vesicles isolated from animals at different stages of maturation and in vitro microperfusion studies using neonatal juxtamedullary proximal convoluted tubules have shown a lower rate of bicarbonate transport, decreased Na^+-K^+-ATPase and NHE activity in immature compared to mature animals (96,97,101).

The postnatal maturation of NHE and the subsequent improvement of bicarbonate transport may be accelerated by adrenocortical steroid stimulation of either NHE and Na^+-K^+-ATPase or direct, receptor-mediated angiotensin II stimulation of NHE. More recently, parallel maturation of apical NHE activity, NHE3 mRNA expression and NHE3 protein levels has been demonstrated, which can be accelerated with glucocorticoids in newborn rabbits, but not with angiotensin II in fetal sheep (102,103). Furthermore, thyroid hormones and the surge in circulating catecholamine levels and increased sympathetic nerve activity at birth have also been claimed to enhance NHE activity (104,105).

As glucocorticoids upregulate α-adrenergic receptor mRNA expression in proximal tubules glucocorticoids may also potentiate the effect of catecholamines to increase NHE activity (106). On the other hand, dopamine inhibits NHE-mediated sodium uptake by proximal tubule segments and tonic inhibition of fetal proximal tubular NHE activity by dopamine has been documented (107).

It is of note that the progressive increase in renal Na^+-H^+ exchange with advancing gestational and postnatal age was described long before the discovery of the NHE system (108).

Another way for sodium entry into the proximal tubular cells is the sodium-dependent phosphate co-transport system (Na-Pi). The transport is electrogenic and involves the co-transport of three sodium ions and one phosphate anion. Three distinct isoforms of mammalian Na-Pi (1–3) have been identified. All are expressed in the proximal tubule cells, but Na-Pi2 is exclusively located in the brush border membrane and has a predominant role in proximal tubular Pi reabsorption. It has been documented that the transport rates of Na-Pi were substantially higher in brush-border membrane vesicles obtained from newborns than those from adults. The high transport capacity of the Na-Pi co-transport system in the newborn kidney, however, is associated with low adaptability to changes in dietary Pi intake. Interestingly, the expression of the Na-Pi mRNA levels in newborns was similar or lower than those in adult rats, suggesting that the increased protein levels and activity of the co-transporter early in life may be accounted for by post-transcriptional regulation. Parathyroid hormone has been shown to inhibit, while growth hormone and insulin-like growth factor increase the Na-Pi-mediated sodium and phosphate uptake (109).

Sodium uptake by the proximal tubule cells can also be achieved by Na-amino acid and Na-glucose co-transporters located in the brush border membrane. Sodium-coupled amino acid and glucose transport are developmentally regulated having low activity during the fetal/neonatal period followed by a steady increase as the maturation progresses. The limited co-transport of Na with amino acids and glucose is responsible for the low threshold of amino acid and glucose reabsorption and contributes to the generalized aminoaciduria and glucosuria frequently seen in early life. On the other hand, it appears to constrain quantitatively important Na influx into the brush-border membrane vesicles, thereby to diminish proximal tubular sodium reabsorption (110).

Molecular Basis of Distal Tubular Sodium Reabsorption

There have been several reports to reveal developmental regulation of sodium transport in the cortical collecting duct (CCD), a nephron segment that plays an important role in determining sodium excretion in the final urine. Vehaskari (94), using isolated perfused rabbit CCD at three different postnatal ages, has found that the maturation of sodium transport occurs in two stages: first the high passive sodium permeability decreases to mature levels during the first two weeks of life, followed by the second stage, an increase in active transport capacity and simultaneous development of mineralocorticoid responsiveness. Vehaskari assumed that the immaturity of active sodium transport may be attributed to intracellular mechanisms that limit transcellular sodium flux. These may include (1) incomplete polarization of the principal cells, (2) decreased basolateral Na^+-K^+-ATPase activity, (3) decreased apical Na permeability due to a decreased number of Na channels, and (4) decreased conductance of the existing channels.

The amiloride-sensitive epithelial sodium channel (ENaC) is made of three homologous subunits, named α, β, and γ ENaC. The α ENaC subunit expressed alone is for channel function and can drive sodium absorption. The β and γ subunits have been demonstrated to stabilize the channel and to allow proper insertion into the membrane. The expression of the three subunits together induces a multiple increase in the amiloride-sensitive sodium flux compared with the α ENaC alone (111). The expression profile of α ENaC mRNA is very similar to that of $\alpha_1 Na^+$-K^+-ATPase mRNA, a constituent of the sodium pump involved in active transepithelial sodium transport. During gestation there is a gradual rise in the renal expression of both α ENaC and α_1 Na^+-K^+-ATPase mRNA, which reaches a plateau after birth. Furthermore, α ENaC mRNA correlates directly with α_1 Na^+-K^+-ATPase mRNA, suggesting that the renal expression of these transporters is regulated by common factors during the perinatal period (112).

Further studies to explore the cellular mechanisms of the limitation of active sodium transport in the distal nephron have shown that in microdissected rat nephron segments all three ENaC mRNA subunits were exclusively detected from the distal convoluted tubule to the outer medullary collecting duct. The levels of their expression, however, proved to be very low during the late fetal period, but they increased rapidly to reach adult level within 24–72 hours after birth. The authors have suggested that the low ENaC subunit gene expression is a potentially limiting factor in Na transport in the very immature kidney only; impaired translation and/or impaired targeted trafficking of the channel protein may also be implicated (113).

To get some more insight into the underlying mechanisms of the low net sodium absorption by the developing CCD, intensive research has been performed on the apical membrane ion conductance and channel expression during the late fetal and early postnatal period. It has been clearly demonstrated that the low rate of sodium absorption in the early neonatal period can be attributed to the paucity of conducting apical ENaCs in principal cells of the CCD and to the lower open probability of these channels in the first then after the second week of life (114).

A markedly increased abundance of the transcripts of all three ENaC subunits has been observed in the last 3–4 days of fetal life in rats. After birth only modest changes could be detected with increasing α and decreasing β and γ subunits. Interestingly, as the kidney matures the expression of the ENaC subunits is redistributed from the inner medullary collecting duct to the CCD (115).

The perinatal upregulation of ENaC activity appears to be related to the perinatal surge of adrenocortical steroid hormones because the trend and time course of the two events run parallel. In contrast to this notion the developmental expression of the three subunits of ENaC did not differ between corticotropin-releasing hormone knockout mice and wild type animals, indicating that the endogenous corticosteroids have no influence on the perinatal expression of ENaC. Interestingly, exogenous, synthetic glucocorticoids (Dexamethasone) significantly enhanced prenatal expression of α-subunit but did not affect the expression of β and γ subunits of renal ENaC (116).

The different response is assumed to be the result of metabolization of the endogenous glucocorticoids by the kidney. In fact, abundant 11 β-hydroxysteroid dehydrogenase type 2 mRNA expression has been noted in fetal mouse kidney, so it is relevant to suggest that this enzyme inactivates endogenous glucocorticoids and by co-localizing with mineralocorticoid receptors is involved in protecting steroid receptors and in controlling glucocorticoid action in developing renal tissues (117).

In addition to the ENaC expression, the ontogenetic expression patterns of other sodium transport proteins have also been examined to define the sodium entry pathways during nephrogenesis. Using high-resolution histochemical techniques and in situ hybridization these transport proteins have been found to begin to be expressed in early nascent tubular segments. Along with the structural differentiation and segmental specialization of this distal nephron, cells committed to active sodium transport exhibit transporters including bumetanide-sensitive Na-K-2Cl co-transporter, Na-Cl co-transporter and Na/Ca exchanger (118). The physiological significance of the transcription of these transport proteins early during development before the excretory function of the kidney is established needs to be defined.

Other Factors Influencing Renal Sodium Handling

In addition to renal immaturity, any increase in GFR, urine output, and fractional sodium excretion contributes to renal salt wasting. Lorenz et al (120) identified three distinct phases of fluid and electrolyte homeostasis in low-birth weight premature infants with or without RDS during the first days of life. The low urine output of the first day (prediuretic phase) is followed by spontaneous diuresis and natriuresis during the second and third days independent of fluid intake (diuretic phase). The onset, duration, and extent of diuresis appear to be variable. The high rate of urine flow and sodium excretions is assumed to be the result of abrupt increases of GFR and fractional sodium excretion subsequent to the reabsorption of residual fetal lung fluid and expansion of extracellular space. During the postdiuretic phase GFR remains unchanged, and urine flow and sodium excretion decrease to values intermediate between those observed in the prediuretic and diuretic phases and begin to vary appropriately in response to changes in fluid intake (119,120).

Premature infants, receiving a high intravenous fluid load, have a high renal sodium loss and an exaggerated sodium deficit. To maintain sodium balance and normal plasma sodium level with intravenous infusions, sodium and fluid intake should be restricted or extra sodium should be given.

Bueva and Guignard (121) also concluded that by providing restricted fluid intake with low sodium (1–2 mEg/kg/day), premature infants with birth weight of

1000–1500 g have fractional sodium excretion not higher than 2.2% and are able to maintain sodium balance. In this group of preterm neonates plasma sodium concentration, however, fell to a level of 132 mEq/L at postnatal age of 15–16 days. In their view the high rate of sodium excretion is iatrogenic in nature and may be due to the liberal fluid intake. The concept, therefore, that salt wasting in preterm neonates is the result of renal immaturity and NaCl supplement should be given to prevent or correct sodium depletion is wrong. In their study fluid intake was 80 mL/kg on the first day and then increased by 20 mL/kg/day to reach 150 mL/kg/day by the end of the first week.

More recently, Delgado et al (122) conducted a longitudinal prospective study of very low birth weight premature infants with gestational age of 23–31 weeks to measure parameters of sodium balance weekly for 5 weeks. Fluid intake did not exceede 150 mL/kg/day in any gestational and postnatal age group and sodium intake was also kept at a relatively low level of less than 4 mEq/kg/day. An inverse relationship was found between fractional sodium excretion and gestational age, and fractional sodium excretion fell progressively in each age group with increasing postnatal age (Fig. 2-5). A state of positive sodium balance was not consistently detected until after ~32 weeks of gestational age. Unfortunately, the postnatal course of plasma sodium was not presented, but the unique value of this report is the measurement of α-ENaC mRNA expression in human kidney homogenates obtained from fetuses of 20–36 weeks' gestation. Most importantly, they could demonstrate for the first time the developmental regulation of the expression of α-ENaC expression, the channel protein that mediates the final excretion of sodium during gestation in humans. They identified a significant inrease of ~25% in α-ENaC mRNA abundance between 20 and 36 weeks of gestational age.

This study is of primary importance to underscore that inefficient sodium handling is an intrinsic feature of the immature kidney, albeit variations in sodium and fluid intake may modify the rate of urinary sodium excretion and subsequently the sodium balance.

As current clinical practice of fluid management of low-birth weight premature infants is quite variable, it is imperative to establish clinical and laboratory parameters that dictate sodium and water intake to meet the optimal needs of infants at various gestational and postnatal ages.

Several approaches have been applied to assess liberal or restricted fluid therapy including determination of urine flow rate, osmolality and sodium excretion, body weight changes with or without plasma sodium levels, and measurements of ECW, TBW and body solids. Occasionally, hormone parameters controlling salt- and water-balance have also been determined. Another approach is to relate fluid therapy to the incidence, severity and mortality of neonatal pathologies known to be associated with fluid-overload. Using different approaches different conclusions could be drawn. However, by integrating the available data, a unified concept may emerge which could be considered for planning neonatal fluid therapy.

However, the renal responses to variations in sodium and water intake are often unpredictable, therefore individualized fluid and electrolyte therapy is needed (Table 2-3).

Renal Sodium Excretion in Response to Salt Loading

The renal response of the newborn to salt loading is blunted compared with that of the adult. Low glomerular filtration rate (GFR) is a limiting factor, although the difference in sodium excretory response between newborns and adults still exists when correction is made for GFR. Studies using free water clearance and the technique of distal nephron blockade have identified the distal nephron as the site where fractional sodium reabsorption increases as development proceeds (123,124).

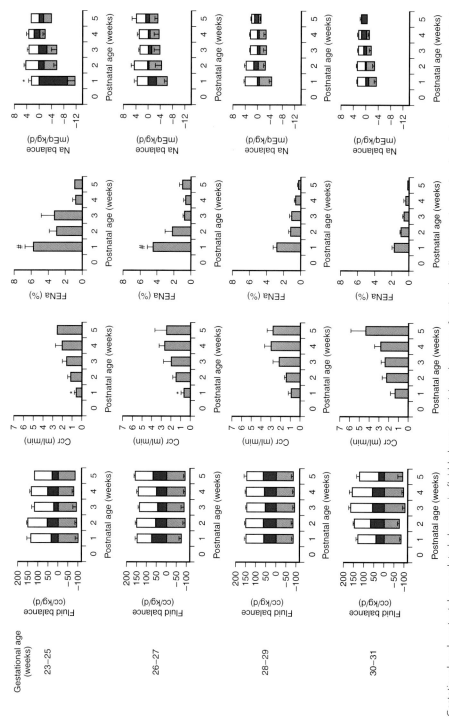

Figure 2-5 Gestational and postnatal age-related changes in fluid balance, creatinine clearance, fractional sodium excretion and sodium balance in premature infants of 23–31 weeks' gestation during the first five weeks of life. (From Delgado MM, Rohatgi R, Khan S, Holzman IR, Satlin LM: Sodium and potassium clearances by the maturing kidney: clinical-molecular correlates. Pediatric Nephrology 18:759–767, 2003, with permission.)

Table 2-3 **Daily Total Fluid Intake in Premature Infants with Birth Weight less than 1500 g during the First 10 Days of Life (mL/kg)**

Age (days)	Iowa	Lausanne	Neonatal Research Network			
			BPD-free survivors		Death or BPD	
			Intake	Weight loss (%)	Intake	Weight loss (%)
1	65–75	80	no data		no data	
2	75–80	100	118	0.4	136	0.1
3	90–95	120	134	3.8	158	2.8
4		140	147	7.3	170	6.7
5		150	154	9.7	171	8.1
6		150	157	8.7	169	7.4
7	120–130	150	156	8.1	165	6.3
8	130	150	153	6.4	163	4.7
9	130	150	152	4.7	159	3.3
10	~135	150	150	3.1	158	1.8

From Bell EF, Acarregui MJ: Restricted versus liberal water intake for preventing morbidity and mortality in preterm infants. Cochrane Database System Review, CD 000503, 2001.

Bueva A, Guignard J-P: Renal function in preterm neonates. Pediatric Research 36:572–577, 1994.

Oh W, Poindexter BB, Perritt R et al: Association between fluid intake and weight loss during the first ten days of life and risk of bronchopulmonary dysplasia in extremely low birth weight infants. Journal of Pediatrics 147:786–790, 2005.

Initial weight loss of no more than 12–15% of birth weight was allowed. In the Neonatal Research Network the study subjects had mean birthweight and gestational age of 736 g and 25.4 weeks in the bronchopulmonary dysplasia (BPD) group and 815 g and 26.7 weeks in the BPD-free survivors group.

The augmented distal tubular sodium transport is assumed to be mediated by the high concentration of plasma aldosterone. This assumption is supported by the diminished response of the renin-angiotensis-aldosterone system to suppression by volume expansion with isotonic saline infusion (125). However, in the newborn dog, most of the increase in sodium load to the distal nephron, which occurs during NaCl expansion, is reabsorbed in the thick ascending limb of the loop of Henle, and it is independent of aldosterone stimulation (126).

When a dose of 0.12 g/kg NaCl is administered orally to premature and term neonates during the first week of life, a significantly higher natriuretic response occurs in premature infants of 29 to 35 weeks' gestation than in term infants. When the natriuretic response to salt challenge is followed in a premature infant until its expected term, the response diminishes to a value characteristic for term neonates. However, the renal capacity to excrete a sodium load is still much lower in premature infants than in children 8–14 years of age (80,127).

The postnatal development of the natriuretic response to salt challenge is accelerated by dietary manipulation. Chronic sodium loading augmented a natriuretic response to acute volume expansion in pre-weaned rats, but the renal response is incomplete and independent of GFR and plasma ANP levels (128).

Infants receiving a high-salt diet before being given a salt load have a greater capacity to excrete sodium than those on a low-salt diet. In some studies sodium is more rapidly excreted when given as $NaHCO_3$ than as NaCl. Others have found no difference in the rate of excretion of sodium as bicarbonate versus sodium as chloride in response to loading doses in the dog. However, the mechanism of natriuresis is probably different. With sodium chloride loading, sodium delivered to the distal nephron is reabsorbed with chloride in the thick ascending limb of Henle's loop, whereas with sodium bicarbonate loading, sodium is reabsorbed in the late distal and cortical collecting tubules in exchange for potassium and H^+ (129).

It is of interest that bicarbonate excretion appears to be largely independent of sodium excretion during the period of spontaneous diuresis. Bicarbonate is effectively retained and the major anion accompanying excreted sodium is chloride, not bicarbonate (130).

Intestinal Sodium Transport

Sodium absorption from the gastrointestinal tract is efficient. Fecal sodium excretion is usually less than 10% of the intake in very-low-birth weight premature infants and does not vary significantly with age over the period of 2–7 postnatal weeks (86).

Al-Dahhan et al (131), investigating the development of intestinal sodium handling, report that stool sodium loss correlates inversely with postconceptional age and parallels urinary sodium excretion, although at much lower absolute values. By contrast, experimental evidence suggests that amiloride-sensitive, electrogenic sodium absorption in the distal colon is more efficient in the newborn than in adult rabbits, and it is assumed to be accounted for by the high circulating aldosterone levels in the neonate (132,133).

Studies on the ontogeny of colonic sodium transport in early childhood have shown the highest sodium absorption rate in preterm infants with gestational age of 30–33 weeks. This decreases in parallel with the fall of plasma aldosterone as gestational and postnatal ages advance. It has been postulated, therefore, that the maturation of colonic sodium absorption precedes that of the renal tubular sodium reabsorption, and it functions as a major self-conserving mechanism that counterbalances urinary sodium loss (134).

DISTURBANCES IN PLASMA SODIUM CONCENTRATIONS

Early-Onset Hyponatremia

Hyponatremia (plasma sodium less than 130 mEq/L), occurring in the first week of life, is designated as an early type of hyponatremia. It is attributed to water retention, but sodium depletion may also contribute. It occurs in association with excessive free water infusion into the mother, with perinatal pathology causing nonosmotic release of antidiuretic hormone (ADH) (135), and with salt-restricted parenteral fluid regimen (136).

Placental permeability to sodium in sheep fetuses increases as gestation progresses so that, prenatally, free water is more likely to be retained early in gestation when ewes are given excess free water (137).

Infants born to mothers on a diet deficient in sodium are also at risk for early hyponatremia (138).

Late-Onset Hyponatremia

This is usually the result of a combination of inadequate sodium intake, renal salt wasting, and free water retention. Accordingly, its incidence, severity, and duration are influenced by the maturity of the neonate and the feeding protocol applied. In the early study by Roy et al (87), when fluid intake was liberal (150–200 mL/kg per day) and only 1.6 mEq/kg per day sodium was given, late hyponatremia occurred in 30–40% of very-low-birth weight infants (Fig. 2-6). When the daily sodium intake was increased to 3 mEq/kg, late hyponatremia was reduced to less than 10% and was practically eliminated when sodium intake was further increased (86,87).

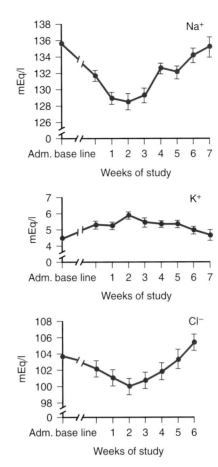

Figure 2-6 Postnatal course of plasma Na+, K+, and Cl- concentrations in very-low-birth weight infants. Admission (ADM) specimen is the baseline specimen at a mean age of 18 days. (From Day GM, Radde IC, Balfe JW, Chance GW: Electrolyte abnormalities in very low birth weight infants. Pediatric Research 10:522–526, 1976, with permission.)

Shaffer and Meade observed lower plasma sodium concentration in infants receiving 1 mEq/kg per day than in those receiving 3 mEq/kg per day sodium over 30 days; however, the pattern of sodium balance remained similar (139).

Lorenz et al (140) maintained plasma sodium in the normal range when they administered a low sodium intake (about 1 mEq/kg per day) and restricted fluid (60 to 80 mL/kg per day), resulting in a weight loss of 13–15%. This approach tested the hypothesis that hyponatremia is accounted for mainly by the high-volume formula intake, natriuresis, and associated water retention. These authors conclude that, given the lack of adverse effects of their low sodium and free water regimen and the absence of hyponatremia, this regimen was appropriate for very-low-birth weight infants. They concluded that no sodium supplement is needed.

Costarino et al (136) compared a salt-restricted parenteral fluid regimen with a sodium-supplemented maintenance regimen (3–4 mEq/kg per day) for the treatment of very-low-birth weight infants during the first 5 days of life. Maintenance sodium intake resulted in a nearly zero sodium balance, whereas sodium-restricted infants continued to excrete urinary sodium at a high rate, which promoted more negative balance. No differences were noted between the two groups in urine output, GFR, urinary sodium excretion, and osmolar clearance. However, serum sodium concentrations were significantly higher in maintenance infants than in restriction infants despite the increased fluid intake in the former. Clinical outcome was not affected by sodium intake except for the lower incidence of bronchopulmonary dysplasia in the sodium-restricted group. The authors conclude that sodium intake should be restricted and the least amount of intravenous fluid should be provided to maintain serum sodium concentration in the normal range. However, their study was limited to the first week of life, and the authors did not obtain reliable information toward defining sodium requirements during the second and third weeks, a period of rapid growth, when late hyponatremia develops. In fact, longitudinal studies reveal that preterm infants on a low-sodium diet, who have renal salt wasting, sustain a protracted sodium loss. In this setting, limiting water intake does not address the sodium deficit; it aggravates volume depletion.

The study by Wilkins (141) argues against sodium restriction; low-birth weight infants excreted excessive amounts of sodium and severe sodium depletion developed during the first 2 weeks, regardless of plasma sodium concentration. However, after some initial increase plasma sodium fell progressively and often culminated in profound and prolonged hyponatremia.

Interestingly, Shaffer et al (142) noted late hyponatremia in association with reduced ECW in 6 out of 18 infants who were born at 32 weeks' gestational age. This finding indicates that endocrine reactions often do not normalize sodium and water balance but lead to sodium chloride losses. Consequently, sodium chloride supplements are needed.

In a randomised controlled trial Hartnoll et al (143,144) compared the effects of early (on 2nd day after birth) and delayed (when weight loss of 6% of birth weight was achieved) sodium supplementation of 4 mmol/kg/day on body composition and sodium balance in infants of 25–30 weeks' gestational age. In the delayed group there was a significant reduction in TBW and ECW by the end of the first week whereas body solids accrued more rapidly in the early group. By day 14 significant differences in body composition were no longer seen. Sodium balance was negative in both groups after the first day and fractional sodium excretion did not differ. It was concluded that early supplementation can delay the physiological water loss, which may cause an inreased risk of continuing oxygen requirement not mediated by alterations in pulmonary artery pressure, but rather by retaining interstitial lung fluid, lowering lung compliance and exacerbating respiratory compromise.

Our own supplementation policy proposes to give extra sodium at a dose of 3–5 mmol/kg/day and 1.5–2.5 mmol/kg/day for 8–21 days and 22–35 days, respectively. Delayed sodium supplementation does not interfere with cardiopulmonary adaptation but ensures positive sodium balance and maintains normal plasma sodium concentrations. Moreover, supplemental sodium prevents the excessive activation of renin-angiotensin-aldosterone system (RAAS), and plasma renin activity, plasma aldosterone concentration and urinary aldosterone excretion remain within the limits characteristic for healthy full-term neonates (145); (Fig. 2-7).

Reduction of flow-dependent urinary sodium excretion (146) and maintaining positive sodium balance by providing restricted fluid intake may carry the risks that the sodium requirements for growth are not met. Moreover, under the conditions of low sodium and fluid intake a positive sodium balance can be achieved by excessive activation of RAAS only, which indicates some extent of volume depletion, marginal somatic stability and still undefined long-term consequences.

Early Hypernatremia

In early hypernatremia, plasma sodium exceeds 150 mEq/L. Repeated administration of hypertonic sodium bicarbonate solution to 'correct' acidosis in critically ill low-birth weight neonates who have compromised renal function is the most common cause of neonatal hypernatremia. This hypernatremia can be reduced or avoided by decreasing the concentration of the sodium bicarbonate given and the amount infused. Very-low-birth weight infants are also at risk for developing

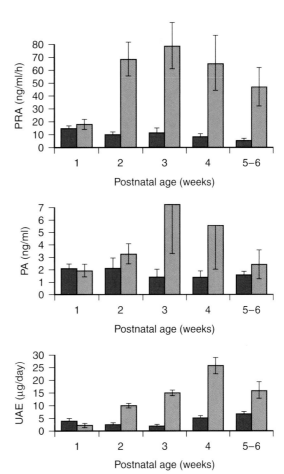

Figure 2-7 Postnatal development plasma renin activity (PRA), plasma aldosterone concentration (PA) and urinary aldosterone excretion (UAE) in premature infants with and without NaCl supplementation during the first six weeks of life. (From Sulyok E, Németh M, Tényi I, Csaba IF, Varga L, Varga F: Relationship between the postnatal development of the renin-angiotensin-aldosterone system and electrolyte and acid-base status of the NaCl-supplemented premature infants. In Spitzer A (Ed.): The kidney during development. Morphology and function (pp 272–281). New York: Masson Publishing, 1982, with permission.)

hypernatremia from extremely high insensible water loss. This is augmented when radiant warmers and phototherapy are used (147) and by the limited ability of the immature kidney to concentrate urine and reabsorb free water (148).

Attempts should be made to reduce insensible water loss, to carefully monitor water balance, and to adjust water intake appropriately to prevent hypernatremia. Hypernatremia occasionally occurs after the first week of life in premature infants who are receiving NaCl supplementation and inadequate free water.

Clinical Consequences of Inadequate Sodium Intake

Premature infants fed breast milk or those fed low-sodium formula and develop renal salt wasting often become sodium depleted and hyponatremic. Premature infants with late hyponatremia generally are asymptomatic. However, some develop apnea and neurological symptoms such as irritability and convulsion.

Sodium chloride makes a major contribution to plasma osmolality. As a result, the fall in plasma sodium is accompanied by a parallel decline in plasma osmolality. A decrease in cell solute content, which occurs in chronic hyponatremia, lowers the increase in cell volume that initially occurs with hyponatremia. The concentrations of intracellular organic osmolytes decrease; these include taurine, myoinositol, phosphocreatine, glutamate, glutamine, and glycerophosphorylcholine. Central

AVP and ANP have also been shown to participate in brain volume regulation. When the brain is exposed to severe hyponatremia AVP accelerates, while ANP reduces cellular water accumulation (149). AVP action is V_1-receptor mediated and it has been claimed to stimulate water flux via AQP4, the brain-specific water channels, directly (150).

It has also been proposed that the V_1-receptor is coupled with the sodium channel and AVP primarily enhances cellular sodium uptake, which is followed by the passive, osmotically-driven channel-mediated water transport. This possibility is supported by the observations that specific blockers of the sodium channel (benzamil, amiloride, amiloride analogues) prevent cellular swelling and an increase in brain water content (151,152). These findings may have relevance to hyponatremic premature infants because, during the period of early or late hyponatremia, preterm infants may encounter increased AVP secretion (153).

During correction of hyponatremia, the reaccumulation of organic osmolytes is delayed following the return of plasma sodium to normal. Rapid correction of hyponatremia may be associated with neurologic lesions, typically designated as central pontine myelinolysis, although sustained deprivation of organic solute alone may also have adverse effects (154).

Central pontine myelinolysis is a rare condition characterized by a symmetrically sited central pontine lesion with a loss of myelin and an absence of inflammation. Its pathogenesis is not clearly defined, however there have been reports implicating apoptosis-mediated death of oligodentrocytes as a significant contributor to the demyelination. Pro-apoptotic markers have been detected in glial cell cytoplasm and there is evidence of activated caspaces to initiate proteolytic cascade (155).

Others have assumed the role of blood-brain barrier disruption, activation of the complement cascade, complement-induced oligodentrocyte lysis and immunological destruction of white matter in the process of demyelinolysis (156). This immune-mediated mechanism is supported by the prevention of blood-brain barrier disruption and of the severe neurological impairment when dexamethasone treatment was applied (157).

Sodium deficiency during gestation in rats is associated with impaired brain growth and alterations in brain cholesterol, protein and RNA content (158). Accordingly, there are data indicating that neonatal sodium deficiency may have unfavorable influences on later development of cognitive and mental functions (159) and severe hyponatremia may be a risk factor for sensorineural hearing loss (160).

Sodium depletion has been associated with retarded growth in height and weight in animals and humans. Young rats with diet-induced sodium deficiency have reduced RNA concentrations and exhibit decreased rates of protein synthesis in skeletal muscle (161).

It has been suggested that ECF volume contraction and hyponatremia reduce growth factor-stimulated Na^+-H^+ exchange activity, decrease muscle intracellular pH, and impair DNA synthesis and cell growth (162). Premature infants with late hyponatremia have been shown to have reduced concentrating performance due to the blunted renal response to AVP. The limited renal tubular sodium reabsorption and the hyponatremic state may hinder the establishment of intrarenal osmotic gradient and impair renal response to AVP, thus preventing excessive water retention and further worsening of hyponatremia (163).

Since Barker et al (164) put forward the hypothesis of fetal origin of some adult diseases many studies have been published to confirm the association of low birth weight and hypertension in adult life. In spite of the great progress that has been made in our understanding of the effect of fetal programming on subsequent organ function and adult disease, the underlying mechanisms still remain to be clearly established. Several lines of evidence have been provided, however, that a reduction in nephron number, enlargement of glomerular volume, alterations in renal sodium handling and adrenocortical hormones are likely to have an impact on blood pressure (165).

It is also to be considered that in low-birth weight premature infants the responses of salt-retaining hormones to renal salt-wasting and sodium depletion, in particular the excessively activated renin-angiotensin-aldosterone system, may have far-reaching consequences on the later course of blood pressure control (166). This assumption awaits exploration.

Clinical Consequences of Excessive Sodium Intake

Excessive use of hypertonic sodium bicarbonate for the correction of severe metabolic acidosis associated with perinatal asphyxia and RDS causes hypernatremia, which increases the risk of neonatal intracranial hemorrhage. The rapid osmotic shift of fluid from ICW leads to cell dehydration, brain shrinkage, and tearing of the cerebral capillaries (167).

In immature animals cerebral cell volume regulation is well developed to maintain brain size in the face of hypernatremic stress. The elevated brain water content is associated with increased concentration of osmoprotective molecules. During development there is a parallel decline in brain water, total electrolyte, and organic osmolyte contents. The percentage contribution of inorganic solutes to osmoprotection is greater than that of organic solutes in immature animals than in adult animals and among the individual organic osmolytes taurine is the most prominent cerebral osmolyte. In support of this notion taurine levels are elevated in the immature brain and cerebral taurine best correlates with brain water content in normonatremic developing animals (12).

High fluid and sodium chloride administration, which offsets the physiological contraction of ECF volume in the first week of life, has severe consequences that include inducing PDA, cardiac failure, BPD, ICH, and NEC. A second problem is that low-birth weight infants, who are fed formula with extra sodium chloride to promote growth, retain salt and water, as evidenced by AVP-mediated reduction in free water clearance (168) and development of delayed-onset peripheral edema, signs of increased intracranial pressure, and congestive heart failure (169).

In full-term newborn infants variations in sodium intake had immediate and long-term effects on blood pressure. Infants kept on low sodium during the first six months of life encountered lower blood pressure at the end of the trial and 15 years later (170).

In view of the widespread untoward clinical consequences of inadequate or excessive sodium intake, sodium supplementation in low-birth weight neonates should be tailored to their individual needs, determined by close monitoring of sodium and water balance and some relevant endocrine parameters. The optimal timing, dosage, and route of sodium supplementation remain to be established.

SODIUM HOMEOSTASIS AND ACID-BASE BALANCE

Recent studies from our laboratory provided evidence that acid-base regulation and renal sodium handling are closely related in the neonatal period (171).

The limited capacity of the immature kidney to excrete H^+ is associated with an obligatory sodium loss. The maturation of renal acidifying processes with increasing gestational and postnatal age results in a progressive increase in renal Na^+-H^+ exchange and in a steady decline in sodium excretion.

Furthermore, metabolic acidosis has been shown to enhance renal sodium excretion and the acidosis-induced urinary sodium loss has been found to follow a developmental pattern; the lower the birth weight and the younger the age of the neonate, the less pronounced was the sodium excretory response.

Renal salt wasting, in turn, has been shown to contribute to the development of late metabolic acidosis, as indicated by:

(a) significantly negative correlation between the renal threshold for bicarbonate reabsorption and urinary sodium excretion;

(b) the similar trend and time course of late metabolic acidosis and late hyponatremia due to the low rate of renal sodium reabsorption in exchange for H^+; and

(c) metabolic acidosis in premature infants was less severe when supplemental NaCl was given to prevent sodium depletion and late hyponatremia.

All these observations are in line with the low activity of renal NHE3 in early life and its steady rise with advancing maturation.

Acknowledgment

This work was supported by the Hungarian Research Foundation (OTKA), no. T 042956 and by the Hungarian Ministry of Health (ETT), no. 50035.

REFERENCES

1. Friis-Hansen B. Body water compartments in children. Changes during growth and related changes in body composition. Pediatrics 28:169–181, 1961.
2. Cassady G. Bromide space studies in infants with low birth weight. Pediatric Research 4:14–24, 1970.
3. Rojas J, Mohan P, Davidson KK. Increased extracellular water volume associated with hyponatremia at birth in premature infants. Journal of Pediatric 105:158–161, 1984.
4. Brans YW, Shannon DL, Hunter MA. Maternal diabetes and neonatal macrosomia: III. Neonatal body water estimates. Early Human Development 8:307–316, 1981.
5. Langman CB, Engle WD, Baumgart S, Fox WW, Polin RA. The diuretic phase of respiratory distress syndrome and its relationship to oxygenation. Journal of Pediatrics 98:462–466, 1981.
6. Shaffer SG, Geer PG, Goetz KL. Elevated atrial natriuretic factor in neonates with respiratory distress syndrome. Journal of Pediatrics 109:1028–1033, 1986.
7. Ziegler EE, O'Donnell AM, Nelson SE, Fomon SJ. Body composition of the reference fetus. Growth 40:329–341, 1976.
8. Bradbury MWB, Crowder J, Desai S, Reynolds JM, Reynolds M, Saunders NR. Electrolytes and water in the brain and cerebrospinal fluid of the foetal sheep and guinea-pig. Journal of Physiology 227:591–610, 1972.
9. Aprison MH, Lukenbill A, Segar WE. Sodium, potassium, chloride and water content of six discrete parts of the mammalian brain. Journal of Neurochemistry 5:150–155, 1960.
10. Stonestreet BS, Oen-Hsiao JM, Petersson KH, Sadowska GB, Patlack CS. Regulation of brain water during acute hyperosmolality in ovine fetuses, lambs, and adults. Journal of Applied Physiology 94:1491–1500, 2003.
11. Widdowson EM, Dickerson JWT. The effect of growth and function on the chemical composition of soft tissues. Biochemical Journal 77:30–43, 1960.
12. Trachtman H, Yancey PH, Gullans SR. Cerebral cell volume regulation during hypernatremia in developing rats. Brain Research 693:155–162, 1995.
13. Nielsen S, Nagelhus EA, Amiry-Moghaddam M, Bourque C, Agre P, Ottersen OP. Specialized membrane domains for water transport in glial cells: high-resolution immunogold cytochemistry of aquaporin-4 in rat brain. Journal of Neuroscience 17:171–180, 1997.
14. Sulyok E, Vajda Z, Dóczi T, Nielsen S. Aquaporins and the central nervous system. Acta Neurochirurgica 146:955–960, 2004.
15. Manley GT, Fujimura M, Ma T, et al. Aquaporin-4 deletion in mice reduces brain edema after acute water intoxication and ischemic stroke. Nature Medical 6:149–1634, 2000.
16. Vajda Zs, Promeneur D, Dóczi T, et al. Increased aquaporin-4 immunoreactivity in rat brain in response to systemic hyponatraemia. Biochemical Biophysical Research Communications 270:495–503, 2000.
17. Han Z, Wax MB, Patil RV. Regulation of aquaporin-4 water channels by phorbol ester-dependent protein phosphorylation. Journal of Biological Chemistry 273:6001–6004, 1998.

18. Vajda Zs, Pedersen M, Füchtbauer E-M, et al. Delayed onset of brain edema and mislocalization of aquaporin-4 in dyshophin-null transgenic mice. Proceedings of National Adademy of Sciences USA 99:13131–13136, 2002.

19. Johansson PA, Dziegielewska KM, Ek CJ. Aqaporin-1 in the choroid plexuses of developing mammalian brain. Cell and Tissue Research 322:353–364, 2005.

20. Wen H, Nagelhus EA, Amiry-Moghaddam M, Agre P, Ottersen OP, Nielsen S. Ontogeny of water transport in rat brain: postnatal expression of the aquaporin-4 water channel. European Journal of Neuroscience 11:935–945, 1999.

21. Štulc J. Placental transfer of inorganic ions and water. Physiological Review 77:805–836, 1997.

22. Wilbur WJ, Power GG, Longo LL. Water exchange in the placenta: a mathematical model. American Journal of Physiology 235:R181–R199, 1978.

23. Konduri GG, Fewell JE. Oligohydramnions. In Brace RA, Ross MG, Robillard JE (Eds.), Fetal and neonatal body fluids (pp. 157–174). New York: Perinatology Press, 1989.

24. Gozzo ML, Noia G, Bargaresi G, et al. Reference intervals for 18 clinical chemistry analytes in fetal plasma samples between 18 and 40 weeks of pregnancy. Clinical Chemistry 44:683–685, 1998.

25. Flexner LD, Cowie DB, Hellman MD, Wilde WS, Vosburg GJ. The permeability of the human placenta to sodium in normal and abnormal pregnancies and the supply of sodium to the human fetus as determined with radioactive sodium. American Journal of Obstetrics and Gynecology 55:469–480, 1948.

26. Curran MA, Nijland MJM, Mann SE, Ross MG. Human amniotic fluid mathematical model: Determination and effect of intramembranous sodium flux. American Journal of Obstetrics and Gynecology 178:484–490, 1998.

27. Štulc J, Štulcová B, Sibley CP. Evidence for active maternal-fetal transport of Na^+ across the placenta of the anaesthetized rat. Journal of Physiology (London) 470:637–649, 1993.

28. Boyd CAR, Chipperfield AR, Steele LW. Separation of the microvillous (maternal) form the basal (fetal) plasma membranes of human term placenta: methods and physiological significance of marker enzyme distribution. Journal of Developmental Physiology 1:361–377, 1979.

29. Brownbill P, Atkinson DE, Glazier JD, Sibley CP, Warhurst GT. Changes in unidirectional maternofetal ^{22}Na clearance (K_{mf}) and Na^+-K^+-ATPase α-subunit expression by the placenta of the anesthetized rat during the last third of gestation (Abstract). Journal of Physiology (London) 476:368P, 1993.

30. Zamora F, Arola LI. (Na^+-K^+)-ATPase activities in rat tissues during pregnancy. Biological Research of Pregnancy 8:89–92, 1986.

31. Speake PF, Mynett KJ, Glazier JD, Greenwood SL, Sibley CP. Activity and expression of Na^+/H^+ exchanger isoforms in the syncytiotrophoblast of the human placenta. Pflügers Archives 450:123–130, 2005.

32. Mahendran D, Byrne S, Donnai P, et al. Na^+ transport, H^+ concentration gradient dissipation and system A amino acid transporter activity in purified microvillons plasma membrane isolated from first trimester human placenta: comparison to the term microvillous membrane. American Journal of Obstetrics and Gynecology 171:1534–1540, 1994.

33. Hughes JL, Doughty IM, Glazier JD, et al. Activity and expression of the Na^+/H^+ exchanger in the microvillous plasma membrane of the syncytiotrophoblast in relation to gestation and small for gestational age birth. Pediatric Research 48:652–659, 2000.

34. Johansson M, Glazier JD, Jansson T, Sibley CP, Powell TL. Na^+/H^+ exchange is reduced in the microvillous membranes isolated form preterm IUGR pregnancies. Placenta 22:A66, 2001.

35. Brunette MG, Leclerc M, Claveau D. Na^+ transport by human placental brush border membranes: are there several mechanisms. Journal of Cellular Physiology 167:72–80, 1996.

36. Zhao H, Hundal HS. Identification and biochemical localization of Na-K-Cl cotransporter in the human placental cell line BeWo. Biochemical Biophysical Research Communications 274:43–48, 2000.

37. Page KR, Ashworth CJ, McArdle HJ, Finch AM, Nwagwu MO. Sodium transport across the chorioallantoic membrane of porcine placenta involves the epithelial sodium channel (ENaC). Journal of Physiology 547:849–857, 2003.

38. Daneshmand SS, Cheung CY, Brace RA. Regulation of amniotic fluid volume by intramembranous absorption in sheep: role of passive permeability and vascular endothelial growth factor. American Journal of Obstetrics and Gynecology 188:786–793, 2003.

39. Roberts TJ, Nijland MJM, Williams L, Ross MG. Fetal diuretic response to maternal hyponatremia: contribution of placental sodium gradient. Journal of Applied Physiology 87:1440–1447, 1999.

40. Kirksey A, Pike RI, Callahan AJ. Some effects of high and low sodium intakes during pregnancy in the rat II. Electrolyte concentrations of maternal plasma, muscle, bone and brain and of placenta, amniotic fluid, fetal plasma and total fetus in normal pregnancy. Journal of Nutrition 77:43–51, 1962.

41. Powell TL, Brace RA. Fetal fluid responses to long-term 5 M NaCl infusion: where does all the salt go? American Journal of Physiology 261:R412–R419, 1991.

42. Gibson KJ, Lumbers ER. Effects of continuous drainage of fetal fluids on salt and water balance in fetal sheep. Journal of Physiology 494:443–450, 1996.

43. Pullano JG, Cohen-Addad N, Apuzzio JJ, Ganesh VL, Josimovich JB. Water and salt conservation in the human fetus and newborn. I. Evidence for a role of fetal prolactin. Journal of Clinical Endocrinology and Metabolism 69:1180–1186, 1989.

44. Riddick DH, Maslar IA. The transport of prolactin by human fetal membranes. Journal of Clinical Endocrinology and Metabolism 52:220–224, 1991.

45. Ertl T, Sulyok E, Bódis J, Csaba IF. Plasma prolactin levels in full-term newborn infants with idiopathic edema: Response to furosemide. Biology of the Neonate 49:15–20, 1986.

46. Ertl T, Sulyok E, Varga L, Csaba IF. Postnatal development of plasma prolactin level in premature infants with and without NaCl supplementation. Biology of the Neonate 44:219–223, 1983.

47. Metcoff J. Synchrony of organ development contributing to water and electrolyte regulation in early life. Clinical Nephrology 1:107–118, 1973.

48. Arant BS. Fluid therapy in the neonate: concept in transition. Journal of Pediatrics 101:387–389, 1982.

49. Shaffer SG, Quimiro CL, Andreson JV, Hall RT. Postnatal weight changes in low birth weight infants. Pediatrics 79:702–705, 1987.

50. Tang W, Ridout D, Modi N. Influence of respiratory distress syndrome on body composition after preterm birth. Archives of Disease in Childhood 77:F28–F31, 1997.

51. Bauer K, Bovermann G, Roithmaier A, Gotz M, Prolss A, Versmold HT. Body composition, nutrition and fluid balance during the first two weeks of life in preterm neonates weighing less than 1500 grams. Journal of Pediatrics 118:615–620, 1991.

52. Bauer K, Cowett RM, Howard GM, van Epp J, Oh W. Effect of intrauterine growth retardation on postnatal weight change in preterm infants. Journal of Pediatrics 123:301–306, 1993.

53. Van der Wagen A, Okken J, Zweens J, Zijlstra WG. Composition of postnatal weight loss and subsequent weight gain in small for dates newborn infants. Acta Paediatrica Scandinavica 74:57–61, 1985.

54. Heimler R, Doumas BT, Jendrzejczak BM, Németh PB, Hoffman RG, Nelin LD. Relationship between nutrition, weight change, and fluid compartments in preterm infants during the first week of life. Journal of Pediatrics 122:110–114, 1993.

55. Cheek DB, Wishart J, MacLennan A, Haslam R. Cell hydration in the normally grown, the premature and the low weight for gestational age infants. Early Human Development 10:75–84, 1984.

56. Thomas JL, Reichelderfer TE. Premature infants: analysis of serum during the first seven weeks. Clinical Chemistry 14:272–280, 1968.

57. Cheek DB. Extracellular volume: its structure and measurement and the influence of age and disease. Journal of Pediatrics 58:103–125, 1961.

58. MacLaurin JC. Changes in body water distribution during the first two weeks of life. Archives of Diseases in Childhood 41:286–291, 1966.

59. Coulter DM, Avery ME. Paradoxical reduction in tissue hydration with weight gain in neonatal rabbit pups. Pediatric Research 14:1122–1126, 1980.

60. Coulter DM. Prolactin: a hormonal regulator of neonatal tissue water reservoir. Pediatric Research 17:665–668, 1983.

61. Tulassay T, Seri I, Rascher W. Atrial natriuretic peptide and extracellular volume contraction after birth. Acta Paediatrica Scandinavica 76:444–446, 1987.

62. Bierd TM, Kattwinkel L, Chevalier RL, et al. Interrelationship of atrial natriuretic peptide, atrial volume, and renal function in premature infants. Journal of Pediatrics 116:753–759, 1990.

63. Sulyok E. Physical water compartments: a revised concept of perinatal body water physiology. Physiological Research 55:133–138, 2005.

64. Ling GN. A revolution in the physiology of the living cell. Malabar, FL: Krieger Publishing Co, 1992.

65. Israelachvili J, Wennerström H. Role of hydration and water structure in biological and colloidal interactions. Nature 379:217–225, 1996.

66. Mulkern RV, Bleier AR, Adzamil IK, Spencer RGS, Sándor T, Jolesz FA. Two-site exchange revisited: a new method for extracting exchange parameters in biological systems. Biophysical Journal 55:221–232, 1989.

67. Berényi E, Szendro Zs, Rózsahegyi P, Bogner P, Sulyok E. Postnatal changes in water content and proton magnetic resonance relaxation times in newborn rabbit tissues. Pediatric Research 39:1091–1098, 1996.

68. Berényi E, Repa I, Bogner P, Dóczi T, Sulyok E. Water content and proton magnetic resonance relaxation times of brain in newborn rabbits. Pediatric Research 43:421–425, 1998.

69. Hällgren R, Samuelsson T, Laurent TC, Moding J. Accumulation of hyaluronan (hyaluronic acid) in the lung in adult respiratory distress syndrome. American Review of Respiratory Diseases 139:682–687, 1989.

70. Allen SJ, Sedin EG, Jonzon A, Wells AF, Laurent TC. Lung hyaluronan during development: a quantitative and morphological study. American Journal of Physiology 260:H1449–H1454, 1991.

71. Sedin EG., Gerdin B, Johnsson H, Jonzon A, Eriksson L, Hällgren R. Hyaluronan and water content in the lung of preterm infants who died less than 24 hours after birth. Pediatric Research 36:37 A, (Abstract), 1994.

72. Sedin EG, Bogner P, Berényi E, Repa I, Nyul Z, Sulyok E. Lung water and proton magnetic resonance relaxation in preterm and term rabbit pups: their relation to tissue hyaluronan. Pediatric Research 48:554–559, 2000.

73. Sulyok E, Nyúl Z, Bogner P, et al. Brain water in fetal and newborn rabbits as assessed by H'-NMR relaxometry: its relation to tissue hyaluronan. Biology of the Neonate 79:62–72, 2001.

74. Hällgren R, Gerdin B, Tufveson G. Hyaluronic acid accumulation and redistribution in rejecting rat kidney graft: Relationship to the transplantation edema. Journal of Experimental Medicine 171:2063–2076, 1990.

75. Fraser JRE, Laurent TC, Laurent UBG. Hyaluronan: Its nature, distribution, function and turnover. Internal Medicine 242:27–33, 1997.

76. Hansell P, Göransson V, Odling C, Gerdin B, Hällgren R. Hyaluronan content in the kidney in different states of body hydration. Kidney International 58:2061–2068, 2000.

77. Sulyok E, Nyul Z. Hyaluronan-related limited concentration by the immature kidney. Medical Hypotheses 65:1058–1061, 2005.

78. Ross B, Cowett RM, Oh W. Renal functions of low birth weight infants during the first two months of life. Pediatric Research 11:1162–1164, 1977.

79. Sulyok E, Heim T, Soltész Gy, Jászai V. The influence of maturity on renal control acidosis in newborn infants. Biology of the Neonate 21:418–435, 1972.

80. Aperia A, Broberger O, Thodenius K, Zetterström R. Developmental study of the renal response to an oral salt load in preterm infants. Acta Paediatrica Scandinavica 63:517–524, 1974.

81. Arant BS. Developmental pattern of renal functional maturation compared in the human neonate. Journal of Pediatrics 92:705–712, 1978.

82. Siegel SR, Oh W. Renal function as a marker of human fetal maturation. Acta Paediatrica Scandinavica 65:481–485, 1976.

83. Bell EF, Acarregui MJ. Restricted versus liberal water intake for preventing morbidity and mortality in preterm infants. Cochrane Database System Review CD 000503, 2001.

84. Oh W, Poindexter BB, Perritt R, et al. Association between fluid intake and weight loss during the first ten days of life and risk of bronchopulmonary dysplasia in extremely low birth weight infants. Journal of Pediatrics 147:786–790, 2005.

85. Sulyok E. The relationship between electrolyte and acid-base balance in the premature infant during early postnatal life. Biology of the Neonate 17:227–237, 1971.

86. Day GM, Radde IC, Bafle JW, Chance GW. Electrolyte abnormalities in very low birthweight infants. Pediatric Research 10:522–526, 1976.

87. Roy RN, Chance CW, Radde IC, Hill DE, Wills DM, Sheepers J. Late hyponatremia in very low birth weight infants (1.3 kilograms). Pediatric Research 10:526–531, 1976.

88. Sulyok E, Németh M, Tényi J, et al. Relationship between maturity, electrolyte balance and the function of the renin-angiotensin-aldosterone system in newborn infants. Biology of the Neonate 35:60–65.

89. Sulyok E, Varga F, Gyory E, Jobst K, Csaba IF. On the mechanism of renal sodium handling in newborn infants. Biology of the Neonate 37:75–79, 1980.

90. Rodriguez-Soriano J, Vallo A, Oliveros R, Castillo G. Renal handling of sodium in premature and full-term neonates: a study using clearance method during water diuresis. Pediatric Research 17:1013–1016, 1983.

91. Sulyok E., Varga F, Gyory E, Jobst K, Csaba IF. Postnatal development of renal sodium handling in premature infants. Journal of Pediatrics 95:787–792, 1979.

92. Leslie GI, Arnold JD, Gyory AZ. Postnatal changes in proximal and distal tubular sodium rabsorption in healthy very low-birth-weight infants. Biology of the Neonate 60:108–113, 1991.

93. Haycock GB, Aperia A. Salt and the newborn kidney. Pediatric Nephrology 5:65–70, 1991.

94. Edelmann CM, Spitzer A. The maturing kidney. A modern view of well-balanced infants with imbalanced nephrons. Journal of Pediatrics 75:509–519, 1969.

95. Schwartz GJ, Evan AP. Development of solute transport in rabbit proximal tubule. III. Na-K-ATPase activity. American Journal of Physiology 246:F845–F852, 1984.

96. Baum M. Neonatal rabbit juxtamedullary proximal convoluted tubule acidification. Journal of Clinical Investigations 85:499–506, 1990.

97. Beck JC, Lipkowitz MS, Abramson RG. Ontogeny of Na/H antiporter activity in rabbit renal brush border membrane vesicles. Journal of Clinical Investigations 87:7067–7076, 1991.

98. Vehaskari VM. Ontogeny of cortical collecting duct sodium transport. American Journal of Physiology 267:F49–F54, 1994.

99. Satlin LM, Palmer LG. Apical Na$^+$ conductance in maturing rabbit principal cell. American Journal of Physiology 266:F57–F65, 1994.

100. Counillon L, Pouysségur J. The expanding family of eukaryotic Na$^+$/H$^+$ exchangers. Journal of Biological Chemistry 275:1–4.

101. Guillery EN, Karniski LP, Mathews MS, Robillard JE. Maturation of proximal tubule Na$^+$/H$^+$ antiproter activity in sheep during transition from fetus to newborn. American Journal of Physiology 267:F537–F545, 1994.

102. Baum M, Quigley R. Glucocorticoids stimulate rabbit proximal convoluted tubule acidification. Journal of Clinical Investigations 91:110–114, 1993.

103. Guillery EN, Karniski LP, Mathews MS, et al. Role of glucocorticoids in the maturation of renal cortical Na$^+$/H$^+$ exchanger activity during fetal life in sheep. American Journal of Physiology 268:F710–F717, 1995.

104. Kinsella JL, Sacktor B. Thyroid hormones increase Na$^+$-H$^+$ exchange activity in renal brush border membranes. Proceedings of National Academy of Sciences USA 82:3606–3610, 1985.

105. Mazursky JE, Segar JL, Smith BA, Merrill DC, Robillard JE. Rapid increase in renal sympathetic nerve activity (RSNA) during the transition form fetal to newborn life (Abstract). Pediatric Research 361A, 1993.

106. Guillery EN, Porter CC, Jose PA, Felder RA, Robillard JE. Developmental regulation of the $\alpha_{1\beta}$-adrenoceptor in the sheep kidney. Pediatric Research 34:124–128, 1993.

107. Gesek FA, Schoolwerth AC. Hormonal interactions with the proximal Na$^+$-H$^+$ exchanger. American Journal of Physiology 258:F514–F521, 1990.

108. Kerpel-Fronius E, Heim T, Sulyok E. The development of the renal acidifying processes and their relation to acidosis in low-birth-weight infants. Biology of the Neonate 15:156–168, 1970.

109. Spitzer A, Barac-Nieto M. Ontogeny of renal phosphate transport and the process of growth. Pediatric Nephrology 16:763–771, 2001.

110. Holtbäck U, Aperia A. Molecular determinants of sodium and water balance during early human development. Seminars in Neonatology 8:291–299, 2003.

111. Canessa CM, Schild L, Buell G, et al. Amiloride-sensitive epithelial Na$^+$ channel is made of three homologous subunits. Nature 367:463–467, 1994.

112. Dagenais A, Kothary R, Berthiaume Y. The α subunit of the epithelial sodium channel in the mouse: developmental regulation of its expression. Pediatric Research 42:327–334, 1997.

113. Vehaskari VM, Hempe JM, Manning J, Aviles DH, Carmichael MC. Developmental regulation of ENaC subunit mRNA levels in rat kidney. American Journal of Physiology 247:C1661–C1666, 1998.

114. Satlin LM, Palmer LG. Apical Na$^+$ conductance in maturing rabbit principal cell. American Journal of Physiology 270:F391–F397, 1996.

115. Watanabe S, Matsushita K, McCray PB, Stokes JB. Developmental expression of the epithelial Na$^+$ channel in kidney and uroepithelia. American Journal of Physiology 276:F304–F314, 1999.

116. Nakamura K, Stokes JB, McCray PB. Endogenous and exogenous glucocorticoid regulation of ENaC mRNA expression in developing kidney and lung. American Journal of Physiology 283:C762–C772, 2002.

117. Brown RW, Diaz R, Robson AC, et al. The ontogeny of 11 β-hydroxysteroid dehydrogenase type 2 and mineralocorticoid receptor gene expression reveal intricate control of glucocorticoid action in development. Endocrinology 137:794–797, 1996.

118. Schmitt R, Ellison DH, Farman N, et al. Developmental expression of sodium entry pathways in rat nephron. American Journal of Physiology 276:F367–F381, 1999.

119. Bidiwala KS, Lorenz JM, Kleinman LI. Renal function correlates of postnatal diuresis in preterm infants. Pediatrics 82:50–58, 1988.

120. Lorenz JM, Kleinman LI, Ahmed G, Makarian K. Phases of fluid and electrolyte homeostasis in the extremely low birth weight infants. Pediatrics 95:484–489, 1995.

121. Bueva A, Guignard J-P. Renal function in preterm neonates. Pediatric Research 36:572–577, 1994.

122. Delgado MM, Rohatgi R, Khan S, Holzman IR, Satlin LM. Sodium and potassium clearances by the maturing kidney: clinical-molecular correlates. Pediatric Nephrology 18:759–767, 2003.

123. Aperia A, Elinder G. Distal tubular sodium reabsorption in the developing rat kidney. American Journal of Physiology 240:F487–F491, 1981.

124. Kleinman LI. Renal sodium reabsorption during saline loading and distal blockade in newborn dog. American Journal of Physiology 228:1407–1408, 1975.

125. Drukker A, Goldsmith DI, Spitzer A, Edelman CM Jr, Blaufox MD. The renin-angiotensin system in newborn dog: deveolopmental pattern of response to acute saline loading. Pediatric Research 14:304–307, 1980.

126. Kleinman LI, Banks RO. Segmental nephron sodium and potassium reabsorption in newborn and adult dogs during saline expansion. Proceedings of the Society for Experimental Biology and Medicine 173:231–237, 1983.

127. Aperia A, Broberger O, Thodenius K, Zetterström R. Renal response to an oral salt load in newborn full-term infants. Acta Paediatrica Scandinavica 61:670–676, 1972.

128. Muchant DG, Tornhill BA, Belmonte DC, Felder RA, Baertschi A, Chevalier R. Chronic sodium loading augments natriuretic response to acute volume expansion in the preweaned rat. American Journal of Physiology 269:R15–R22, 1995.

129. Lorenz JM, Kleinman LI, Disney TA. Lack of anion effect on volume expansion natriuresis in the developing canine kidney. Journal of Developmental Physiology 8:395–410, 1986.

130. Ramiro-Tolentino SB, Markarian K, Kleinman LI. Renal bicarbonate excretion in extremely low birth weight infants. Pediatrics 98:256–261, 1996.

131. Al-Dahhan J, Haycock GB, Chantler C, Stimmler L. Sodium homeostasis in term and preterm monates II. Gastrointestinal aspects. Archives of Disease in Childhood 58:343–345, 1983.

132. O'Loughlin EV, Hunt DM, Kreutzmann D. Postnatal development of colonic electrolyte transport in rabbits. American Journal of Physiology 258:G447–G453, 1990.

133. Cho JH, Musch MW, Bookstein CM, McSwine RL, Rabenau K, Chang EB. Aldosterone stimulates intestinal Na$^+$ absorption in rats by increasing NHE3 expression in proximal colon. American Journal of Physiology 247:C586–C594, 1998.

134. Jenkins HR, Fenton TR, McIntosh N, Dillon MJ, Milla PJ. Development of colonic sodium transoport in early childhood and its regulation by aldosterone. Gut 31:194–197, 1990.

135. Rees L, Brook CGD, Shaw JCL, Forsling MR. Hyponatraemia in the first week of life in preterm infants. Part 1. Arginine vasopressin secretion. Archives of Disease of Childhood 59:414–422, 1984.

136. Costarino AT, Gruskay JA, Corcoran L, Polin RA, Baumgart S. Sodium restriction versus daily maintenance replacement in very low birth weight premature neonates: a randomized, blind therapeutic trial. Journal of Pediatrics 120:99–106, 1992.

137. Boyd KDH, Canning JF, Stacey TE, et al. Steady state ion distribution and feto-maternal ion fluxes across the sheep placenta. Placenta (Suppl 2):229–234, 1981.

138. Lelong-Tissier M-C, Retbi J-M, Dehan M, Vial M, Frydman R, Gabilan JC. Hyponatremie maternofoetale carentielle par regime desodé au cours d'une grosesse multiple. Archives Francaises de Pédiatric 34:64–70, 1977.

139. Shaffer SG, Meade VM. Sodium balance and extracellular volume regulation in very low birth weight infants. Journal of Pediatrics 115:285–290, 1989.

140. Lorenz JM, Kleinman LI, Kotagal UR, Reller MD. Water balance in very low-birth-weight infants: relationship to water and sodium intake and effect on outcome. Journal of Pediatrics 101:423–432, 1982.

141. Wilkins BH. Renal function in sick very low birth weight infants: 3. Sodium, potassium and water excretion. Archives of Disease in Childhood 67:1154–1161, 1992.
142. Shaffer SG, Bradt SK, Meade VM, Hall RT. Extracellular fluid volume changes in very low-birth-weight infants during first 2 postnatal months. Journal of Pediatrics 111:124–128, 1987.
143. Hartnoll G, Bétrémieux P, Modi N. Randomised controlled trial of postnatal sodium supplementation on body composition in 25 to 30 week gestational age infants. Archives of Disease in Childhood 82:24–28, 2000.
144. Hartnoll G, Bétrémieux P, Modi N. Randomised controlled trial of postnatal sodium supplementation in infants of 25-30 weeks gestational age: effects on cardiopulmonary adaptation. Archives of Disease in Childhood 85:29–32, 2001.
145. Sulyok E, Németh M, Tényi I, Csaba IF, Varga L, Varga F. Relationship between the postnatal development of the renin-angiotensin-aldosterone system and electrolyte and acid-base status of the NaCl-supplemented premature infants. In Spitzer A (Ed.), The kidney during development. Morphology and function (pp. 272–281). New York: Masson Publishing USA, Inc., 1982.
146. Satlin LM, Sheng S, Woda CB, Kleyman TR. Epithelial Na$^+$ channels are regulated by flow. American Journal of Physiology Renal Physiology 280:F1010–F1018, 2001.
147. Bell EF, Heidrich GA, Cashore WJ, Oh W. Combined effect of radiant warmer and phototherapy on insensible water loss in low-birth-weight infants. Journal of Pediatrics 94:810–813, 1979.
148. Rees L, Shaw JCL, Brook CDG, Forsling ML. Hyponatraemia in the first week of life in preterm infants. Part II. Sodium and water balance. Archives of Disease in Childhood 59:423–429, 1984.
149. Vajda Zs, Pedersen M, Dóczi T, et al. Effects of centrally administered arginine vasopressin and atrial natriuretic peptide on the development of brain edema in hyponatremic rat. Neurosurgery 49:697–705, 2001.
150. Gunnarson E, Zelenina M, Aperia A. Regulation of brain aquaporins. Neuroscience 129:947–955, 2004.
151. Ecelbarger CA, Kim G-H, Terris J, et al. Vasopressin-mediated regulation of epithelial sodium channel abundance in rat kidney. American Journal of Physiology, Renal Physiology 279:F46–F53, 2000.
152. Machida K, Nonoguchi H, Wakamatsu S, et al. Acute regulation of epithelial sodium channel gene by vasopressin and hyperosmolality. Hypertension Research 26:629–634, 2003.
153. Sulyok E, Kovács L, Lichardus B, et al. Late hyponatremia in premature infants: role of aldosterone and arginine vasopressin. Journal of Pediatrics 106:990–994, 1985.
154. Lien Y-HH, Shapiro JI, Chan L. Study of brain electrolytes and organic osmolytes during correction of chronic hyponatremia. Implications for the pathogenesis of central pontine myelinolysis. Acta Neuropathology 103:590–598, 1991.
155. DeLuca GC, Nagy Zs, Esiri MM, Davey P. Evidence for a role for apoptosis in central pontine myelinolysis. Acta Neuropathology 103:590–598, 2002.
156. Baker EA, Tian Y, Adler S, Verbalis JG. Blood-brain barrier disruption and complement activation in the brain following rapid correction of chronic hyponatremia. Experimental Neurology 165:221–230, 2000.
157. Sigamura Y, Murase T, Takefuji S, et al. Protective effect of dexamethasone on osmotic-induced demyelination in rats. Experimental Neurology 192:178–183, 2005.
158. Bursey RG, Watson ML. The effect of sodium restriction during gestation on offspring brain development in rats. American Journal of Clinical Nutrition, 37, 43–51.
159. Aviv A, Kobayashi T, Higashino H, Bauman JW Jr, Yu SS. Chronic sodium deficit in the immature rats: its effect on adaptation to sodium excess. American Journal of Physiology 242:E241–E247, 1982.
160. Ertl T, Hadzsiev K, Vincze O, Pytel J, Szabó I, Sulyok E. Hyponatremia and sensorineurtal hearing loss in preterm infants. Biology of the Neonate 79:109–112, 2001.
161. Wassner SJ. Altered growth and protein turnover in rats fed sodium deficient diet. Pediatric Research 26:608–613, 1989.
162. Ray PE, Lyon RC, Ruley EJ, Holliday MA. Sodium or chloride deficiency lowers muscle intracellular pH in growing rats. Pediatric Nephrology 10:33–37, 1996.
163. Kovács L, Sulyok E, Lichardus B, Michajlovskij N, Bircak J. Renal response to arginine vasopressin in premature infants with late hyponatraemia. Archives of Diseases in Childhood 61:1030–1032, 1986.
164. Barker DJP. The developmental origins of adult disease. Journal of American College of Nutrition 23:588–595.
165. Luyckx VA, Brenner BM. Low-birth-weight, nephron number, and kidney disease. Kidney International 68 Supplement, 97:S68–S72, 2005.
166. Sulyok E, Németh M, Tényi I, et al. Postnatal development of renin-angiotensin-aldosterone system, RAAS, in relation to electrolyte balance in premature infants. Pediatric Research 13:817–820, 1979.
167. Simmons MA, Adock EW, Bard H. Hypernatremia and intracranial hemorrhage in neonates. New England Journal of Medicine 291:6–10, 1974.
168. Sulyok E, Rascher W, Baranyai Zs, Ertl T, Kerekes L. The influence of NaCl supplementation on vasopressin secretion and renal water excretion in premature infants. Biology of the Neonate 64:201–208, 1993.
169. Hornich H, Amiel-Tison C. Retention hydrosaline chez les enfants de faible poids de naissnace. Archives Francaises de Pédiatrie 34:206–218, 1977.
170. Geleijnse JM, Hofman A, Witteman JCM, Hazebraek AAJM, Valkenburg HA, Grobbe DE. Long-term effects of neonatal sodium restriction on blood pressure. Hypertension 29:913–917, 1997.
171. Sulyok E, Varga F. Renal aspects of neonatal sodium homeostasis. Acta Paediatrica Hungarica 24:23–35, 1983.

Chapter 3

Potassium Metabolism

John M. Lorenz, MD

Normal Metabolism
Developmental Physiology
Clinical Relevance

NORMAL METABOLISM

Total body potassium (K) in an adult male is about 50 mmol/kg of body weight and is influenced by age, sex, and, very importantly, muscle mass. Approximately 98% of the total body K is found in the intracellular fluid (ICF) space at a concentration of 100–150 mmol/L, depending on the cell type. This high intracellular $[K^+]$ is essential for many basic cellular processes. In plasma water, the concentration of K is only 3.5–5 mmol/L. (In interstitial fluid water, with which ICF K is in equilibrium, $[K^+]$ is 7–8% higher due to the Gibbs-Donnan equilibrium.) This steep $[K^+]$ gradient from the ICF to extracellular fluid (ECF) compartment is maintained by active transport of K into the cell in exchange for sodium, which is mediated by sodium-potassium-triphosphatase (Na^+,K^+-ATPase) in the cell membrane. Most of the total body K is contained in muscle. This gradient is the major determinate of the resting membrane potential across the cell membrane, affecting muscle excitability and contractility.

Figure 3-1 shows the distribution and regulation of total body K in the normal adult.

K homeostasis requires appropriate internal distribution of K and maintenance of an appropriate external K balance. Regulation of the internal K balance refers to the regulation of the critical concentration K gradient across cell membranes. Regulation of the external K balance refers to the regulation of total body K content. While maintenance of total body K balance is dependent on excretion of K, predominantly by the kidney, this is a relatively slow process. In the adult, daily K intake (~ 100 mmol/day) exceeds the total K content of the ECF and only $\sim 50\%$ of oral K load is excreted in the following 4–6 hours. Of the retained K, 80–90% is rapidly transported from the ECF to the ICF space. Thus, life-threatening hyperkalemia would result were it not for the temporary, but rapid, extracellular to intracellular translocation of the transient excess of K.

Regulation of Internal K Balance (1)

The regulation of K distribution across cell membranes is critical for cellular function. Uptake of K into cells is active in exchange for Na driven by Na^+,K^+-ATPase, whereas the efflux of K from the cell is passive and depends on the type, density and open probability of K specific channels in various cell types. Figure 3-2 illustrates the factors affecting internal K balance. An increase in plasma [K+] decreases the

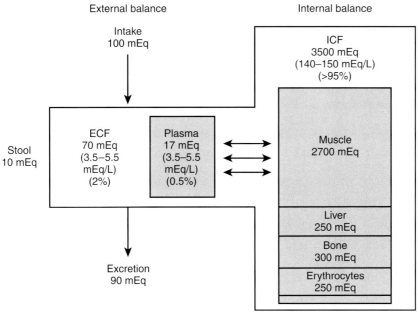

Figure 3-1 Total body K distribution and regulation in a 70 kg adult under normal conditions. (From Williams ME, Epstein FH: Internal exchanges of potassium. In Seldin DW, Giebisch G (Eds): The Regulation of Potassium Balance (pp. 3–29). New York: Raven Press, 1989, with permission.)

concentration gradient against which the Na^+,K^+-ATPase pump must operate and thereby favors cellular uptake of K. A decrease in plasma [K^+] decreases cellular K uptake by increasing this concentration gradient.

Insulin stimulates the cellular uptake of K by hepatocytes and muscle cells, independent of its affect on glucose transport, by inducing an increase in Na^+,K^+-ATPase activity. Beta-adrenergic stimulation promotes K uptake by hepatocytes, skeletal, and cardiac muscle via beta-2 receptors. Conversely, beta-adrenergic blockade impairs cellular uptake of K. Insulin and the beta-adrenergic system are

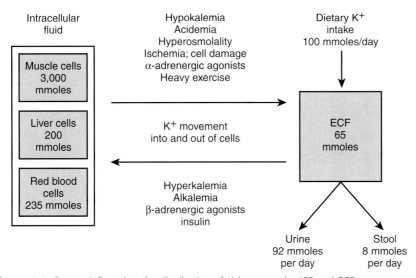

Figure 3-2 Factors influencing the distribution of K between the ICF and ECF compartments. (After Schafer J: Renal regulation of potassium, calcium and magnesium. In Johnson LR (Ed.): Essential Medical Physiology (pp. 437–446). Amsterdam/Boston: Elsevier Academic Press, 3rd edn, 2003, with permission.)

important components of the extrarenal defense against hyperkalemia and act in both physiological and pathological concentrations. Alpha-adrenergic receptor stimulation promotes efflux of K from hepatocytes. The role of aldosterone in modulating internal K balance is uncertain.

Acute administration or the production of acid with an associated anion to which the cell membrane is relatively impermeable (i.e., exogenous hydrochloric acid, ammonium chloride or endogenous acidosis of uremia) promotes K efflux from cells (2). In this situation, K and sodium (Na) exit the cell in exchange for the excess ECF protons, which are buffered intracellularly, in order to maintain electroneutrality across the cell membrane. However, with organic acidemia (e.g., lactic acidemia), the associated anion diffuses into the cell more freely and thus is not associated with K efflux. During respiratory acidosis the increment in plasma [K+] for any given change in pH is greater than with organic acidemia, but less than with mineral acidemia. An increase in the diffusion of bicarbonate (HCO_3) into cells as the result of an increase in plasma [HCO_3^-], independent of ECF pH, may be associated with the concomitant uptake of K. Respiratory alkalosis does not promote much shift of K across cell membranes.

The shift of water out of cells with severe ECF hyperosmolarity increases the intracellular [K^+], promoting K efflux from cells. Impairment of Na^+,K^+-ATPase activity by hypoxia (or loss of Na^+,K^+-ATPase activity with cell death) results in the movement of K out of the cell down its concentration gradient.

Regulation of External K Balance

Total body K content is a reflection of the balance between K intake and output. K intake depends on the quantity and type of intake. Under normal conditions the average adult takes in about 50–100 mmol of K per day, about the same amount as Na. K output occurs through three primary routes: urine, gastrointestinal tract, and skin.

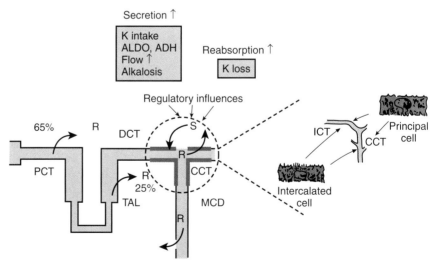

Figure 3-3 Summary of K transport along the nephron. Arrows demonstrate the direction of net K transport. The percentages of the filtered K load remaining at specific nephron sites are shown. The collecting duct system is indicated by the hatched portion of the nephron. R, reabsorption; S, secretion; PCT, Proximal convoluted tubule; TAL, thick ascending limb of the loop of Henle; DCT, distal convoluted tubule; ICT, initial connecting tubule; CCT, cortical collecting tubule; MCD, medullary collecting duct; ALDO, aldosterone; ADH, antidiuretic hormone. (From Giebisch G, Wang W: Potassium transport from clearance to channels to pumps. Kidney Int 49: 1624, 1996, with permission.)

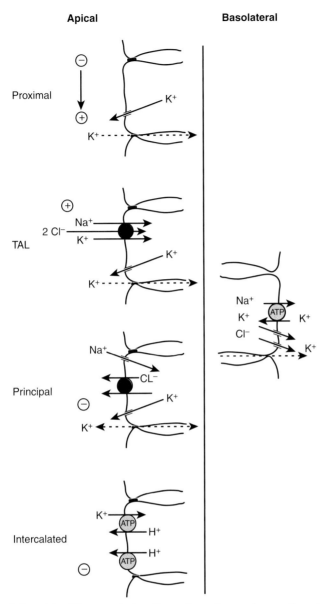

Figure 3-4 Cell models of K transport along the nephron. Transport across the apical membrane is different in each nephron segment or cell type, but basolateral membrane transport is similar. TAL, thick ascending limb of the loop of Henle. (From Giebisch G, Wang W: Potassium transport from clearance to channels to pumps. Kidney Int 49: 1624, 1996, with permission.)

Renal K Excretion (3)

The kidney is the major excretory organ for K and primarily responsible for the regulation of external K balance. K is freely filtered across the glomerulus. As shown in Fig. 3-3, 60–70% of the filtered K is reabsorbed in the proximal tubule. Reabsorption in this tubular segment is the result of solvent drag (dependent on active Na transport and a high permeability of the paracellular pathway to K) and by the positive transepithelial voltage in the second half of this segment (Fig. 3-4). Net K reabsorption continues in the loop of Henle. In the thick ascending limb of the loop of Henle, K is reabsorbed across the apical cell membrane by means of a Na$^+$,K$^+$-Cl co-transporter. This co-transporter is driven by the electrochemical gradient generated by Na$^+$,K$^+$-ATPase in the basolateral membrane, which favors Na entry across the luminal membrane (Fig. 3-4). Reabsorption in this nephron segment results in the delivery of only 10% of the filtered K to the distal renal tubule (Fig. 3-3). Thus, the balance of regulated, active K secretion and regulated, active K reabsorption in the distal tubule, specifically in the late distal tubule and cortical collecting tubule (CCT), determines the magnitude of renal K excretion (4). Principle cells are responsible for K secretion and intercalated cells are responsible for K reabsorption in the late distal tubule and CCT.

K secretion by principle cells is effected by the active exchange of K for Na across the basolateral membrane, driven by Na$^+$,K$^+$-ATPase (Fig. 3-4 and Fig. 3-5). A lumen negative voltage is generated across the late distal tubule and CCT by the apical entry of Na into the principle cell down its concentration gradient via epithelial sodium channels (ENaCs), driven by the extrusion of Na from the principle cell across the basolateral membrane by Na$^+$,K$^+$-ATPase. Intracellular K passively diffuses down a favorable electrochemical gradient via K channels in the apical membrane. Under baseline conditions, K transverses the apical membrane of the principle cell via an ATPase sensitive, small conductance (SK) channel with a high open probability. Maxi-K channels are high conductance K channels in the apical membrane, but are present at low density and low opening probability under baseline conditions. SK channels are responsible for baseline K secretion, whereas flow dependent K secretion (see below) is thought to be mediated by maxi-K channels. The magnitude of transport of K across the principle cell, then, is determined by the electrochemical gradient across the late distal tubule and CCT and the permeability of the apical membrane of the principle cell to Na and K. The latter are a function of the number and open probability of ion specific apical membrane channels. Therefore, K secretion in the late distal tubule and CCT is regulated by factors that affect the electrochemical gradient or apical membrane permeability to Na or K. Since urinary K excretion is largely the result of K secretion in the late distal tubule and CCT under most conditions, these factors then determine urinary K excretion.

An acute increase in plasma [K$^+$] as the result of K intake produces a more favorable electrochemical gradient for K secretion in the late distal tubule and CCT, increases the density of SK channels, and stimulates aldosterone secretion. Aldosterone stimulates K secretion in the late distal tubule and CCT by increasing the density of ENaCs and increasing Na$^+$,K$^+$-ATPase activity in the basolateral membrane of principle cells. Na$^+$,K$^+$-ATPase activity is coupled to SK density in

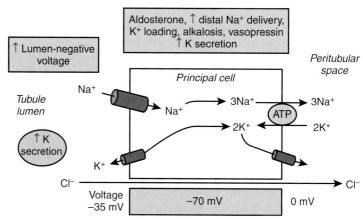

Figure 3-5 Cell model of a principle cell with overview of factors known to regulate K secretion. (From Giebisch GH: A trail of research on potassium. Kidney Int 62:1498, 2002, with permission.)

the apical membrane—increased pump activity increases SK density and decreased pump activity decreases SK density. A chronic increase in K intake results in increased capacity of the principle cell for K secretion—a process referred to as K adaptation. It results from an increase in the density of SK channels, increased activity of ENaCs, and increased Na^+,K^+-ATPase activity in the basolateral membrane. These changes are independent of aldosterone, but depend on increased plasma $[K^+]$.

K secretion is strongly stimulated by an increase in the tubular fluid flow rate in the late distal tubule and CCT. This is the result of both a more favorable electrochemical gradient and increased permeability of the luminal membrane to K. The higher the tubular flow rate, the slower the rise in $[K^+]$ along the late distal tubule and CCT as secreted K is more rapidly diluted in the greater volume of tubular fluid transversing the late distal tubule and CCT. Any associated increase in Na delivery to the late distal tubule and CCT also increases the concentration gradient driving Na across the apical membrane. High tubular flow rates also increase the permeability of the principle cell membrane to K by activating maxi-K channels (5).

Acute metabolic acidosis reduces K secretion by decreasing $[K^+]$ in the principle cell, which reduces the electrochemical gradient for K secretion, and by increasing tubular fluid acidity, which inhibits apical SK activity. The effect of chronic metabolic acidosis is complex; it depends on associated changes in filtered chloride (Cl) and HCO_3, distal tubular flow rate, and aldosterone. Acute respiratory and metabolic alkalosis stimulate K secretion in the late distal tubule and CCT by increasing tubular fluid pH. The latter increases the permeability of the apical membrane of the principle cell to K by increasing the duration that SK channels remain open. A K-Cl co-transporter in the apical membrane may also be involved in the increase in K secretion in response to metabolic alkalosis. While mediating only a modest amount of K secretion at physiological tubular fluid $[Cl^-]$, this co-transporter is activated when the tubular fluid $[HCO_3^-]$ or pH rises (6). Metabolic alkalosis also stimulates the basolateral uptake of K.

Vasopressin has both apical and peritubular sites of action on the principle cell that stimulate K secretion. It may stimulate SK channels and K-Cl co-transporters in the apical membrane. It is unlikely that vasopressin is involved in the physiological regulation of urinary K excretion. However, it may sustain K excretion in the face of reductions in distal tubular flow rate, e.g. during extracellular volume contraction.

Intercalated cells in the late distal tubule and CCT primarily function in H^+/HCO_3^- transport. However, under conditions of chronic K depletion, intercalated cells reabsorb K, by the active exchange of a single K^+ for a proton catalyzed by hydrogen, potassium-triphosphatase in the apical membrane (Fig. 3-4). K depletion increases the activity of the hydrogen, potassium-triphosphatase in the apical membrane, decreases apical membrane K permeability (channel not shown in Fig. 3-4), reducing the back leak K into the lumen down its electrochemical gradient, and increases basolateral membrane K permeability. Both metabolic acidosis and Na depletion also increase K^+-H^+ exchange across the apical membrane of the intercalated cell.

Intestinal K Excretion

Under normal conditions loss of K through the gastrointestinal tract is only 5–10% of dietary intake. The bulk of dietary K intake is reabsorbed in the small intestine. Analogous to the kidney, gastrointestinal K output is primarily a balance of regulated, active K secretion and regulated, active K reabsorption in the colon. Active K secretion in the colon is driven by basolateral uptake of K via Na^+,K^+-ATPase. Movement of K across the apical membrane, down its electrochemical concentration gradient, occurs via a Na-K-2Cl co-transporter. K reabsorption is active, mediated by a colonic apical K^+-ATPase. Aldosterone, glucocorticoids, epinephrine, and prostaglandins increase stool K content. Indomethacin and K depletion reduce it.

Intestinal K excretion assumes a significant role in maintaining external K balance in severe renal insufficiency, when as much as 30–80% of K intake may be excreted in the feces.

Sweat Gland K Excretion

Human excretory sweat $[K^+]$ is 5–10 mmol/L, so K losses from the skin in sweat are negligible under baseline conditions.

Plasma [K⁺]

Extracellular fluid (ECF) $[K^+]$ is a function of both internal and external K balance. Since the ICF K pool is 50 fold that of the ECF, changes in internal K balance can result in acute, dramatic, life threatening changes in ECF $[K^+]$. On the other hand, changes in ECF $[K^+]$ as the result of changes in external K balance usually occur more slowly and are buffered by homeostatic changes in internal K balance. As a result, plasma $[K^+]$ concentration is a late indicator of changes in external K balance.

DEVELOPMENTAL PHYSIOLOGY

Unlike the adult, in whom K homeostasis requires that the external K balance be zero, the external K balance must be positive for the growth of the fetus and neonate. Change in fetal/neonatal total body K content during development is shown in Fig. 3-6. This is a reflection, at least in part, of an increase in muscle mass and ICF $[K^+]$ in muscle during development (7). K metabolism in the fetus and neonate reflects this K requirement.

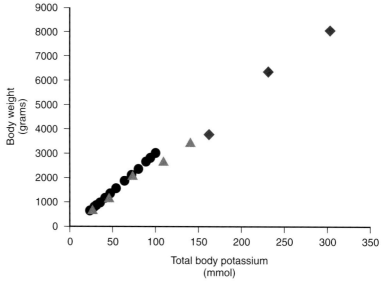

Figure 3-6 Total body K versus body weight. ●, calculated as 0.0716 × body weight (g)0.906, derived from neutron activation analysis of cadavers (live births nutritionally adequate mothers surviving 1–10 days (Ellis KJ: Body composition of the neonate. In RM Cowett (Ed.): Principles of Neonatal-Perinatal Metabolism (pp. 1077–1095). New York, 1998); ▲, chemical analysis of cadavers (Widdowson EM, Dickerson JWT: Chemical composition of the body. In Comar CL, Bonner F (Eds): Mineral Metabolism, Vol 2, Part A (pp. 2–247). New York/London: Academic Press, 1964); ◇, sequential TBK by whole body 40K counting in 76 breast or formula fed, normally growing, term infants at 0.5, 3, and 6 months of age (Butte NF, Hopkinson JM, Wong WW, Smith EO, Ellis KJ: Body composition during the first two years of life: an updated reference. Pediatr Res 47:578–585, 2000).

Fetus

K is actively transported across the placenta from the mother to the fetus. The plasma $[K^+]$ in the canine fetus nearly always exceeds maternal plasma $[K^+]$ under basal conditions (8). Human fetal plasma $[K^+]$ is also higher than that of the mother's at term, but not significantly so at 16–22 weeks (9). Thus, maternal-placental-fetal K metabolism is appropriately geared towards supplying the fetus with the K necessary for growth.

The fetus is also buffered against maternal K deficiency. Despite a 35% decrease in plasma $[K^+]$ and 28% decrease in intercellular $[K^+]$ of skeletal muscle in pregnant female dogs fed a K deficient diet throughout gestation, there was no difference in fetal plasma $[K^+]$, fetal total body K, fetal dry weight, or litter size at near term compared to controls (8). Despite a 50% decrease in plasma $[K^+]$ and 30% decrease in intercellular $[K^+]$ of skeletal muscle of rat dams fed a K deficient diet from days 2–5 to day 21 of gestation, there was no change in fetal plasma $[K^+]$ and only a 10% decrease in fetal TBK at 22 days of gestation (10). Similar results were found when acute K deficiency was induced in rat dams at 14 or 16 days of gestation by peritoneal dialysis with isotonic $NaHCO_3$ (11). On the other hand, the fetus does not seem to be buffered against excess maternal K. Serum $[K^+]$ of pups of rat dams infused with KCl to maintain serum $[K^+] > 10$ mmol/L for two hours also exceeded 10 mmol/L (10).

Neonate

Internal K Metabolism

There are no data regarding whether there are quantitative differences between the newborn and adult in the effect of factors controlling the distribution of K between the ICF and ECF spaces. However, studies in newborns confirm that β-catecholamine (12) and insulin administration stimulate the movement of K from the ECF to ICF space (13,14).

Renal K Metabolism

Clearance studies in preterm infants and newborn dogs, micropuncture studies in developing rodents, and in vitro microperfusion studies of single nephron segments in the developing rabbit confirm that the distal nephron plays a major role in the regulation of renal K excretion, as is the case in adults. In the newborn dog, urinary K excretion is largely the result of amiloride-sensitive K secretion under basal conditions and during K loading. Amiloride is known to selectively block sodium conductance across the luminal membrane in the distal tubule. This then suggests that urinary K excretion under basal and K loaded conditions is largely the result of K secretion in the distal nephron (as is the case in the adult) and that the cellular mechanisms of K secretion in this segment are similar to those in the adult.

Even low birth weight (and presumably preterm) infants are capable of urinary K excretion at a rate in excess of the rate of K filtration across the glomerulus during K and/or $NaHCO_3$ loading in the first month of life, indicating net tubular K secretion (15). However, the rate of K excretion per unit body or kidney weight during exogenous K loading is lower in the immature than mature animal (16). In newborn infants, K secretion (as indicated indirectly by the calculated transtubular K concentration gradient in the distal nephron) was lower in preterm infants (mean GA 29.3 ± 2.7 weeks) in the first two weeks of life than in term infants under basal conditions, but similar to that in 1–2 week old term infants during 3–5 weeks of life (17). There was also a significant positive correlation between K secretion and postmenstrual age in the preterm infants. However, the relevance of these results to the developmental changes in K secretory capacity is unclear, since no information is provided about the rate of K administration. In general, the limited K secretory capacity of the immature distal nephron is clinically relevant only under conditions of K excess.

Data in newborn dogs suggest that K secretion in response to K loading is not limited by basolateral Na^+, K^+-ATPase activity (18,19). In vivo studies in suckling rats indicate that $[Na^+]$ in distal tubular fluid is greater than 35 mmol/L (as in adult rats) and, therefore, should not restrict K secretion (20,21). Plasma aldosterone concentration is higher in preterm and term infants than in adults (22,23) and the density of aldosterone binding sites, receptor affinity, and degree of nuclear binding of hormone–receptor are similar in immature and mature rats (23). However, clearance studies in the fetus and neonate and the immature and mature rat demonstrate a relative insensitivity of the immature kidney to aldosterone (22–24), presumably due to a post receptor phenomenon. Studies in developing rabbits suggest that K secretion in the CCT in this species is limited by a paucity of SK channels (25). In a study of single nephrectomy specimens from 20–36 week' gestational infants, steady-state expression of mRNA encoding the SK channel did not change during this period and was only approximately a third of that in nephrectomy specimens from 7-month-old subjects (26). This could be expected to result in a decreased K secretory capacity of the immature distal tubule. Woda et al (5) have also shown the lack of response to increased tubular flow rate in the developing rabbit as a result of the delayed expression of maxi-K channels. However, the kaliuresis associated with postnatal diuresis/natriuresis in preterm infants (27) and the development of hypokalemic hypochloremic metabolic alkalosis in association with loop diuretic therapy in the newborn (see below) suggest that this finding may not be relevant to the human infant.

On the other hand, K reabsorption increased in parallel to the increase in the filtered K load with increasing gestational age in a study of infants at 23–31 weeks of gestation on days 4–5 of life, so that urinary K excretion remained low and unchanged over this period of gestation (28).

Intestinal K Metabolism

There are no data regarding whether there are differences between the newborn and adult in intestinal K transport. While the neonatal intestine is certainly capable of reabsorbing dietary K, the capacity of the neonatal colon for net K secretion is unknown. One study of fecal K excretion found that intestinal K excretion, controlled for body weight, was similar in parenterally fed infants with a mean gestational age of 27 weeks and mean postnatal age of 4.8 days compared to that of enterally fed infants with mean gestational ages of 32 or 39 weeks and similar postnatal ages (29). However, significant differences in plasma $[K^+]$ and in the magnitude and route of K intake during the study period, as well as the absence of data about K intake prior to and during the study period, preclude conclusions regarding developmental changes in intestinal K homeostasis.

CLINICAL RELEVANCE

Perturbations in internal or external K balance on usual K intakes (1–3 mmol/kg/day) are unusual in the neonate except under few circumstances.

Hyperkalemia

Spurious Hyperkalemia

Hyperkalemia in the neonatal intensive care unit is most commonly spurious secondary to red cell hemolysis in the whole blood sample.

Non-oliguric Hyperkalemia

Plasma [K$^+$] rises in the first 24–72 hours after birth in very premature infants, even in the absence of exogenous K intake or renal failure (27,30,31). This increase results from the transcellular movement of K from the ICF space to the ECF space. This shift occurs at a time when the renal K excretion is restricted by the low GFR and relatively low fractional excretion of Na, which limits sodium and water delivery to the distal nephron (27). The reason for and appropriateness of this shift are not understood. However, it is known to result in hyperkalemia in 25% to 50% of infants weighing less than 1000 g at birth or born at less than 28 weeks' gestation (27,32–37). The magnitude of this shift correlates roughly with the degree of prematurity, but it does not seem to occur (or at least is not clinically significant) after 30–32 weeks' gestation (34). The most effective strategy for managing non-oliguric hyperkalemia when renal secretory capacity is so restricted is to stimulate the movement of K back from the ECF to ICF space with albuterol inhalation (12) or insulin (13,14) therapy.

Even without albuterol or insulin therapy, plasma [K$^+$] falls with the onset of physiologic diuresis and natriuresis, as the associated increase in delivery of water and Na to the distal nephron results in marked kaliuresis. In fact, many infants with non-oliguric hyperkalemia will become hypokalemic after the onset of diuresis and natriuresis if K administration is not initiated as plasma [K$^+$] declines (27).

Renal Failure

As in adults, acute severe reduction in GFR severely reduces water and Na delivery to the distal nephron and thus restricts K secretion.

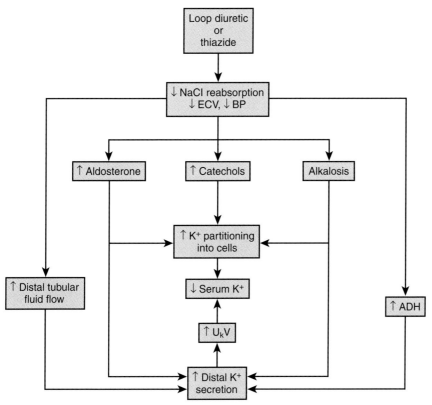

Figure 3-7 Effects of loop and thiazide diuretics on internal K balance and K transport in the distal nephron. (From Wilcox CS: Diuretics and potassium. In Seldin DW, Giebisch G (Eds): Regulation of Potassium Balance (pp. 325–345). New York, Raven Press, 1989, with permission.)

Hypokalemia

Loop and Thiazide Diuretics

Hypokalemia commonly results from loop and diuretic therapy (Fig. 3-7) (38). This is primarily the result of the stimulation of distal K secretion by the increased delivery of water and Na delivery. However, increases in aldosterone, catecholamines, vasopressin, and alkalosis (caused by contraction of the ECF) also results in enhanced cellular uptake of K from the ECF space.

Alkalosis

The predominant cause of hypokalemia with metabolic or respiratory alkalosis is negative external K balance. An increase in plasma $[HCO_3{}^-]$ also produces a rapid decrease in plasma $[K^+]$, which is due to enhanced cellular uptake of K from the ECF space.

REFERENCES

1. Rosa RM, Eckstein FH. Extrarenal potassium metabolism. In: Seldin DW, Giebisch G (Eds.): The Kidney: Physiology and Pathophysiology (pp. 1515–1574). New York, Raven Press, 2000.
2. Androgúe HF, Madias NE. Changes in plasma potassium concentration during acid and base disturbances. Am J Med 71:454, 1981.
3. Giebisch G. Challenges to potassium metabolism: internal distribution and external balance. Wein Klin Wochenschr 166:353, 2004.
4. Berliner RW. Renal mechanisms for K excretion. Harvey Lect 55:141–171, 1961.
5. Woda CB, Bragin A, Kleyman TR, et al. Flow-dependent K^+ secretion in the cortical collecting duct is mediated by a maxi-K channel. AJP 49:F793, 2001.
6. Amorim JBO, Bailey MA, Musa-Aziz R, et al. Role of luminal anion and pH in distal potassium secretion. Am J Physiol 284:F381, 2003.
7. Dickerson JWT, Widdowson EM. Chemical changes in skeletal muscle during development. Biochem J 74:247, 1960.
8. Servano CV, Talbert LM, Welt LG. Potassium deficiency in the pregnant dog. J Clin Invest 43:27, 1964.
9. Bengtsson B, Gennser G, Nilsson E. Sodium, potassium, and water content of human fetal, neonatal, and maternal plasma and red blood cells. Acta Paediatr Scand 59:192, 1970.
10. Dancis J, Springer D. Fetal homeostasis in maternal malnutrition: potassium and sodium deficiency in rats. Pediatr Res 4:345, 1970.
11. Stewart EL, Welt LG. Protection of the fetus in experimental potassium depletion. Am J Physiol 200:824, 1961.
12. Singh DS, Sadiq HF, Noguchi A, et al. Efficacy of albuterol inhalation in treatment of hyperkalemia in premature infants. J Pediatr 141:16, 2002.
13. Malone TA. Glucose and insulin versus cation-exchange resin for the treatment of hyperkalemia in very low birth weight infants. J Pediatr 118:121, 1991.
14. Hu PS, Su BH, Peng CT, et al. Glucose and insulin infusion versus kayexalate for early treatment of non-oliguric hyperkalemia in very-low-birth-weight infants. Acta Paediatr Taiwan 40:314, 1999.
15. Tudvad F, McNamara MA, Barnett HL. Renal response of premature infants to administration of bicarbonate and potassium. Pediatrics 13:4, 1964.
16. Lorenz JM, Kleinman LI, Disney TA. Renal response of the newborn dog to potassium loading. Am J Physiol 251:F513, 1986.
17. Nako Y, Ohki Y, Harigaya A, et al. Transtubular potassium concentration gradient in preterm neonates. Pediatr Nephrol 13:880, 1999.
18. Lorenz JM, Manuli MA, Browne LE. Chronic potassium supplementation of newborn dogs increases cortical Na, K-ATPase but not urinary potassium excretion. J Dev Physiol 13:181, 1990.
19. Lorenz JM, Manuli MA, Browne LE. The role of cortical Na,K-ATPase in distal nephron potassium secretion by the immature canine kidney. Pediatr Res 30:457, 1991.
20. Aperia A, Elinder G. Distal tubular sodium reabsorption in the developing rat kidney. Am J Physiol 240:F487, 1981.
21. Lelievre-Pegorier M, Merlet-Benichou C, Roinel N, et al. Developmental pattern of water and electrolyte transport in rat superficial nephrons. Am J Physiol 245:F15, 1983.
22. Sulyok E, Nemeth M, Tenyi I, et al. Relationship between maturity, electrolyte balance, and the function of the renin-angiotensin-aldosterone system in newborn infants. Bio Neonate 35:60, 1979.
23. Stephenson G, Hammet M, Hadaway G, et al. Ontogeny of renal mineralocorticoid receptors and urinary electrolyte responses in rats. Am J Physiol 247:F665, 1984.
24. Van Acker KJ, Sharpe SL, Deprettere AJ, et al. Renin-angiotensin-aldosterone system in the healthy infant and child. Kidney Int 16:196, 1979.

25. Benchimol C, Zavilowitz B and Satlin LM. Developmental expression of ROMK mRNA in rabbit cortical collecting duct. Pediatr Res 47:46, 2002.

26. Satlin LM. Developmental regulation of expression of renal potassium secretory channels. Curr Opin Nephrol Hyperten 13:445, 2004.

27. Lorenz JM, Kleinman LI, Markarian K. Potassium metabolism in extremely low birth weight infants in the first week of life. J Pediatr 131:81, 1997.

28. Delgado MM, Rohati R, Khan S, et al. Sodium and potassium clearances by the maturing kidney: clinical-metabolic correlates. Pediatr Nephrol 18:759, 2003.

29. Verma RP, John E, Fornell L, Vidyasasgar D. Fecal sodium and potassium losses in low birth weight infants. Indian J Pediatr 60:631, 1993.

30. Usher R. The respiratory distress syndrome of prematurity. I. Changes in potassium in the serum and the electrocardiogram and effects of therapy. Pediatrics 24:562, 1959.

31. Sato K, Kondo T, Iwao H, et al. Internal potassium shift in premature infants: cause of nonoliguric hyperkalemia. J Pediatr 126:109, 1995.

32. Gruskay J, Costarino AT, Polin RA, et al. Nonoliguric hyperkalemia in the premature infant weighing less than 1000 grams. J Pediatr 113:381, 1988.

33. Fukada Y, Kojima T, Ono A, et al. Factors causing hyperkalemia in premature infants. Am J Perinatology 6:76, 1989.

34. Sato K, Kondo T, Iwao H, et al. Sodium and potassium in red blood cells of premature infants during the first few days: risk of hyperkalemia. Acta Paediatr Scand 80:899, 1991.

35. Shaffer SG, Kilbride HW, Hayes LK, et al. Hyperkalemia in very low birth weight infants. J Pediatr 121:275–279, 1992.

36. Stefano JL, Norman ME, Morales MC et al. Decreased erythrocyte Na+-K+-ATPase activity associated with cellular potassium loss in extremely low birth weight infants with nonoliguric hyperkalemia. J Pediatr 122:276–284, 1993.

37. Stefano JL, Norman ME. Nitrogen balance in extremely low birth weight infants with nonoliguric hyperkalemia. J Pediatr 123:632, 1993.

38. Wilcox CS: Diuretics and potassium. In Seldin DW, Giebisch G (Eds.): The Regulation of Potassium Balance (pp. 325–345). New York, Raven Press, 1989.

Chapter 4

Acid-base Homeostasis in the Fetus and Newborn

Istvan Seri, MD, PhD

Regulation of Acid-base Homeostasis: Respiratory Acidosis
Regulation of Acid-base Homeostasis: Metabolic Acidosis
Regulation of Acid-base Homeostasis: Respiratory Alkalosis
Regulation of Acid-base Homeostasis: Metabolic Alkalosis
Normal Acid-base Balance and Growth
Summary

This chapter provides information on the regulation of fetal and neonatal acid base balance with a focus on the elimination of the acid load by the placenta, the lungs and the kidneys and briefly discusses the impact of acid-base disturbance on fetal and postnatal growth.

Hydrogen ion concentration is tightly regulated by the intra- and extracellular buffer systems and respiratory and renal compensatory mechanisms. The normal range of hydrogen ion concentration in the extracellular fluid is between 35 mEq/L and 45 mEq/L, which translates to a pH of 7.35 to 7.45. Under physiologic circumstances, volatile and fixed acids generated by normal metabolism are excreted and the pH remains stable (1). Carbonic acid is the most common volatile acid produced, and is readily excreted by the lungs in the form of carbon dioxide. Fixed acids, such as lactic acid, ketoacids, phosphoric acid and sulfuric acid, are buffered principally by bicarbonate in the extracellular compartment. The bicarbonate used in this process is then regenerated by the kidneys in a series of transmembrane transport processes linked to the excretion of hydrogen ions in the form of titratable acids (phosphate and sulfate salts) and ammonium. Several aspects of the regulation of acid-base homeostasis are developmentally regulated in the fetus and neonate and thus differ from those in children and adults. These developmentally regulated differences of acid-base homeostasis and their impact on fetal and postnatal growth are reviewed in this chapter.

REGULATION OF ACID-BASE HOMEOSTASIS: RESPIRATORY ACIDOSIS

In postnatal respiratory acidosis, unlike in fetal respiratory acidosis, immediate activation of the pulmonary compensatory mechanism leads to enhanced elimination of carbon dioxide and the resulting fall in carbon dioxide concentration increases the pH toward normal. The rapid activation of the respiratory compensatory mechanism is a result of the free movement of carbon dioxide across the blood–brain barrier (2) leading to instantaneous changes in cerebrospinal fluid (CSF) and cerebral interstitial fluid hydrogen ion concentrations.

Correction of Fetal Respiratory Acidosis

Fetal respiratory acidosis develops when prolonged maternal hypoventilation occurs with maternal asthma, airway obstruction, narcotic overdosing, maternal anesthesia, and magnesium sulfate toxicity. Fetal breathing movements increase, and the fetal kidneys exert a maturation-dependent limited response by reclaiming more bicarbonate in an attempt to restore the physiologic 20:1 ratio of bicarbonate-to-carbonic acid, resulting in a return of the pH toward normal (3). In the fetus, the renal compensation only has some limited physiologic significance when respiratory acidosis develops due to prolonged maternal hypoventilation.

Correction of Postnatal Respiratory Acidosis

In the clinical setting, acute neonatal respiratory acidosis develops most frequently in preterm infants with respiratory distress syndrome. Although stimulation of the respiratory center in the brain by elevated interstitial carbon dioxide concentration immediately increases respiratory rate and depth, carbon dioxide elimination by the lungs is usually limited because of immaturity and parenchymal disease. As in the fetus, the kidneys reclaim more bicarbonate in response to respiratory acidosis. Especially during the first few weeks of postnatal life, however, renal compensation is limited by the developmentally regulated immaturity of renal tubular functions.

REGULATION OF ACID-BASE HOMEOSTASIS: METABOLIC ACIDOSIS

As in respiratory acidosis, the pulmonary gas exchange serves as the *immediate* regulator of acid-base homeostasis when metabolic acidosis develops. However, since bicarbonate crosses the blood–brain barrier by active transport mechanisms (4) and since the central respiratory drive is triggered by the low steady-state values of CSF and not plasma bicarbonate (2), a full activation of the respiratory acid-base regulatory system only occurs a few hours after the development of metabolic acidosis. This is different from the above-described truly immediate activation of the respiratory acid-base regulatory system by respiratory acidosis.

Fetoplacental Elimination of Metabolic Acid Load

Fetal respiratory and renal compensation in response to changes in fetal pH is limited by the level of maturity and the surrounding maternal environment. However, although the placentomaternal unit performs most compensatory functions (3), the fetal kidneys have some, though limited, ability to contribute to the maintenance of fetal acid-base balance.

The most frequent cause of fetal metabolic acidosis is fetal hypoxemia owing to abnormalities of uteroplacental function or blood flow, or both. Primary maternal hypoxemia or maternal metabolic acidosis secondary to maternal diabetes mellitus, sepsis, or renal tubular abnormalities is an unusual cause of fetal metabolic acidosis.

The pregnant woman, at least in late gestation, maintains a somewhat more alkaline plasma environment compared to that of non-pregnant controls. This pattern of acid-base regulation in pregnant women is present during both resting and after maximal exertion and may serve as a protective mechanism from sudden decreases in fetal pH. Maintenance of the less acidic environment during pregnancy appears to be achieved through reduced plasma carbon dioxide and weak acid concentrations (3,5).

The placenta plays an essential role in the maintenance of fetal acid-base balance when metabolic acidosis develops. As mentioned earlier, fetal metabolic acidosis most frequently occurs when abnormal uteroplacental function or blood flow results in fetal hypoxemia. Fetal hypoxemia then causes a shift to anaerobic metabolism and large quantities of lactic acid accumulate. As hydrogen ions are buffered by the extracellular and intracellular buffering systems of the fetus, pH drops as plasma bicarbonate decreases. Because of the unhindered diffusion of carbon dioxide through the placenta (3), restoration of normal fetal pH initially occurs through elimination of the volatile element of the carbonic acid-bicarbonate system via the maternal lungs. However, as lactate and other fixed acids cross the placenta more slowly (3), the onset of maternal renal compensation of fetal metabolic acidosis is delayed. In addition, if fetal oxygenation improves, the products of anaerobic metabolism are also metabolized by the fetus.

As there is no physiologic significance to respiratory compensation of metabolic acidosis in utero, the finding that the respiratory control system in the fetus is much less sensitive to changes in pH than in the neonate (6) has little practical importance. Yet, a decrease in the fetal pH stimulates breathing movements in the fetus (7,8).

Finally, as for the role of the fetal kidneys in the maintenance of acid-base balance, available evidence indicates that the fetal kidneys excrete both inorganic (9–11) and organic acids (12) and are also able to generate bicarbonate (13,14). Studies in fetal sheep have found age-dependent increases in glomerular filtration rate (GFR), and urinary titratable acid, ammonium and net acid excretion (9). A positive relationship also exists between changes in GFR and bicarbonate, sodium and chloride excretions (9,11). Yet, the adaptive capacity of the fetal kidney to changes in fetal acid-base balance is limited. In fetal sheep, the hydrochloric acid infusion-induced metabolic acidosis results in increases in titratable acid, ammonium and net acid excretion without significant changes in GFR or renal tubular bicarbonate absorption (11). However, as mentioned earlier, under certain conditions such as volume depletion (13) or recovery from mild hypocapnic hypoxia (14), the fetal kidney has the ability to increase bicarbonate reabsorption. It is also important to note that the vast majority of these data have been obtained in animal models and that there is only very limited information available concerning renal acidification by the human fetus (15). In addition, the physiologic importance of the adaptive fetal renal responses is limited compared to that in the postnatal period because the acid load excreted in the fetal urine remains within the immediate fetal environment and needs to be eliminated by the placenta or metabolized by the fetus.

Indeed, amniotic fluid acid base status and electrolyte composition have been shown to affect the fetus. When the effects of amnion infusion of physiologic saline to those of lactated Ringer were compared in the fetal sheep, significant increases in fetal plasma sodium and chloride concentrations were noted only in the physiologic-saline infusion group (16). In addition, fetal arterial pH decreased in the physiologic-saline group and the change in the fetal pH was directly related to the changes in plasma chloride concentrations. However, despite the significant changes in plasma sodium and chloride concentrations and pH, fetal plasma electrolyte composition and acid-base balance remained in the physiologic range, leaving these findings with little clinical significance (16).

Postnatal Elimination of Metabolic Acid Load

The most frequent causes of increased anion-gap (lactic acid) metabolic acidosis in the neonate are hypoxemia or ischemia secondary to perinatal asphyxia;

vasoregulatory disturbances and/or myocardial dysfunction caused by immaturity, sepsis, or asphyxia; severe lung disease with or without pulmonary hypertension; certain types of structural heart disease and volume depletion. Severe metabolic acidosis caused by a neonatal metabolic disorder is rare but should always be considered. Preterm neonates frequently present with a mild to moderate normal anion-gap acidosis, which almost always is the consequence of the low renal bicarbonate threshold of the premature kidney (17–19). However, the use of carbonic anhydrase inhibitors and parenteral alimentation, as well as the maturation related decreased sensitivity to aldosterone have also been suggested to contribute to the development of normal anion-gap acidosis in the neonate (17,20,21).

As mentioned earlier, in metabolic acidosis caused by the accumulation of lactic acid, hydrogen ions are buffered by the intra- and extracellular buffering systems and plasma bicarbonate concentration decreases and pH drops. Restoration of pH toward normal initially occurs through elimination of the volatile element of the carbonic acid-bicarbonate system via the lungs. This process may be severely compromised in the sick preterm and term neonate with parenchymal lung disease.

The principal mechanism of renal compensation is the regulation of renal tubular bicarbonate and acid secretion in response to changes in extracellular pH. Although full activation of this system requires at least 2–3 days, changes in renal acidification may be seen as early as a few hours following the development of the acid-base disturbance. Although renal compensation is the ultimate mechanism that adjusts the hydrogen ion content of the body, this compensatory function is also affected by the immaturity of the neonatal kidneys (19,22). Both renal hemodynamic and tubular epithelial factors play a role in the limited renal compensatory capacity of the newborn.

Renal blood flow (RBF) significantly increases after the immediate postnatal period and some of the renal vasodilatory mechanisms are functionally mature as early as the 24th week of gestation (23). Similar to RBF, GFR is also low in the immediate postnatal period and increases as a function of both gestational and postnatal age (24,25). Indeed, the low GFR is considered as the primary hemodynamic factor limiting the ability of the neonate to adequately handle an acid load (19,22).

In addition, net renal acid excretion is regulated by several tubular epithelial functions (19,26). In the proximal tubule, the following four transport mechanisms regulate active acid extrusion and transepithelial bicarbonate reabsorption: the H^+-ATPase, the electrogenic $Na^+/3HCO_3^-$ cotransporter, the Na^+,K^+-ATPase-driven secondary active Na^+/H^+ antiporter, and the Na^+,K^+-ATPase-driven tertiary active Na^+-coupled organic ion transporter (26). Because approximately 85–90% of the filtered bicarbonate is reabsorbed in the proximal tubule (19,26), the function of these proximal tubular transporters determines the renal threshold for bicarbonate reabsorption. The bicarbonate threshold is 18 mEq/L in the premature infant and 21 mEq/L in the term infant, and it reaches adult levels (24–26 mEq/L) only after the first postnatal year (17,18). In the extremely low gestational age neonate, however, the renal bicarbonate threshold may be as low as 14 mEq/L. Because renal carbonic anhydrase is present and active during fetal life (27), and because its activity is similar in the 26-week-old extremely immature neonate to that of the adult (28), a developmentally regulated immaturity in the function of the above described proximal tubular transporters is most likely responsible for the low bicarbonate threshold during early development. Indeed, both the activity and the hormonal responsiveness of the proximal tubular Na^+,K^+-ATPase is decreased in younger compared to older animals (29).

In addition to immaturity, medications used in critically ill neonates may also affect proximal tubular bicarbonate reabsorption. For example, via inhibition of the proximal tubular Na^+/H^+ antiporter (30), dopamine may potentially decrease the low bicarbonate threshold of the neonate (31). Carbonic anhydrase inhibitors also decrease proximal tubular bicarbonate reabsorption by limiting bicarbonate formation and hydrogen ion availability for the Na^+/H^+ antiporter. By acting on several transport proteins along the nephron, furosemide directly increases urinary excretion of titratable acids (phosphate and sulfate salts) and ammonium (32). On the other hand, by inhibition of the activation of aldosterone receptors, spironolactone indirectly decreases hydrogen ion excretion in the distal tubule.

Under physiologic circumstances, the distal nephron reabsorbs the remaining 10–15% of the filtered bicarbonate via transport mechanisms similar to those of the proximal tubule (26). However, the distal tubule lacks the carbonic anhydrase enzyme (26). Net hydrogen ion secretion in the distal nephron continues after the reabsorption of virtually all bicarbonate via active extrusion of hydrogen and the ability of the distal tubular epithelium to maintain large transepithelial concentration gradients for hydrogen and bicarbonate (26). Aldosterone is one of the most important hormones influencing distal tubular acidification. By affecting the function of several different transport mechanisms aldosterone stimulates net hydrogen ion excretion in the distal nephron. However, the premature neonate has a developmentally regulated relative insensitivity to aldosterone (17,21).

Hydrogen ions are excreted in the urine in the form of titratable acids (phosphate and sulfate salts) and as ammonium salts, which are formed by the combination of hydrogen with ammonia (26). Because the major constituent of titratable acid in urine is $H_2PO_4^-$, drugs that decrease proximal tubular phosphate reabsorption, and thus increase the delivery of phosphate to the distal nephron, may increase the renal acidification capacity of the neonate. Indeed, by inhibiting proximal tubular phosphate reabsorption, dopamine has been shown to increase the excretion of titratable acids in preterm infants (33). In addition, urinary excretion of titratable acid and ammonium increases as a function of gestational and postnatal age (19). However, because effective urinary acidification is usually acquired by the age of one month even in premature infants, postnatal distal tubular hydrogen ion secretion is inducible independent of the gestational age at birth (34).

In summary, the renal response to metabolic acidosis in the immediate postnatal period consists of attenuated increases in GFR, proximal tubular bicarbonate reabsorption, and distal tubular net acid secretion. However, a significant improvement in the overall renal response occurs after the first postnatal month, even in the premature infant (22).

REGULATION OF ACID-BASE HOMEOSTASIS: RESPIRATORY ALKALOSIS

Correction of Fetal Respiratory Alkalosis

Rather than causing fetal respiratory alkalosis, acute maternal hyperventilation may lead to the development of fetal metabolic acidosis. The fetal acidosis under these circumstances is the consequence of the acute decrease in placental blood flow caused by the maternal hypocapnia-induced significant uterine vasoconstriction (35). In these cases, restoration of maternal carbon dioxide levels rapidly corrects both the abnormal uterine blood flow and the acid-base abnormality in the fetus.

The physiologic hyperventilation of the pregnant woman causes a compensatory decrease in maternal serum bicarbonate concentration to approximately 22 mM (3) without any apparent effect on the fetus (see above).

Correction of Postnatal Respiratory Alkalosis

Neonatal respiratory alkalosis occurs most often in the febrile non-ventilated neonate or in cases with iatrogenic hyperventilation of the intubated preterm or term infant. Rarely, respiratory alkalosis may be the presenting sign of a urea cycle disorder during the first days of postnatal life because the rising ammonia level may initially stimulate the respiratory center in the brain. As for the renal compensation of respiratory alkalosis, both urinary bicarbonate reabsorption and distal tubular net acid excretion decrease and thus extracellular pH tends to return toward normal. This renal compensation plays an important although somewhat limited role in neonatal respiratory alkalosis.

REGULATION OF ACID-BASE HOMEOSTASIS: METABOLIC ALKALOSIS

Correction of Fetal Metabolic Alkalosis

Although metabolic alkalosis is a very rare fetal condition, it may occur in hyperemesis gravidarum. As a result of the significant and lasting hydrogen chloride losses, maternal renal compensation results in retention of bicarbonate to maintain maternal anionic balance. Because bicarbonate is transported slowly across the placenta, the development of fetal metabolic alkalosis lags behind that of the mother. On the other hand, the maternal respiratory compensation (hypoventilation with the ensuing hypercapnia) tends to restore normal pH in the fetus as carbon dioxide is rapidly transported across the placenta.

Correction of Postnatal Metabolic Alkalosis

Metabolic alkalosis most frequently develops in the preterm neonate receiving prolonged diuretic treatment for bronchopulmonary dysplasia. Although there is little evidence that chronic diuretic management results in improved medium- or long-term pulmonary outcome, the majority of neonatologists use this treatment modality. If total body chloride and potassium content is not appropriately maintained during chronic diuretic administration, severe metabolic 'contraction' alkalosis may develop, which also results in poor growth. The respiratory response is a decrease in the rate and depth of breathing to increase carbon dioxide retention. This response may be interpreted as a sign of worsening pulmonary condition in the ventilated preterm neonate and may inappropriately trigger an increase in ventilatory support. Thus, respiratory compensation of metabolic alkalosis may be ineffective if the intubated neonate is subjected to iatrogenic over-ventilation on the mechanical ventilator. As for the neonatal renal compensation for metabolic alkalosis, urinary bicarbonate reabsorption and distal tubular net acid excretion fall, resulting in a return of the extracellular pH toward normal.

Finally, metabolic alkalosis can also result from a non-diuretic administration-related loss of extracellular fluid containing disproportionally more chloride than bicarbonate. During the diuretic phase of normal postnatal adaptation, preterm and term newborns tend to retain relatively more bicarbonate than chloride (36). The obvious benefits of allowing this physiologic extracellular volume contraction to occur clearly outweigh the clinical importance of a mild contraction alkalosis developing during postnatal adaptation. Thus, no specific treatment is needed in these cases, especially since, with the stabilization of the extracellular volume status and the renal function with time, acid-base balance rapidly returns to normal.

NORMAL ACID-BASE BALANCE AND GROWTH

Growth is most accelerated during fetal life. The normal fetus grows from a weight of 0.22 g at the 8th week of gestation to 3400 g at 40 weeks' completed gestation (37). The estimated energy density of each gram of body weight gained (or lost) is 23 kJ (5.6 kcal). However, in premature infants, especially if they are critically ill and/or growth restricted, the energy density of the new tissue is estimated to be higher than 5.6 kcal/g (38). For instance, in small-for-gestational-age infants at approximately 5 weeks after birth, the total energy expenditure is estimated to be 20% greater than in appropriate-for-gestational-age controls (39).

Fetal growth can be negatively affected by several fetal and placento-maternal conditions. Proven fetal conditions affecting fetal growth include certain genetic conditions and infection of the fetus (40). Placento-maternal conditions with demonstrated influence on fetal growth are primary placental insufficiency and maternal diseases, nutritional status or substance abuse leading to secondary placental insufficiency, decreased fetal nutrient availability or direct fetal toxicity or a combination of these harmful effects on fetal well-being (40).

Although, there is little direct evidence available to demonstrate an impact of chronic fetal acid-base abnormality on fetal growth, a recent hypothesis implicates a mild shift in the fetal acid-base status as the primary pathological factor for intrauterine growth restriction caused by placental insufficiency of any etiology (41). From 18 weeks' post-conception, growth restricted fetuses exhibit a greater degree of mild acidemia than their appropriately growing counterparts (42). This acidemia is attributed to the reduced perfusion and mild hypoxemia facing the growth-restricted fetus as a result of the placental insufficiency. According to this hypothesis, the small initial reduction in the pH negatively affects nitric oxide production in the fetus and it is the decreased availability of nitric oxide that then plays a major role in the ensuing growth restriction (41).

The following findings are in support of this hypothesis. As locally formed nitric oxide regulates tissue perfusion and thus oxygen delivery and tissue growth itself, it has been suggested to play a pivotal role in regulation of growth in the fetus (40,41). In addition to its effect on oxygen delivery to the tissues, nitric oxide is an anabolic factor. Indeed, it is necessary for normal growth of several tissues including the bone and muscle and for the action of different hormones such as the parathyroid hormone, vitamin D and estrogen known to be of importance in fetal growth and development (43,44).

Interestingly, the enzyme responsible for generating nitric oxide from L-arginine, the constitutive nitric oxide synthase (cNOS) is sensitive to changes in pH and its activity decreases even with a mild shift in the pH toward acidosis (45). Thus, a vicious cycle may develop in growth restricted fetuses, as the initial decrease in blood flow and pH caused by placental insufficiency may lead to decreased cNOS activity and thus nitric oxide production. Decreased nitric oxide production, in turn, leads to further decreases in tissue perfusion and thus in pH, exacerbating the decrease in local nitric oxide production (41).

In addition to being the source of locally generated nitric oxide, L-arginine also serves as the source polyamines and L-proline. These compounds are generated by the arginase enzyme and are important when growth and tissue repair processes predominate. The function of this enzyme is also pH dependent (46) and the proposed decrease in its activity in the growth retarded fetus may contribute to further impairment of fetal growth.

Based on this information, it seems that elevating the pH in the fetus toward normal and supplementing L-arginine to the mother may be a plausible approach to attenuate the impact on fetal growth of the placental insufficiency-induced decreased fetal oxygen delivery. However, due to the inherent difficulties associated with attempts to effectively control fetal pH, no clinical trial has as yet attempted this combined approach.

As for the neonate, the syndrome of late metabolic acidosis of prematurity is an example of how postnatal growth can be affected by alterations in the acid-base balance. This entity was first described in the 1960s, in which otherwise healthy premature infants after a few weeks developed mild-to-moderate anion-gap acidosis and decreased growth rate. All of these infants were receiving high-protein cow's milk formulas, and demonstrated increased net acid excretion compared to controls. This type of late metabolic acidosis is now rarely seen, probably because of the use of special premature formulas and the changes made to regular formulas now containing a decreased casein-to-whey ratio and lower fixed acid loads.

The diuretic administration-induced hypochloremic metabolic alkalosis is another example of the impact of acid-base balance on postnatal growth. This phenomenon is also associated with growth failure and may be a contributing factor of poor outcome in infants with bronchopulmonary dysplasia (47). The growth failure is most likely caused by the decrease in cell proliferation and diminished DNA and protein synthesis in response to intracellular alkalosis (48). Chronic decrease in total body sodium resulting in a negative sodium balance may further hinder the growth of these infants (49). Aggressive chloride and potassium supplementation with relatively limited sodium supplementation decreases the risk for the development of clinically significant severe contraction alkalosis associated with chronic diuretic use in these patients.

SUMMARY

This chapter has reviewed the available information and the gaps in our knowledge on how fetal and neonatal acid base balance is regulated and the impact of alterations in acid-base balance on some aspects of fetal and postnatal growth. In the future, a better understanding of the role of growth factors and their interaction with the fetal acid-base status may result in improved early management of the growth restricted fetus. This, in turn, may decrease the negative impact of growth restriction on brain- and other organ-development.

REFERENCES

1. Masoro EJ. An overview of hydrogen ion regulation. Arch Intern Med 142:1019, 1982.
2. Sorensen SC. The chemical control of ventilation. Acta Physiol Scand 361:1, 1971.
3. Blechner JN. Maternal-fetal acid-base, physiology. Clin Obstet Gynecol 36:3, 1993.
4. Vogh BP, Maren TH. Sodium, chloride, and bicarbonate movement from plasma to cerebrospinal fluid in cats. Am J Physiol 228:673, 1975.
5. Kemp JG, Greer FA, Wolfe LA. Acid-base regulation after maximal exercise testing in late gestation. J Appl Physiol 83:644, 1997.
6. Blechner JN, Meshia G, Barron DH. A study of the acid-base balance of fetal sheep and goats. Q J Exp Physiol 45:60, 1960.
7. Jansen A, Shernick V. Fetal breathing and development of control of breathing. J Appl Physiol 70:143L, 1991.
8. Molteni RA, Melmed MH, Sheldon RE, Jones MD, Meschia G. Induction of fetal breathing by metabolic acidemia and its effect on blood flow to the respiratory muscles. Am J Obstet Gynecol 136:609, 1980.
9. Kesby GJ, Lumbers ER. Factors affecting renal handling of sodium, hydrogen ions, and bicarbonate in the fetus. Am J Physiol 251:F226, 1986.
10. Hill KJ, Lumbers ER. Renal function in adult and fetal sheep. Dev Physiol 10:149, 1988.
11. Kesby GJ, Lumbers ER. The effects of metabolic acidosis on renal function of fetal sheep. J Physiol 396:65, 1988.
12. Elbourne I, Lumbers ER, Hill KJ. The secretion of organic acids and bases by the ovine fetal kidney. Exp Physiol 75:211, 1990.

13. Robillard JE, Sessions C, Burmeister L, Smith FG. Influence of fetal extracellular volume contraction on renal reabsorption of bicarbonate in fetal lambs. Pediatr Res 11:649, 1977.

14. Gibson KJ, McMullen JR, Lumbers ER. Renal acid-base and sodium handling in hypoxia and subsequent mild metabolic acidosis in fetal sheep. Clin Exper Pharmacol Physiol 27:67, 2000.

15. Blechner JN, Stenger VG, Eitzman DV, Prystowsky H. Effects of maternal metabolic acidosis on the human fetus and newborn infant. Am J Obstet Gynecol 9:46, 1967.

16. Shields LE, Moore TR, Brace RA. Fetal electrolyte and acid-base responses to amnioinfusion: lactated Ringer's versus normal saline in the ovine fetus. J Soci Gynecol Invest 2:602, 1995.

17. Sulyok E, Nemeth M, Tenyi I, Csaba IF, Varga F, Gyory E, Thurzo V. Relationship between maturity, electrolyte balance and the function of the renin-angiotensin-aldosterone system in newborn infants. Biol Neonate 35:60, 1979.

18. Avner ED. Normal neonates and the maturational development of homeostatic mechanisms. In Ichikawa I (Ed.): Pediatric Textbook of Fluids and Electrolytes (pp. 107–118). Baltimore, MD: Williams & Wilkins, 1990.

19. Jones DP, Chesney RW. Development of tubular function. Clin Perinatol 19:33, 1992.

20. Brewer ED. Disorders of acid-base balance. Pediatr Clin North Am 37:429, 1990.

21. Stephenson G, Hammet M, Hadaway G, Funder JW. Ontogeny of renal mineralocorticoid receptors and urinary electrolyte responses in the rat. Am J Physiol 247:F665, 1984.

22. Guignard JP, John EG. Renal function in the tiny premature infant. Clin Permatol 13:377, 1986.

23. Seri I, Abbasi S, Wood DC, Gerdes JS. Regional hemodynamic effects of dopamine in the sick preterm infant. J Pediatr 133:728, 1998.

24. Fawer CL, Torrado A, Guignard J. Maturation of renal function in full-term and premature neonates. Helv Paediatr Acta 34:11, 1979.

25. Guignard JP, Torrado A, Da Cunha O, Gautier E. Glomerular filtration rate in the first three weeks of life. J Pediatr 87:268, 1975.

26. Hamm LL, Alpern RJ. Cellular mechanisms of renal tubular acidification. In Sedin DW, Giebisch G (Eds.): The Kidney: Physiology and Pathophysiology, 2nd ed (pp 2581–2626). New York: Raven Press, 1992.

27. Robillard JP, Sessions C, Smith FG. In vivo demonstration of renal carbonic anhydrase activity in the fetal lamb. Biol Neonate 34:253, 1978.

28. Lonnerholm C, Wistrand PJ. Carbonic anhydrase in the human fetal kidney. Pediatr Res 17:390, 1983.

29. Fryckstedt J, Svensson LB, Linden M, Aperia A. The effect of dopamine on adenylate cyclase and Na+,K+ -ATPase activity in the developing rat renal cortical and medullary tubule cells. Pediatr Res 34:308, 1993.

30. Felder CC, Campbell T, Albrecht F, Jose PA. Dopamine inhibits Na+/H+ exchanger activity in renal BBMV by stimulation of adenylate cyclase. Am J Physiol 259:F297, 1990.

31. Seri I. Cardiovascular, renal, and endocrine actions of dopamine in neonates and children. J Pediatr 126:333, 1995.

32. Hropot M, Fowler N, Karlmark B, Giebisch G. Tubular action of diuretics: distal effects on electrolyte transport and acidification. Kidney Int 28:477, 1985.

33. Seri I, Rudas G, Bors Zs, Kanyicska B, Tulassay T. Effects of low-dose dopamine on cardiovascular and renal functions, cerebral blood flow, and plasma catecholamine levels in sick preterm neonates. Pediatr Res 34:742, 1993.

34. Stonestreet BS, Rubin L, Pollak A, Cowett RM, Oh W. Renal functions of low birth weight infants with hyperglycemia and glucosuria produced by glucose infusions. Pediatrics 66:561, 1980.

35. Moya F, Morishima HO, Shnider SM, James L. Influence of maternal hypoventilation on the newborn infant. Am J Obstet Gynecol 91:76, 1965.

36. Ramiro-Tolentino SB, Markarian K, Kleinman LI. Renal bicarbonate excretion in extremely low birth weight infants. Pediatrics 98:256-261, 1996.

37. Appendix 2. Avery's Diseases of the Newborn. Taeusch HW, Ballard RA, Gleason CA (Eds): 8th edn (p.1574) Philadelphia, PA: Elsevier/Saunders, 2005.

38. Davies PSW. Energy requirements for growth and development in infancy. Am J Clin Nutr 68:939S, 1998.

39. Davies PSW, Clough H, Bishop N, Lucas A, Cole TJ, Cole J. Total energy expenditure in small-for-gestational-age infants. Arch Dis Child 74:F208, 1996.

40. Hay WW, Catz CS, Grave GD, Yaffe SJ. Workshop summary: Fetal growth: its regulation and disorders. Pediatrics 99:585, 1997.

41. Stearns MR, Jackson CGR, Landauer JA, Frye SD, Hay WW, Burke TJ. Small for gestational age: A new insight? Medical Hypotheses 53:186, 1999.

42. Nicolaides KH, Economides DL, Soothill PW. Blood gasses, pH and lactate in appropriate- and small-for-gestational-age fetuses. Am J Obstet Gynecol 161:996, 1989.

43. Kaiser FE, Dirighi M, Muchnick J, Morley JE, Patrick P. Regulation of gonadotropins and parathyroid hormone by nitric oxide. Life Sci 59:987, 1996.

44. Evans CH, Stefanovic-Racic M, Lancaster J. Nitric oxide and it role in orthopedic disease. Clin Orthoped Rel Res 312:275, 1995.

45. Fleming I, Hecker M, Busse R. Intracellular alkalinization induced by bradykinin sustains activation of the constitutive nitric oxide synthase in endothelial cells. Circ Res 74:1220, 1994.

46. Kuhn NJ, Ward S, Piponski M, Young TW. Purification of human hepatic arginase and its manganese (II)-dependent and pH-dependent interconversion between active and inactive forms: A possible pH-sensing function of the enzyme on the ornithine cycle. Arch Biochem Biophys 320:24, 1995.

47. Perlman JF, Moore V, Siegel MJ, Dawson J. Is chloride depletion an important contributing cause of death in infants with bronchopulmonary dysplasia? Pediatrics 77:212–216, 1986.

48. Heinly MM, Wassner SJ. The effect of isolated chloride depletion on growth and protein turnover in young rats. Pediatr Nephrol 8:555–560, 1994.

49. Sulyok E, Kovacs L, Lichardus B, Michajlovskij N, Lehotska V, Nemethova V, Varga L, Ertl T. Late hyponatremia in premature infants: role of aldosterone and arginine vasopressin. J Pediatr 106:990–994, 1985.

Section III

The Kidney: Normal Development and Hormone Modulators

Chapter 5

Glomerular Filtration Rate in Neonates

Jean-Pierre Guignard, MD • Jean-Bernard Gouyon, MD

Development of Glomerular Filtration
Assessment of GFR
Conditions and Factors that Impair GFR
Prevention of Oliguric States due to Low GFR

Ultrafiltration of plasma across permselective capillaries is the first step in urine formation. This process starts with the development of the metanephros, around the 10th week of gestation. The rate of glomerular filtration (GFR) increases progressively throughout fetal and postnatal life, to reach 'adult' mature levels by 1 year of life. During the period of maturation, the function of the kidney is characterized by elevated renal vascular resistance (RVR), low arterial renal perfusion pressure, and low renal blood flow (RBF). The ultrafiltration process is maintained by a delicate balance between vasoconstrictor and counteracting vasodilator forces. This balance can be easily disturbed by various factors, resulting in transient or permanent impairment in GFR. This chapter briefly reviews the maturation of glomerular filtration, discusses the techniques available to assess GFR in the neonate, and describes factors and agents that can impair, or protect, the maturing glomerular filtration.

DEVELOPMENT OF GLOMERULAR FILTRATION

Glomerular ultrafiltration depends upon the net ultrafiltration pressure, which is the difference between the hydrostatic and oncotic pressures across glomerular capillaries. The low perfusion pressure and low glomerular plasma flow account, at least in part, for the low levels of GFR present during gestation. For any given ultrafiltration pressure, GFR will depend on the rate at which plasma flows through the glomerular capillaries, as well as on the ultrafiltration coefficient (K_f). K_f is a function of the total capillary surface area and of the permeability per unit of surface area.

During the last months of gestation, GFR increases in parallel with gestational age, up to the end of nephrogenesis around the 35th week of gestation (1). This pattern of development reflects both an increase in the number of nephrons, and the growth of existing nephrons. From the 35th week of gestation, the development of GFR slows down up to the time of birth (Fig. 5-1). Postnatal maturation of renal function is characterized by a striking increase in GFR, the value of which doubles within the first two weeks of life (Fig. 5-2)(1). The velocity of this increase is somewhat slower in the most premature infants. An increase in the glomerular

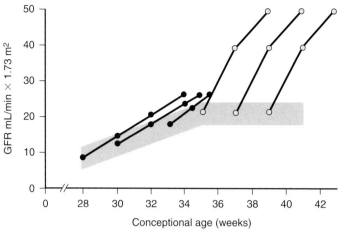

Figure 5-1 Development of GFR as a function of conceptional age during the last 3 months of gestation and the first month of postnatal life. The shaded area represents the range of normal values. The postnatal increase in GFR observed in preterm (●-●) and term neonates (○-○) is schematically represented. (After Guignard JP, John EG: Renal function in the tiny, premature infant. Clin Perinatol 13:377, 1986.)

capillary surface area represents the main factor responsible for the postnatal increase in GFR. Additional maturational changes that may contribute to the post-natal maturation of GFR include: (a) an increase in pore size and glomerular hydraulic permeability; (b) an increase in the effective ultrafiltration pressure; and (c) a decrease in both afferent and efferent arteriolar resistance (2).

Vasoactive Factors

Several vasoactive agents and hormones modulate GFR and RBF (2). By acting on the arcuate arteries, the interlobular arteries, the afferent and the efferent arterioles, they regulate the glomerular hydrostatic pressure and the glomerular transcapillary

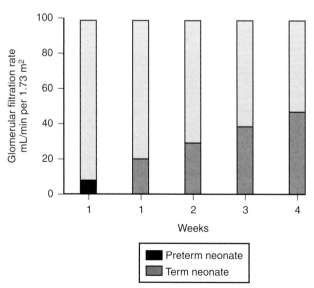

Figure 5-2 Postnatal increase in glomerular filtration rate (GFR) in term and preterm infants. The upper part of each column represents the deficit between the neonate's glomerular filtration rate and mature levels (100 mL/min per 1.73 m²). Note that at the end of the first month of life, the human neonate is in a state of relative renal insufficiency, as compared to adults. (After Guignard JP, John EG: Renal function in the tiny, premature infant. Clin Perinatol 13:377, 1986.)

Table 5-1 Vasoactive Factors Regulating the Glomerular Microcirculation

Vasoconstrictors	Vasodilators
Circulating hormones • Catecholamines • Angiotensin II • Vasopressin • Glucocorticoids Paracrine + autocoïds • Endothelin • Thromboxan A_2 • Leukotrienes • Adenosine	Circulating hormones • Dopamine Paracrine + autocoïds • Nitric oxide • Acetylcholine • $PGI_2 + PGE_2$ • Bradykinin • Adenosine

hydraulic pressure gradient. These agents can also modify the ultrafiltration coefficient by two mechanisms: (a) a change in the capillary filtration area by contracting the mesangial cells; (b) a change in hydraulic conductivity by decreasing the number and/or size of the filtration slit pores. The main vasoactive forces modulating single nephron GFR (SNGFR) are listed in Table 5-1. Two vasoactive systems, the renin-angiotensin system and the prostaglandins (Fig. 5-3) play key roles in the protection of the stressed kidney.

Angiotensin II (Angio II)

This octapeptide is a very potent vasoconstrictor of the afferent and efferent arterioles, acting on two types of receptors, the AT_1 and the AT_2 receptor subtypes. The AT_1 receptors are widely distributed and appear to mediate most of the biologic effects of Angio II. The exact role of the AT_2 receptors remains uncertain. Angio II acts on both pre- and post-glomerular resistance, but appears to predominantly vasoconstrict the efferent arteriole, thereby increasing the glomerular capillary hydrostatic pressure while decreasing glomerular plasma flow rate (3). This mechanism serves to maintain GFR when the renal perfusion pressure decreases to low levels. The action of Angio II on the efferent arteriole is counterbalanced by intrarenal adenosine, an agent modulating the tubuloglomerular feedback mechanism. When both Angio II and adenosine are overstimulated, their combined action results in afferent vasoconstriction (4).

Prostaglandins (PGs)

The renal prostaglandins are potent vasoactive metabolites of arachidonic acid (5). Under normal conditions, the renal prostaglandins are present in low concentrations and exert only minor effects on the renal circulation and GFR. The vasodilator

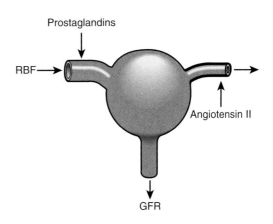

Figure 5-3 The physiological regulation of GFR depends on two main factors: the afferent vasodilator prostaglandins and the efferent vasoconstrictor angiotensin II. RBF, renal blood flow; GFR, glomerular filtration rate.

prostaglandins are however of major importance in protecting renal perfusion and GFR when vasoconstrictor forces are activated, as for instance during hypotensive, hypovolemic and sodium depletion states or during congestive heart failure. The prostaglandins protect GFR by vasodilating the afferent arterioles, and by dampening the renal vasoconstrictor effects of Angio II, endothelin, and sympathetic nerve stimulation on the afferent arteriole (5).

Maturational Aspects of the Renin-angiotensin and Prostaglandins Systems

THE RENIN-ANGIOTENSIN SYSTEM

Renin is found as early as the 5th week in the mesonephros and by the 8th week in the metanephros. The plasma renin concentration and activity generated by the fetal kidney are elevated (6). The plasma renin activity further increases after birth before slowly decreasing through infancy. The factors controlling renin release (macula densa, baroreceptor, sympathetic nervous system and hormonal mechanisms) are active in the fetus (6).

Elevated levels of Angio II are present in the fetus and remain high in the neonatal period. While AT_2 receptors predominate during embryonic and fetal life, they rapidly decline after birth (7). AT_1 receptors predominate after birth and are found in glomeruli, macula densa and mesangial cells, resistance arteries and vasa recta (8). In addition to its AT_1-mediated vasoconstrictor effects, Angio II promotes growth of the renal vasculature (7). Blockade of the AT_1 receptors with losartan during fetal life interferes with normal renal development and results in vascular malformations, cystic dilatation of the tubules and a decrease in the number of glomeruli (9). Blockade of AT_1 receptor by losartan in newborn rabbits induces a drop in GFR, without affecting RBF (10), thus illustrating the major role of Angio II in regulating and protecting GFR in kidneys perfused at low systemic arterial pressures.

THE PROSTAGLANDINS

Cyclooxygenases 1 and 2 (COX-1 and COX-2) are expressed in the fetal renal vasculature, glomeruli and collecting ducts. COX-2 activity is highest after birth (11). Interference with prostaglandins synthesis during fetal life leads to renal dysgenesis with cortical dysplasia, cystic tubular dilatation and impaired nephrogenesis (12). COX-2 is probably involved in this pathogenesis (13). While the PGs do probably not regulate GFR in normal conditions, interference with PGs synthesis may have deleterious effects in conditions associated with renal hypoperfusion.

ASSESSMENT OF GFR

Different methods, using various markers, have been used to assess GFR in neonates. The most common measurement of GFR is based on the concept of 'clearance,' which relates the quantitative urinary excretion of a substance per unit time to the volume of plasma that, if 'cleared' completely of the same contained substance, would yield a quantity equivalent to that excreted in the urine. The clearance C of a substance x is expressed by the formula:

$$C = U_X \bullet V/P_X,$$

where U_X represents the urinary concentration of the substance, V the urine flow rate, and P_X the plasma concentration. For its clearance to be equal to the rate of glomerular filtration, a substance must have the following properties: (a) it must be freely filterable through the glomerular capillary membranes, that is, not be bound to plasma proteins or sieved in the process of ultrafiltration; (b) it must not be excreted by an extrarenal route; and (c) it must be biologically inert and neither reabsorbed nor secreted by the renal tubules. Several substances, endogenous or exogenous, have been claimed to have the above properties: inulin, creatinine, iohexol, ethylenediaminetetra-acetic acid (EDTA), diethylenetriaminepenta-acetic acid (DTPA) and sodium iothalamate. The experimental evidence that this is true has been produced only for inulin.

Glomerular Markers

Several endogenous or exogenous markers have been used to assess GFR (Table 5-2). The markers used in neonates are described below:

Inulin

Inulin, an exogenous starch-like fructose polymer extracted from Jerusalem artichokes, has an Einstein-Stokes radius of 1.5 nm, and a molecular weight (MW) of approximately 5.2 kDa. It diffuses, as would a spherical body of such radius. Inulin is inert, it is not metabolized, not reabsorbed and not secreted by the renal tubular cells. Its clearance, consequently, reflects the rate of filtration only. Estimates of inulin clearance provide the basis for a standard reference against which the route or mechanisms of excretion of other substances can be ascertained.

INULIN AS A MARKER OF GFR IN THE NEONATE

The hypothesis that inulin may not be freely filtered by the immature glomerular barrier has never been confirmed, neither in animal nor in human studies (14). Inulin has been used as a marker of GFR in human neonates, using three different techniques to measure or estimate its clearance: (a) the urinary UV/P clearance; (b) the constant infusion technique without urine collection and (c) the single injection (plasma disappearance curve) technique.

Creatinine

Creatinine, the normal metabolite of creatine phosphate present in skeletal muscle, has a molecular weight of 113 Da. The renal excretion of endogenous creatinine is fairly similar to that of inulin in humans and several animal species. However, in addition to being filtered through the glomerulus, creatinine is secreted in part by the renal tubular cells.

Overestimation of GFR by creatinine clearance is usually more evident at low GFRs. As GFR falls progressively during the course of renal disease, the renal tubular secretion of creatinine contributes an increasing fraction to urinary excretion, so that creatinine clearance may substantially exceed the actual GFR. Secretion of creatinine into the gut plays a role in this phenomenon.

While creatinine has been used for decades, the methods available for its chemical determination are still biased by various interfering substances (15). Improvement in measuring creatinine has been achieved by the use of newer techniques such as high-performance liquid chromatography (HPLC), the gas

Table 5-2	Characteristics of the Glomerular Markers					
	Inulin	Creatinine	Iohexol	DTPA	EDTA	Iothalamate
Molecular weight (Da)	5200	113	811	393	292	637
Elimination half-life (min)	70	200	90	110	120	120
Plasma protein binding (%)	0	0	< 2	5	0	< 5
Space of distribution	EC	TBW	EC	EC	EC	EC

DTPA, diethylenetriaminepenta-acetic acid; EC, extracellular space; EDTA, ethylenediaminetetra-acetic acid; TBW, total body water.

chromatography-isotope dilution mass spectrometry (Gc-IDSM) and the HPLC-IMSD coupled technique (15).

Gas chromatography-isotope-dilution mass spectrometry (Gc-IDMS) is now considered the method of choice for measuring true creatinine. It has an excellent specificity and low relative SD (less than 0.3%) (15). A method coupling HPLC with IDMS for the direct determination of creatinine has been developed recently (16). The procedure is simple and speedy. It appears to offer the same advantage as the Gc-IDMS technique.

While accurate and reproducible assessment of creatinine is mandatory, the calibration of its measurement is not yet standardized to a gold standard in most places, thereby leading to substantial variations between laboratories (15).

CREATININE AS A MARKER OF GFR IN THE NEONATE

The handling of creatinine by the immature kidney is unique, creatinine apparently undergoing glomerular filtration and partial tubular reabsorption. In newborn rabbits, the urinary clearance of creatinine underestimates the concomitantly measured clearance of inulin (17). This phenomenon is only present in the first postnatal days and is probably explained by the passive reabsorption of the filtered creatinine across immature leaky tubules. When water is reabsorbed along the nephron, the concentration of filtered creatinine rises so that creatinine back-diffuses into the blood according to its concentration gradient, thus raising its plasma concentration. The clearance of creatinine has also been shown to underestimate true GFR in very low birth-weight (VLBW) human neonates, thus suggesting the occurrence of the same phenomenon in the human immature kidney (18).

The use of creatinine as a marker of GFR in neonates is not only hampered by its specific handling by the immature kidney, but also as previously mentioned, by technical difficulties related to its chemical determination. The Jaffe reaction is indeed affected by interfering substances such as bilirubin, leading to spurious overestimation of the true plasma creatinine.

Iohexol

Iohexol is a non-ionic agent with a MW of 821 Da that appears to be eliminated exclusively by glomerular filtration. A significant correlation has been observed between the urinary clearance of iohexol and that of inulin in children (19). Large studies to validate iohexol as a true glomerular marker are not yet available. Iohexol has not been validated in neonates.

Iothalamate Sodium

Iothalamate sodium has a molecular weight of 637 Da. It can be used as ^{125}I-radiolabeled or without radioactive label, its plasma concentration then being assessed by X-ray fluorescence or by HPLC or, more recently, by capillary electrophoresis. It is only minimally bound to proteins and its renal handling has some similarities with that of inulin. Critical studies have however unequivocally demonstrated that iothalamate is actively secreted by the renal tubules, and perhaps also undergoes tubular reabsorption in humans and animal species (20). The agreement between iothalamate and inulin clearances appears to be a fortuitous cancellation of errors between tubular excretion and protein binding of the agent. The substance does not consequently appear suitable for accurate estimation of GFR. The use of iothalamate has not been properly validated in neonates. Radiolabeled iothalamate should not be used in the first month of life.

^{99m}Tc-DTPA and ^{51}Cr-EDTA

The use of radiolabeled markers is not recommended during the neonatal period. This group of markers will thus not be discussed here.

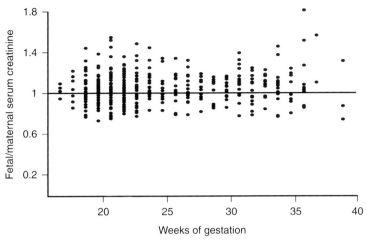

Figure 5-4 Relation between fetal cord and maternal serum creatinine during gestation. The ratio of the fetal to maternal serum creatinine remains close to 1 throughout gestation, indicating free diffusion of creatinine across the placental barrier. (After Guignard JP, Drukker A: Why do newborn infants have a high plasma creatinine? Pediatrics 103(4):e49, 1999.)

Techniques Used to Assess GFR in Neonates

The Plasma Concentration

The use of the plasma creatinine (P_{creat}) concentration to estimate GFR presents specific problems in the neonate. The neonate's creatininemia is elevated at birth, reflecting the maternal plasma creatinine concentration. A near perfect equilibrium between the maternal and fetal plasma creatinine concentrations has indeed been shown to occur throughout gestation (Fig. 5-4) (18). In preterm infants, the elevated plasma creatinine further increases transiently to reach a peak value between the second and fourth day of postnatal life (Fig. 5-5) (21,22). Peak plasma creatinine concentrations as high as 195–247 µmol/L in 23–26 weeks gestational age (GA) neonates, and 99–140 µmol/L in 33–40 weeks GA neonates have been recorded (Table 5-3) (22). This transient increase in the very low birthweight neonates' postnatal plasma creatinine concentration is probably the consequence of creatinine reabsorption across leaky tubules, as suggested by studies in piglets and newborn rabbits (17,18). It accounts for the observation that when measured during the first week of life, the P_{creat} is highest in the most premature infants (23).

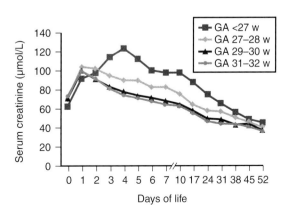

Figure 5-5 Changes in serum creatinine in preterm neonates during the first 52 h of postnatal life. Peak increases are observed on day 4 in the most premature infants. (After Gallini F, Maggio L, Romagnoli C et al: Progression of renal function in preterm neonates with gestational age ≤32 weeks. Pediatr Nephrol 15:119, 2000.)

Table 5-3   Changes in Plasma Creatinine over Time for Different Gestation Groups

Group gestation age (week)	Birth creatinine (μmol/L)*	Peak plasma creatinine (μmol/L)*	Time to peak plasma creatinine (h)*
23–26	67–92	195–247	40–78
27–29	65–89	158–200	28–51
30–32	60–69	120–158	25–40
33–45	67–79	99–140	8–23

*Range intervals. After Miall LS, Henderson MJ, Turner, AJ et al: Plasma creatinine rises dramatically in the first 48 hours of life in preterm infants. Pediatrics 6:104, 1999.

Urinary Clearance (UV/P)

INULIN

The method based on the urinary clearance of inulin is the reference method. Measurement of the urinary clearance of this exogenous marker is cumbersome, however, because it requires its constant intravenous infusion and the precise collection of urine. The method has been used in early developmental studies (1) to define the maturation of GFR in relation to gestational and postnatal age (Fig. 5-1 and Fig. 5-2).

CREATININE

The urinary clearance of creatinine has been claimed to approximate the urinary clearance of inulin in both preterm and term neonates. In premature infants, a creatinine to inulin clearance ratio below 1 has often been observed, suggesting that tubular reabsorption of creatinine also occurs in premature humans, as it does in immature animals (17). Developmental studies based on the urinary clearance of creatinine have produced valuable information on the maturation of GFR (1,23–25).

The Constant Infusion Technique without Urine Collection

The constant infusion technique (26) assumes that the rate of infusion of a marker *(x)* needed to maintain constant its plasma concentration is equal to the rate of its excretion. After equilibration of the marker in its distribution space, the excretion rate must thus be equal to the rate of infusion *(IR)*, hence the derived clearance formula:

$$C_x = U_x \bullet V/P_x = IR_x \bullet P_x$$

The flow rate of the test solution containing the marker is expressed in mL/min per 1.73 m^2, so is the clearance C of the marker x.

The constant infusion technique, without urine collection, is attractive and has been used in newborn infants. The results obtained in short term (a few hours) infusion studies have produced conflicting results. When inulin was constantly infused for 24 h, the results obtained by this technique were in reasonable agreement with those obtained by the traditional urinary clearance (27,28). As a whole, the infusion technique has the advantage of avoiding the need for urine collection, but presents with the main disadvantage of requiring careful time-consuming supervision of the long-duration infusion of inulin.

The Single Injection (Plasma Disappearance Curve) Technique

The mathematical model for this technique is an open two-compartment system. The glomerular marker is injected in the first compartment, equilibrates with the second compartment, and is excreted from the first compartment by glomerular filtration. The plasma disappearance curve of the marker follows two consecutive patterns. In the first phase, the agent diffuses in its distribution space and its plasma concentration falls rapidly. In the second phase, when the equilibration has been reached the slope of the decline of the plasma concentration of the marker basically reflects its urinary excretion rate.

The plasma disappearance curve method has occasionally been used in neonates. A large overestimation of GFR by the single injection technique has been repeatedly observed; it was ascribed to incomplete equilibration of inulin in its distribution space during the study period (28,29).

Estimation of Creatinine Clearance from its Plasma Concentration without Urine Collection

The concentration of endogenous markers such as creatinine increases when GFR decreases. The increase in plasma creatinine is not linear however. Several attempts have thus been made to develop reliable methods that will allow a correct estimate of creatinine clearance (eC_{creat}) from its plasma concentration alone, without urine collection. A formula has been developed for children (30,31), which allows an estimate of creatinine clearance (eC_{creat}) derived from the patient's creatinine plasma concentration and body length:

$$eC_{creat} = k \bullet Length/P_{creat}$$

Where k is a constant, L represents the body length and P_{creat} the plasma creatinine concentration. This formula is based on the assumption that creatinine excretion is proportional to body length and inversely proportional to plasma creatinine (31). The value of the constant k can be obtained from the formula $k = eC_{creat} \bullet P_{creat}/Length$. When Length is expressed in cm and P_{creat} in mg (%), the resulting eC_{creat} is expressed in mL/min per 1.73 m^2. Under steady state conditions, k should be directly proportional to the muscle component of body weight, which corresponds reasonably well to the daily urinary creatinine excretion rate.

The Schwartz formula has been used in neonates (31). The mean value of k, calculated in 118 low birth weight infants with a corrected age of 25–105 weeks, was 0.33 ± 0.01. It rose to 0.45 in full-term infants up to 18 months (31). In spite of a large scatter of normal values, the formula was claimed to be useful, because it correlated well with the inulin single-injection technique (31). It is only unfortunate that the $k \bullet Length/P_{creat}$ formula has not been validated in neonates by comparing its results with those given by the standard $U \bullet (V/P)$ inulin clearance. The accuracy of the $k \bullet Length/P_{creat}$ formula, as an estimate of GFR, has indeed been questioned. In a study in infants younger than 1 year of age, the k value ranged from 0.17 to 0.82 [15–72 when P_{creat} in μmol/L], and factor k was found to vary markedly with the state of hydration (32). The $k \bullet Length/P_{creat}$ formula may be more informative clinically than P_{creat} alone because the creatinine value, in addition to renal function, is critically dependent on the percentage of muscle mass. Caution should be exercised, however, when using the formula as an estimate of GFR in studies aimed at defining renal pathophysiologic mechanisms in neonates.

The Special Case of Cystatin C: A Non Classical Glomerular Marker!

Cystatin C, a non-glycosated 13-kDa basic protein, is a proteinase inhibitor involved in the intracellular catabolism of proteins (33). It is produced by all nucleated cells, freely filtered across the glomerular capillaries, almost completely reabsorbed and catabolized in the renal proximal tubular cells (34). Being reabsorbed, cystatin C is not a classical marker of glomerular filtration, as strictly defined (see Assessment of GFR). When using the particle-enhanced immunonephelometry assay for its determination in blood, no interference from bilirubin, hemoglobin, triglycerides and rheumatoid factor could be observed (35). Cystatin C has been claimed to be a reliable marker of GFR, independent of inflammatory conditions, muscle mass and gender (36,37). In children aged 1.8–18.8 years with various levels of GFR, serum Cystatin C has been found to be broadly equivalent (38) or even superior (39) to P_{creat} as an estimate of GFR. A very large recent study of 8058 inhabitants of Groeningen questions, however, the advantages of cystatin C (40). In this study, male gender, older age, greater weight, higher serum C-reactive protein levels and cigarette smoking were all independently associated with higher cystatin C levels after adjusting for creatinine clearance. Cystatin C has also been shown to be a poor marker of GFR in pregnancy (41), in renal transplant patients and/or in patients receiving corticosteroids (42–44) as well as in intensive care patients (45). In a recent study in children cystatin C has also been shown to be less reliable than the Schwartz formula in distinguishing impaired from normal GFR (46).

Cystatin C as a Marker of GFR in Neonates

The handling of cystatin C by the immature kidney is not known. Cystatin C does not appear to cross the placental barrier, and there is no correlation between maternal and neonatal serum cystatin C levels (47). Cystatin C concentrations are highest at birth, and then decrease to stabilize after 12 months of age (47) (Fig. 5-6). Cystatin C is significantly higher in premature infants as compared to term infants (36,48). In the study by Randers et al (37), mean values of 1.63 ± 0.26 mg/L ($x \pm SD$) were recorded during the first month of life, and of 0.95 ± 0.22 mg/L during months 1–12, and 0.72 ± 0.12 mg/L after the first year of life.

The claim has been made (a) that the concentration of cystatin C offers a greater sensitivity and reliability than creatinine in detecting an abnormal GFR in newborn infants, and (b) 'that unlike creatinine, cystatin C can be used to assess GFR of the newborn and even the fetus' (49). Such a statement is somewhat ill-founded and there are numerous reasons to refute this conclusion:

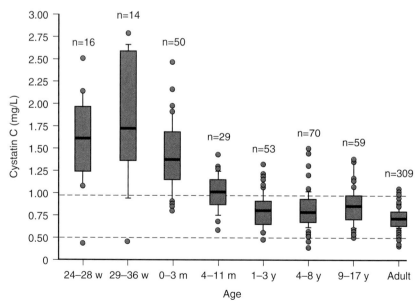

Figure 5-6 Box plot distributions showing plasma cystatin C values across the age groups. Dotted lines indicate 95% confidence interval of adult range. Preterm babies born between 24–36 weeks of gestation were 1 day old. (After Finney H, Newman DJ, Thakkar H et al: Reference ranges for plasma cystatin C and creatinine measurements in premature infants, neonates, and older children. Arch Dis Child 82:71, 2000.)

(a) the handling of cystatin C by the immature kidney is not known;

(b) the scatter of the serum cystatin C concentrations in neonates is very large, so that it is unlikely that a useful formula will be established to reliably estimate GFR at this age;

(c) because cystatin C is filtered and then reabsorbed and catabolized by the proximal tubular cells, its plasma concentation will obviously be influenced by changes in the rate of degradation of cystatin C by injured renal proximal tubular cells;

(d) the claim that cystatin C is a valuable marker of GFR has not been validated by comparison to the gold standard, either in neonates or in children;

(e) the production and concentration of cystatin C may be influenced by factors other than GFR, such as the serum C-reactive protein levels, thyroid dysfunction or corticosteroid administration;

(f) measurement of cystatin C is considerably more expensive than that of creatinine, by a factor of at least 12 (49).

Conclusion: Assessment of Renal Function in Neonates: Which Method for Which Purpose?

Developmental Studies

When the purpose of performing clearance studies is to obtain basic information on the physiological maturation of GFR, the use of reliable methods is mandatory. The urinary clearance of inulin remains the method of choice. This method requires timed-urine collection, by bladder catheterization or bag. The urinary clearance of creatinine also requires timed-collection of urine, and blood sampling in the middle of the urinary collection period. Valuable information has been obtained by this technique. The need for urine collection can be avoided by using the constant inulin infusion technique. In this case, inulin needs to be constantly infused for at least 24 h, requiring careful supervision. When respecting the protocol strictly (27,28), useful information can be obtained by this technique.

Other non-validated methods for measuring GFR should be avoided, as they are unnecessarily complex without providing indisputable data.

Clinical Purposes

Simpler techniques can be used to estimate GFR for clinical purposes. When interpreted with caution, the serum creatinine concentrations can provide crude but valid information on the neonates' renal function. The transient 'physiological' increase in plasma concentrations occurring during the first days of very premature infants should be taken into account when interpreting such concentrations. The data published by Miall et al (22) and Gallini et al (21) should be used as reference values for creatinine levels in very low birth weight infants. In doing so, sequential measurements of the plasma concentration of creatinine can provide useful information on the putative presence of renal insufficiency.

When a rough estimate of creatinine clearance is needed, the Schwartz formula adapted for neonates (31) can be used. The formula is simple, and only requires measurement of the neonate's plasma creatinine and body length. The formula has indeed been shown to provide useful data on the level of GFR. The value of $0.33 +/- 0.01$ for constant k (when creatinine is expressed in mg%, and 29 when it is expressed in µmol/L) will of course only be valid if the reference values for creatinine are the same in the laboratory where creatinine is tested and in the laboratory where the value of factor k has been calculated (31). Ideally, each laboratory should define its own value for constant k in a selected group of patients.

The use of more sophisticated techniques for clinical purpose is not justified. Such is the case for the single injection technique of inulin or iothalamate, and for the plasma cystatin C concentration. The information they give is not accurate enough to justify their complexity. They will not provide information that cannot be obtained by the simple Schwartz formula.

CONDITIONS AND FACTORS THAT IMPAIR GFR

In human neonates, the major risk factors for developing acute renal insufficiency are severe respiratory disorders and perinatal exposure to PGs synthesis inhibitors (50–53).

Perinatal Asphyxia

Perinatal asphyxia is defined as a condition leading to progressive hypoxemia, hypercapnia and metabolic acidosis. The pathogenesis of the hypoxia-induced vasomotor nephropathy has been studied in newborn rabbits and lambs. In the rabbit model, isolated hypoxemia induces intense renal vasoconstriction with a consequent decrease in GFR and in the filtration fraction (FF), and to a lesser extent in RBF. The observed decrease in FF suggests efferent arteriolar vasodilation, presumably as a consequence of intrarenal activation of adenosine (54), an endogenous vasoactive agent known to vasodilate the efferent arteriole and to decrease the intraglomerular pressure. The hypothesis that adenosine plays a key role in mediating the hypoxemic renal vasoconstriction was supported by the fact that theophylline, a non-specific antagonist of adenosine cell surface receptors, prevented the drop in GFR induced by hypoxemia in newborn rabbits (54). Such an effect was not observed when enprofylline, a xanthine devoid of adenosine antagonistic properties, was administered instead of theophylline (55). Clinical studies using prophylactic theophylline in high-risk asphyxiated neonates seem to confirm the putative beneficial effect of theophylline in protecting GFR (see Theophylline below).

Non-steroidal Antiinflammatory Agents (NSAIDs)

Exposure to PGs synthesis inhibitors during fetal development can lead to severe renal dysgenesis. Increased activity of the vasodilator PGs present during development is necessary to protect the function of the immature kidney. By blunting the effect of vasodilator PGs on the afferent arteriole, PGs synthesis inhibitors can impair GFR in both the fetus and neonate. Indomethacin is sometimes used in pregnant women with polyhydramnios, to reduce fetal urine output and consequently the production of amniotic fluid (56). It should be realized that this 'obstetrical' benefit is achieved by producing a state of renal insufficiency in the fetus. Decreased GFR has been demonstrated in neonates whose mother had been administered indomethacin shortly before birth (57) as well as in neonates administered indomethacin for the closure of PDA (58). This deleterious effect is usually transient, renal function normalizing within 30 days (59), but may have deleterious consequences for the elimination of drugs such as vancomycin, aminoglycosides and digoxin, which are excreted mainly by glomerular filtration.

Ibuprofen, a COX non-selective inhibitor like indomethacin, has been claimed to be safer than the latter for the newborn kidney (60). The efficacy and renal side effects of ibuprofen and indomethacin have been compared in two recent meta-analyses (61,62). While the efficacy of the two drugs in closing the ductus arteriosus was similar, ibuprofen appeared to have fewer renal side effects than indomethacin. Ibuprofen-treated neonates presented with higher urine output (+0.74 mL/kg per min), and a lower increase of serum creatinine concentration (+0.44 ± 0.10 µmol/L).

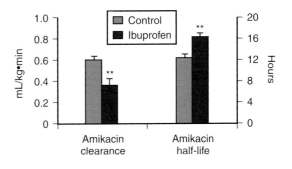

Figure 5-7 Effect of prophylactic ibuprofen on the pharmacokinetics of amikacin. The decrease in amikacin clearance and the increase in amikacin half-life reflect the decrease in GFR induced by ibuprofen. (After Allegaert K, Cossey V, Langhendries JP et al: Effects of co-administration of ibuprofen-lysine on the pharmacokinetics of amikacin in preterm infants during the first days of life. Biol Neonate 86:207, 2004.)

In contrast, in a recent well-controlled clinical study, the prophylactic administration of either acetylsalicylic acid (4×11 mg/kg per day for two days) or ibuprofen (10 mg/kg and 5 mg/kg at 24 h and 48 h, respectively) was associated with similar decreases in the clearance of amikacin administered concomitantly (63,64) (Fig. 5-7). Amikacin being eliminated almost exclusively by glomerular filtration, a decrease in its clearance indicates a decrease in GFR. This observation casts doubt on the renal innocuousness of ibuprofen. This doubt is supported by experimental studies failing to demonstrate a difference between various NSAIDs, including the non-specific COX inhibitors aspirin, indomethacin and ibuprofen. All agents acutely decreased GFR and RBF when administered to newborn rabbits (65,66).

Differences in the renal side effects of indomethacin and ibuprofen, if they do exist, may depend on the ratio of their respective activities on the two-cyclooxygenase isoenzymes COX-1 and COX-2, indomethacin-inhibiting COX-1 more than COX-2. This hypothesis does not fit well, however, with the observation made in newborn rabbits that the preferential COX-2 inhibitor nimesulide induced the same renal vasoconstriction as the non-selective inhibitors (67). If real, the potential advantage of using ibuprofen may have to be counterbalanced by a slight increase in the occurrence of chronic lung disease at 28 days of age (62).

Angiotensin Converting Enzyme Inhibitors (ACEIs) and Angio II Receptor Antagonists (ARAs)

ACEIs and ARAs are potent hypotensive agents that act by interfering with the formation or the action of Angio II. When administered to the hypertensive mother early in pregnancy, they can induce renal dysgenesis (68). When administered later in pregnancy or to the neonate after birth, these agents can induce renal failure (69). In high-risk hypertensive neonates with bronchopulmonary dysplasia, whose renin-angiotensin system is overstimulated beyond the neonatal period, the administration of captopril has resulted in dramatic falls in blood pressure and episodes of prolonged oliguria and seizures (69). Inhibitors and antagonists of the renin-angiotensin system must not be administered to pregnant mothers and should be administered with caution to sick neonates.

PREVENTION OF OLIGURIC STATES DUE TO LOW GFR

Furosemide in Oliguric Neonates

Furosemide, a potent loop natriuretic agent, is commonly used to improve urine output in oliguric neonates, in the hope of increasing diuresis and improving renal blood flow and GFR. This hope is based on the fact that furosemide stimulates the production of vasodilator prostaglandins. The natriuretic and the diuretic response to furosemide are highly variable and depend largely on the level of GFR. Furosemide indeed acts from within the tubular lumen, which it reaches by glomerular filtration and tubular secretion. When a diuretic response is present, it carries the risk of inducing hypovolemia, with consequent vasoconstriction of the kidney. In the newborn rabbit, torasemide, a loop diuretic with close similarities to furosemide, increased sodium and water excretion without modifying RBF and GFR (70,71). When given to immature animals undergoing hypoxemic vasomotor nephropathy, torasemide still improved sodium excretion and diuresis, but was without effect on renal perfusion and GFR (71).

The administration of furosemide to preterm neonates with respiratory distress syndrome (RDS) has produced conflicting results. While furosemide usually induces diuresis and a transient improvement in pulmonary function, a critical review of published data did not support the routine administration of furosemide (or any diuretic) to preterm infants with RDS (72). Although it may stimulate PGs production, furosemide is sometimes administered to indomethacin-treated preterm infants presenting with oliguria, with an apparent benefit. A recent critical review also concluded, however, that there was not enough evidence to recommend the administration of furosemide to preterm infants treated with indomethacin for PDA (73). Clearly, furosemide should not be used to treat oliguric neonates, but primarily those presenting with edematous states and congestive heart failure.

Dopaminergic Agents (Dopamine, Dopexamine) in Oliguric Neonates

Low doses of dopamine, the so-called 'renal' doses (0.5–2.5 µg/kg per min) have been widely used in the hope that its selective actions on DA_1 dopaminergic receptors in the vascular bed would induce renal vasodilation and improve GFR in the newborn infant. Increases in urine output, sodium excretion and creatinine clearance have been initially described following the administration of renal doses of dopamine to sick neonates or to oliguric neonates treated with indomethacin (74). In the latter group, dopamine (5 µg/kg per min) increased urine output without affecting blood pressure, and decreased the pulsatility index in the renal artery. These results were considered as reflecting a dopamine-induced increase in renal blood flow (74).

Because of the great overlap in the response to dopamine and significant interindividual variability, the benefit of dopamine is difficult to ascertain, and detrimental effects following dopamine have been described (75). Noteworthy is the fact that: (a) all studies in favor of the renal doses of dopamine were uncontrolled (74–77); (b) early favorable results in indomethacin-treated preterm infants (74) have not been confirmed by the meta-analysis of three randomized trials (73); and (c) experiments in newborn rabbits also failed to demonstrate an increase in RBF and GFR following the administration of dopamine (4 µg/kg per min and 10 µg/kg per min) or dopexamine (4 µg/kg per min and 10 µg/kg per min), a dopaminergic agonist devoid of any alpha-adrenergic effect (78). Dopexamine also failed to improve renal function in newborn rabbits presenting with hypoxemic vasomotor nephropathy (79).

In view of its potential side effects (worsening of the hypothyroid state of the preterm infant, decrease in growth hormone and prolactin secretion, cardiac arrhythmia, constriction of pulmonary, renal and peripheral vasculature) and the doubt cast on their efficacy, dopamine and dopaminergic agents should not be used with the aim of improving GFR.

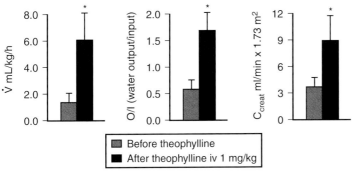

Figure 5-8 Changes in urine flow rate (V), water input/output ratio and creatinine clearance (C_{creat}) following theophylline administration in high-risk neonates with compromised renal function. (After Huet F, Semama D, Grimaldi M et al: Effects of theophylline on renal insufficiency in neonates with respiratory distress syndrome. Intensive Care Med 21:511, 1995.)

Theophylline

Low-dose theophylline (0.5–1 mg/kg), a xanthine derivative with strong adenosine antagonistic properties, has been shown to prevent the hypoxemia-induced vasoconstriction in both newborn and adult rabbits (54). It probably does so by blunting the efferent arteriolar adenosine-mediated vasodilation induced by hypoxia. A marked improvement in both urinary water excretion and GFR following theophylline administration was first observed in high-risk neonates with oliguric renal insufficiency (Fig. 5-8) (80). Later studies confirmed this observation. A double-blind placebo-controlled study showed that theophylline (single dose of 8 mg/kg) given early after birth significantly improved renal dysfunction in term-neonates presenting with severe perinatal dysfunction (81). Two recent placebo-controlled studies in severely asphyxiated term-neonates demonstrated that a single dose of theophylline (5 mg/kg or 8 mg/kg) given in the first hours of life significantly improved renal function and creatinine clearance, without affecting the central nervous system (82,83). Improvement in renal function has also been observed in a controlled study in preterm neonates with RDS. The intravenous administration of a low dose of theophylline (1 mg/kg for 3 days) resulted in lower levels of serum creatinine, increased urine output and decreased the occurrence of oligoanuria (84). Interestingly enough, in the neonatal rabbit model, the specific adenosine A_1 receptor antagonist DPCPX does not offer the same protection as theophylline during a hypoxemic stress (85).

While the use of the non-specific adenosine antagonist theophylline appears to offer significant protection for the stressed kidney, additional studies are required before recommending the routine use of theophylline for preventive or curative purposes in neonates with perinatal asphyxia or RDS.

REFERENCES

1. Guignard JP, John EG. Renal function in the tiny, premature infant. Clin Perinatol 13:377, 1986.
2. Kon V, Ichikawa I. Glomerular circulation and function. In Avner ED, Harmond P, Niaudet P (Eds.): Pediatric Nephrology, 5th edn (pp 25–45). Philadelphia: Lippincott Williams & Wilkins, 2004.
3. Arendshorst WJ, Brännström K, Ruan X. Actions of angiotensin II on the renal microvasculature. J Am Soc Nephrol 10:S149, 1999.
4. Guignard JP, Gouyon JB, John E. Vasoactive factors in the immature kidney. Pediatr Nephrol 5:443, 1991.
5. Morris JL, Rosen DA, Rosen KR. Nonsteroidal anti-inflammatory agents in neonates. Paediatr Drug 5:385, 2003.

6. Gomez RA, Pupilli C, Everett AD. Molecular and cellular aspects of renin during kidney ontogeny. Pediatr Nephrol 5:80, 1991.

7. Norwood VF, Craig MR, Harris JM, et al. Differential expression of angiotensin II receptors during early renal morphogenesis. Am J Physiol 272:R662, 1997.

8. Tufro-McReddie A, Harrison JK, Everett AD, et al. Ontogeny of type 1 angiotensin II receptor gene expression in the rat. J Clin Invest 91:530, 1993.

9. Tufro-McReddie A, Romano LM, Harris JM, et al. Angiotensin II regulates nephrogenesis and renal vascular development. Am J Physiol 269:F110, 1995.

10. Prévot A, Mosig D, Guignard JP. The effects of losartan on renal function in the newborn rabbit. Pediatr Res 51:728, 2002.

11. Khan KN, Paulson SK, Verburg KM, et al. Pharmacology of cyclooxygenase-2 inhibition in the kidney. Kidney Int 61:1210, 2002.

12. Kömoff M, Wang JL, Cheng HF, et al. Cyclooxygenase-2-selective inhibitors impair glomerulogenesis and renal cortical development. Kidney Int 57:14, 2000.

13. Norwood VF, Morham SG, Smithies O. Postnatal development and progression of renal dysplasia in cyclooxygenase-2 null-mice. Kidney Int 58:2291, 2000.

14. Coulthard MG, Ruddock V. Validation of inulin as a marker for glomerular filtration in preterm babies. Kidney Int 23:407, 1983.

15. Myers GL, Miller WG, Coresh J, et al. Recommendations for improving serum creatinine measurement: a report from the Laboratory Working Group of the National Kidney Disease Education Program. Clin Chem 52:169, 2006.

16. Stokes P, O'Connor G. Development of a liquid chromatography-mass spectrometry method for high-accuracy determination of creatinine in serum. J Chromatogr B Analyt Technol Biomed Life Sci 794:125, 2003.

17. Matos P, Duarte-Silva M, Drukker A, Guignard JP. Creatinine reabsorption by the newborn rabbit kidney. Pediatr Res 44:639, 1998.

18. Guignard JP, Drukker A. Why do newborn infants have a high plasma creatinine? Pediatrics 103(4):e49, 1999.

19. Lindblad HG, Berg HB. Comparative evaluation of iohexol and inulin clearance for glomerular filtration rate determinations. Acta Paediatr 83:418, 1994.

20. Odlind B, Hallgren R, Sohtell M, et al. Is 125I iothalamate an ideal marker for glomerular filtration? Kidney Int 27:9, 1985.

21. Gallini F, Maggio L, Romagnoli C, et al. Progression of renal function in preterm neonates with gestational age ≤32 weeks. Pediatr Nephrol 15:119, 2000.

22. Miall LS, Henderson MJ, Turner AJ, et al. Plasma creatinine rises dramatically in the first 48 hours of life in preterm infants. Pediatrics 6:104, 1999.

23. Bueva A, Guignard JP. Renal function in preterm neonates. Pediatr Res 36:572, 1994.

24. Stonestreet BS, Bell EF, Oh W. Validity of endogenous creatinine clearance in low birthweight infants. Pediatr Res 13:1002, 1979.

25. Coulthard MG, Hey EN, Ruddock V. Creatinine and urea clearances compared to inulin clearance in preterm and mature babies. Early Hum Dev 11:11, 1985.

26. Cole BR, Giangiacomo J, Ingelfinger JR, et al. Measurement of renal function without urine collection. A critical evaluation of the constant-infusion technique for determination of inulin and para-aminohippurate. N Engl J Med 287:1109, 1972.

27. vd Heijden AJ, Grose WF, Ambagtsheer JJ, et al. Glomerular filtration rate in the preterm infant: the relation to gestational and postnatal age. Eur J Pediatr 148:24, 1988.

28. Coulthard MG. Comparison of methods of measuring renal function in preterm babies using inulin. J Pediatr 102:923, 1983.

29. Fawer CL, Torrado A, Guignard JP. Maturation of renal function in full-term and premature neonates. Helv Paediatr Acta 34:11, 1979.

30. Counahan R, Chantler C, Ghazali S, et al. Estimation of glomerular filtration rate from plasma creatinine concentration in children. Arch Dis Child 51:875, 1976.

31. Schwartz GJ, Brion LP, Spitzer A. The use of plasma creatinine concentration for estimating glomerular filtration rate in infants, children, and adolescents. Pediatr Clin North Am 34:571, 1987.

32. Haenggi MH, Pelet J, Guignard JP. Estimation of glomerular filtration rate by the formula GFR = K × T/Pc. Arch Pediatr 6:165, 1999.

33. Olafsson I. The human cystatin C gene promotor: Functional analysis and identification of heterogeneous mRNA. Scand J Clin Lab Invest 55:597, 1995.

34. Tenstad O, Roald AB, Grubb A. Renal handling of radiolabelled human cystatin C in the rat. Scand J Clin Lab Invest 56:409, 1996.

35. Erlandsen EJ, Randers E, Kristensen JH. Evaluation of the N Latex Cystatin C assay on the Dade Behring Nephelometer II system. Scand J Clin Lab Invest 59:1, 1999.

36. Finney H, Newman DJ, Thakkar H, et al. Reference ranges for plasma cystatin C and creatinine measurements in premature infants, neonates, and older children. Arch Dis Child 82:71, 2000.

37. Randers E, Krue S, Erlandsen EJ, et al. Reference interval for serum cystatin C in children. Clinical Chemistry 45:1856, 1999.

38. Stickle D, Cole B, Hock K, et al. Correlation of plasma concentrations of cystatin C and creatinine to inulin clearance in a pediatric population. Clin Chem 44:1334, 1998.

39. Bökenkamp A, Domanetzki M, Zinck R, et al. Reference values for cystatin C serum concentrations in children. Pediatr Nephrol 12:125, 1998.

40. Knight EL, Verhave JC, Spiegelman D, et al. Factors influencing serum cystatin C levels other than renal function and the impact on renal function measurement. Kidney Int 65:777, 2004.

41. Akbari A, Lepage N, Keely E, et al. Cystatin-C and beta trace protein as markers of renal function in pregnancy. BJOG 112:575, 2005.

42. Podraacka L, Feber J, Lepage N, et al. Intra-individual variation of cystatin C and creatinine in pediatric solid organ transplant recipients. Pediatr Transplant 9:28, 2005.

43. Mendiluce A, Bustamante J, Martin D, et al. Cystatin C as a marker of renal function in kidney transplant patients. Transplant Proc 37:3844, 2005.

44. Bökenkamp A, van Wijk JAE, Lentze MJ, et al. Effects of corticosteroid therapy on serum cystatin C and beta 2-microglobulin concentrations. Clin Chem 48:1123, 2002.

45. Wulkan R, den Hollander J, Berghout A. Cystatin C unsuited to use as a marker of kidney function in the intensive care unit. Crit Care 9:531, 2005.

46. Martini S, Prévot A, Mosig D, Guignard JP. Glomerular filtration rate: measure creatinine and height rather than cystatin C! Acta Paediatr 92:1052, 2003.

47. Cataldi L, Mussap M, Bertelli N, et al. Cystatin C in healthy women at term pregnancy and in their infant newborns: relationship between maternal and neonatal serum levels and reference values. Am J Perinatol 16:287, 1999.

48. Harmoinen A, Ylinen E, Ala-Houhala M, et al. Reference intervals for cystatin C in pre-and full-term infants and children. Pediatr Nephrol 15:105, 2000.

49. Filler G, Bökenkamp A, Hofmann W, et al. Cystatin C as a marker of GFR: history, indications, and future research. Clin Biochem 38:1, 2005.

50. Toth-Heynh P, Drukker A, Guignard JP. The stressed neonatal kidney: From pathophysiology to clinical management of neonatal vasomotor nephropathy. Pediatr Nephrol 14:227, 2000.

51. Gouyon JB, Guignard JP. Management of acute renal failure in newborns. Pediatr Nephrol 14:1037, 2000.

52. Choker G, Gouyon JB. Diagnosis of acute renal failure in very preterm infants. Biol Neonate 86:212, 2004.

53. Cataldi L, Leone R, Moretti U, et al. Potential risk factors for the development of acute renal failure in preterm newborn infants: A case-control study. Arch Dis Child Fetal Neonatal Ed 90:F514, 2005.

54. Gouyon JB, Guignard JP. Theophylline prevents the hypoxemia-induced renal hemodynamic changes in rabbits. Kidney Int 33:1078, 1988.

55. Gouyon JB, Arnaud M, Guignard JP. Renal effects of low-dose aminophylline and enprofylline in newborn rabbits. Life Sci 42:1271, 1988.

56. Abhyankar S, Salvi VS. Indomethacin therapy in hydrammios. J Postgrad Med 46:176, 2000.

57. vd Heijden AJ, Provoost AP, Nauta J, et al. Renal function impairment in preterm neonates related to intrauterine indomethacin exposure. Pediatr Res 24:644, 1988.

58. Catterton Z, Sellers B Jr, Gray B. Inulin clearance in the premature infant receiving indomethacin. J Pedriatr 96:737, 1980.

59. Akima S, Kent A, Reynolds GJ, et al. Indomethacin and renal impairment in neonates. Pediatr Nephrol 19:490, 2004.

60. Van Overmeire B, Smets K, Lecoutere D, et al. A comparison of ibuprofen and indomethacin for closure of patent ductus arteriosus. N Engl J Med 343:674, 2000.

61. Thomas RL, Parker GC, Van Overmeire B, et al. A meta-analysis of ibuprofen versus indomethacin for closure of patent ductus arteriosus. Eur J Pediatr 164:135, 2005.

62. Ohlsson A, Walia R, Schah S. Ibuprofen for the treatment of patent ductus arteriosus in preterm and/or low birth weight infants. Cochrane Database Syst Rev 2: CD003481, 2003.

63. Allegaert K, Cossey V, Langhendries JP, et al. Effects of co-administration of ibuprofen-lysine on the pharmacokinetics of amikacin in preterm infants during the first days of life. Biol Neonate 86:207, 2004.

64. Allegaert K, Vanhole C, de Hoon J, et al. Nonselective cyclo-oxygenase inhibitors and glomerular filtration rate in preterm neonates. Pediatr Nephrol 20:1557, 2005.

65. Guignard JP. The adverse renal effects of prostaglandin-synthesis inhibitors in the newborn rabbit. Semin Perinatol 26:398, 2002.

66. Chamaa NS, Mosig D, Drukker A, et al. The renal hemodynamic effects of ibuprofen in the newborn rabbit. Pediatr Res 48:600, 2000.

67. Prevot A, Mosig D, Martini S, et al. Nimesulide, a cyclooxygenase-2 preferential inhibitor, impairs renal function in the newborn rabbit. Pediatr Res 55:254, 2004.

68. Cunniff C, Jones KL, Phillipson J, et al. Oligohydramnios sequence and renal tubular malformation associated with maternal enalapril use. Am J Obstet Gynecol 162:187, 1990.

69. Tack ED, Perlman JM. Renal failure in sick hypertensive premature infants receiving captopril therapy. J Pediatr 112:805, 1988.

70. Dubourg L, Mosig D, Drukker A, et al. Torasemide is an effective diuretic in the newborn rabbit. Pediatr Nephrol 14:476, 2000.

71. Dubourg L, Drukker A, Guignard JP. Failure of the loop diuretic torasemide to improve renal function of hypoxemic vasomotor nephropathy in the newborn rabbit. Pediatr Res 47:504, 2000.

72. Brion LP, Soll RF. Diuretics for respiratory distress syndrome in preterm infants. Cochrane Database Syt Rev 2: CD001454, 2001.

73. Barrington K, Brion LP. Dopamine versus no treatment to prevent renal dysfunction in indomethacin-treated preterm newborn infants. Cochrane Database Syst Rev 3: CD003213, 2002.

74. Seri I, Abbasi S, Wood DC, et al. Regional hemodynamic effects of dopamine in the indomethacin-treated preterm infant. J Perinatol 22:300, 2002.

75. Lauschke A, Teichgraber UK, Frei U, Eckhardt KU. "Low-dose" dopamine worsens renal perfusion in patients with acute renal failure. Kidney Int 65:1416, 2004.

76. Prins I, Plotz FB, Uiterwaal CS, et al. Low-dose dopamine in neonatal and pediatric intensive care: a systematic review. Intensive Care Med 27:206, 2001.

77. Lynch SK, Lemley KV, Polak MJ. The effect of dopamine on glomerular filtration rate in normotensive, oliguric premature neonates. Pediatr Nephrol 18:649, 2003.

78. Jaton T, Thonney M, Gouyon JB, et al. Renal effects of dopamine and dopexamine in the newborn anesthetized rabbit. Life Sci 50:195, 1992.

79. Jaton T, Thonney M, Guignard JP. Failure of dopexamine to protect the hypoxemic newborn rabbit kidney. Dev Pharmacol Ther 17:161, 1991.

80. Huet F, Semama D, Grimaldi M, et al. Effects of theophylline on renal insufficiency in neonates with respiratory distress syndrome. Intensive Care Med 21:511, 1995.

81. Jenik AG, Ceriani Cernadas JM, Gorenstein A, et al. A randomized, double blind, placebo-controlled trial of the effects of prophylactic theophylline on renal function in term neonates with perinatal asphyxia. Pediatrics 105(4):e45, 2000.

82. Bakr AF. Prophylactic theophylline to prevent renal dysfunction in newborns exposed to perinatal asphyxia—a study in a developing country. Pediatr Nephrol 20:1249, 2005.

83. Bhat MA, Shah ZA, Makhdoomi MS, Mufti MH. Theophylline for renal function in term neonates with perinatal asphyxia: A randomized, placebo-controlled trial. J Pediatr 149:e180–e184, 2006.

84. Cattarelli D, Spandrio M, Gasparoni A, et al. A randomized, double blind, placebo controlled trial of the effect of theophylline in prevention of vasomotor nephropathy in very preterm neonates with respiratory distress syndrome. Arch Dis Child Fetal Neonatal Ed 91:F80, 2006.

85. Prévot A, Mosig D, Rijtema M, et al. Renal effects of adenosine A1-receptor blockade with 8-cyclopentyl-1, 3-dipropylxanthine in hypoxemic newborn rabbits. Pediatr Res 54:400, 2003.

Chapter 6

The Developing Kidney and the Fetal Origins of Adult Cardiovascular Disease

Umberto Simeoni, MD • Farid Boubred, MD •
Christophe Buffat, PharmD • Daniel Vaiman, PhD

Developmental Origins of Health and Disease

Nephron Number Reduction

**Molecular Mechanisms Involved in the Developmental Origins of
Cardiovascular Disease**

Conclusion

Since the pioneering work of David Barker and colleagues (1), worldwide epidemiological studies have demonstrated that low birth weight is associated with an increased risk of death due to coronary heart disease (2–4). The path between early development and adult disease has been shown to involve arterial hypertension and metabolic disorders, such as insulin-resistance and hyperlipidemia, the elements of 'metabolic syndrome' or 'X syndrome' (5,6). The concept of the developmental origins and programming of adult disease is now widely understood, as evidence of the relationship between early growth and development and disease occurring in the long term is growing.

Studies on blood pressure and early growth show that in both children and adults there is an inverse relationship between birth weight and arterial blood pressure: blood pressure is increased by reduced birth weight, the size of this effect ranging between 1–3 mmHg/kg of birth weight (7). Such findings have been replicated with various animal models of intrauterine growth restriction (IUGR), in guinea pig (8), sheep (9) and particularly rat (10–12). The developing kidney has been shown to be one key organ involved in the programming of hypertension in adulthood, due in particular to the definitive reduction in the total number of nephrons, which is a characteristic of low birth weight (13–15).

While evidence of the early programming of cardiovascular function and disease is provided by studies including subjects whose low birth weight is likely to be caused principally by IUGR, recent studies raised the issue of the long term consequences of low or very low birth weight due to preterm birth. Premature birth has been shown to be associated with elevated arterial blood pressure in adulthood independent of birth weight (16–19).

The aim of this review is to summarize current knowledge on the physiological, structural and molecular mechanisms by which the kidney is involved in the developmental origins of arterial hypertension, and to discuss the potential impact of such findings on care and follow-up of low birth weight subjects and patients.

DEVELOPMENTAL ORIGINS OF HEALTH AND DISEASE

Key concepts have been proposed to understand both epidemiologic findings and animal experimental data on the early influences that control long term health and diseases.

The early origins of adult diseases hypothesis has been developed by Barker and colleagues after they characterized a relationship between increased coronary heart disease mortality rates with decreasing birth weight in a cohort of men and women whose characteristics at birth were known, in Hertfordshire, UK(1). According to this concept, environmental factors, in particular nutrition, act early during fetal and postnatal life to program the risk for later cardiovascular and metabolic disease in adulthood. Common risk factors for cardiovascular disease, such as arterial hypertension, hyperlipidemia, type 2 diabetes and the components of the metabolic syndrome, a major cause of mortality in developed countries, are thus at least in part associated with early life environment.

The Thrifty Phenotype Hypothesis

The thrifty phenotype hypothesis has been the principal mechanistic frame proposed to explain that an adverse fetal respiratory and nutritional environment results in an adaptive response designed to protect key fetal organs and systems, such as the brain and the heart, to the detriment of others, resulting in a physiologic programming that then enables the newborn to adapt and thrive under scarce environmental conditions. Such an adaptive response to fetal chronic stress, however, results in detrimental effects such as type 2 diabetes mellitus when the postnatal environment is abundant, instead of restricted (20). Immediate fetal and neonatal survival advantage is thus balanced by unfavorable long term consequences. However, the thrifty phenotype theory may show its limits when taking into account that not only low birth weight due to intrauterine growth restriction, but also to preterm birth (16–19,21), is associated with long term functional alterations such as increased arterial blood pressure or insulin resistance. Indeed, new paradigms are needed as premature birth most frequently is not associated with chronic fetal distress.

The Role of Altered Growth during Fetal Life and Infancy and Later Growth Acceleration

The idea that a poor environment during fetal and infantile life, contrasting later with more affluent nutritional conditions, may favor disease and premature death is supported by studies relating infantile mortality rates and mortality due to coronary heart disease in adulthood within specific areas in Norway (22).

Late infancy seems a key period in programming the risk of adult disease by switching from poor growth early in life to a more favorable nutrition. Low weight at birth, but also at the age of 1 year has been shown to be associated with higher rates of cardiovascular mortality (2). Studies in Finland show that low birth weight, associated with later catch-up growth after the age of two, are associated with increased rates of death from coronary heart disease (23). In parallel to low birth weight, longitudinal studies and nutritional intervention studies on premature babies suggested that postnatal growth, especially accelerated weight gain, may play an important role in programming later cardiovascular diseases (7,24–30). Infants with low birth weight often show accelerated rates of growth in infancy and early childhood, a phenomenon known as catch-up growth. The critical 'window' when catch-up growth contributes to higher blood pressure in adulthood is still in discussion. Many studies have shown that increased weight gain in early childhood (5–7 years) is independently associated with increased blood pressure levels in adulthood, while others have suggested that body mass index in pre-adolescents (11–15 years), which is predicted by early postnatal growth, contributes to cardiovascular disease in adults.

The role of weight gain in the first months of postnatal life is a matter of considerable interest. In a nutritional intervention study, Lucas et al have shown that increased weight gain during the first two weeks of postnatal life was associated with elevated diastolic blood pressure in adolescents born preterm (29). In some populations, reduced infant growth seems to confer additional cardiovascular risk that is predicted by birth weight, and may independently affect blood pressure in adulthood. In a young adult population study in Hong Kong, those who were thinner and, independently, those who had gained less body mass between 6–18 months, had higher systolic blood pressure (30). The authors suggested that the poor infant growth may be due to living disadvantages and a higher burden of infectious diseases. Similar results have been observed in 11–12 year-old Jamaican children who were stunted in early infancy (6–24 months) (28). However, such a relationship has not been observed in other studies (24,25). The fact that an impairment of fetal growth and/or growth during early infancy, followed by an accelerated postnatal growth, may contribute to elevated blood pressure in adulthood, suggests that postnatal adaptations in growth are responsible for higher levels of blood pressure later. The role of postnatal nutrition on programming later systemic hypertension has been confirmed by animal models (31,32). Studies in our laboratory show that arterial blood pressure is elevated in adult rats exposed to early postnatal overfeeding (obtained by reduction of litter size during the suckling period). Such an effect is amplified by a high caloric diet in young adult rats born with intrauterine growth restriction (Boubred et al 2007, unpublished data).

It thus appears that the early programming of durable physiologic alterations and risk of disease is likely to occur at critical periods of early life, during a sensitive window covering fetal life and infancy. Such critical periods allow developmental plasticity, i.e., the ability of a single genotype to produce different phenotypes, to take place (33).

Being born small at birth may reflect a process that involves adaptive responses. However, small size at birth may also induce responses that intervene as consequences of the process, and are defective in nature. For example, low birth weight, whether due to intrauterine growth restriction or to preterm birth, is associated with a reduction in the constitutive nephron endowment. As far as its consequences are known, congenital nephron number reduction is not likely to reflect an adaptive response, but simply an arrest in nephron development that may induce long term renal and vascular physiologic changes of utmost importance.

NEPHRON NUMBER REDUCTION

Experimental studies and human findings provide evidence for a pathogenic link between low nephron number and systemic hypertension and renal function deterioration. In animals as well as in humans, a reduction in nephron number leads to the development of hypertension and progressive renal failure. It has been shown that in some individuals born with a solitary kidney or with severe degrees of oligomeganephronia, hypertension and renal disease develop (34). Interestingly, in a recent autopsy study, patients with essential hypertension had a significantly lower nephron number and higher glomerular volume than sex and age-matched normotensive patients (15). Such findings have been reproduced in recent

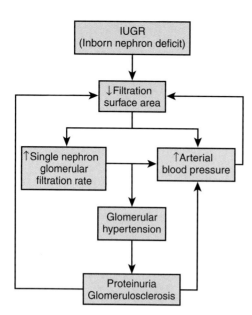

Figure 6-1 Pathogenesis of elevated blood pressure and reduced glomerular function associated with decreased birth weight and nephron endowment. (After Brenner BM, Garcia DL, Anderson S: Glomeruli and blood pressure. Less of one, more the other? Am J Hypertens 1:335-47, 1988.)

experimental studies of reduced nephron mass. Reduction of nephron mass by nephrectomy during nephrogenesis is associated with arterial hypertension and alteration of glomerular filtration rate in adulthood (35,36). Nephrogenesis is achieved in the human before delivery, up to the 34th week of gestation and is influenced by the fetal environment. It is clearly established that an adverse fetal environment results in fetal growth restriction, alters nephron formation and is responsible for a reduced total number of nephrons (37). Such nephron number deficit is considered permanent throughout life despite improved postnatal nutrition. Studies on necropsies of human fetuses and newborns, and experimental studies in various animal species have shown that the total number of nephrons is proportional to birth weight and is reduced by approximately 30–40% when IUGR is present (37,38). Hughson et al have shown in an autopsy study a relationship between birth weight and nephron number and an adaptive increase in glomerular volume (39).

However, little is known regarding glomerulogenesis in preterm infants. It has been postulated that nephrogenesis may be impaired when part of it has to develop 'ex-utero', contributing to the susceptibility of preterm infants to hypertension in adulthood. In an autopsy study of 56 extremely premature infants, whose birth weights were, in the majority, appropriate for gestational age, Rodriguez et al found that nephrogenesis was considerably decreased compared to term controls, and radial glomerular count number correlated with gestational age. However, markers of active glomerulogenesis were absent in longer surviving extremely low birth weight infants, as in term controls whose nephrogenesis was terminated. Signs of impaired nephrogenesis were furthermore accentuated in patients who suffered from renal failure (40).

As postulated by Brenner and co-workers, nephron deficit as a result of intra-uterine growth restriction leads to reduced filtration surface area and glomerular single nephron hyperfiltration, which is responsible over a long time for glomerular injury, long term proteinuria, glomerulosclerosis, progressive deterioration of renal function and finally hypertension (14) (Fig. 6-1). Compensatory glomerular hemodynamic changes associated with increased single-nephron glomerular filtration rate (SNGFR) initiate and perpetuate injury following inborn nephron deficit. In response to reduced nephron number, remaining nephrons undergo an adaptation in structure and function, including nephron hypertrophy (an increase in glomerular volume) and increases in SNGFR to meet excretory demands. Such compensatory adaptation, which at first appears beneficial, may have a harmful long-term effect. Recent experimental studies have shown that other mechanisms may be involved in such adaptive changes. Both renal expression of and responsiveness to the renin-angiotensin system are up-regulated during early adulthood in intrauterine growth restricted rats, further increasing the systemic blood pressure needed to maintain sodium and water balance (41).

In general, hypertension occurs because of reduced GFR, and the inability of the kidney to maintain sodium and water balance at a normal pressure. The effects on renal function of accelerated weight gain, favored by high caloric and protein intakes, are not completely known but they may contribute to an alteration in renal function in adulthood. It has been known for a long time that a high protein intake in rats is associated with an adaptive, elevated glomerular filtration rate and renal hypertrophy, which result over a long time in glomerular damage, especially when renal mass is reduced (42,43).

Little is known about the effects of low birth weight and renal function in adult humans. It has been shown in south-eastern USA that low birth weight contributes to the early onset of end-stage renal disease, but more studies are needed to confirm and detail the renal consequences of low birth weight in humans (44). Recently, Keijzer-Veen MG et al, in a prospective follow-up study of young adults born preterm in the Netherlands, have shown that renal function was altered in those born with intrauterine growth restriction (21).

MOLECULAR MECHANISMS INVOLVED IN THE DEVELOPMENTAL ORIGINS OF CARDIOVASCULAR DISEASE

Nephron formation during embryonic and fetal life occurs through the epithelial differentiation of mesenchymal cells within the nephrogenic blastema, induced by the adjacent ureteric bud branch division. It is thus not surprising that the expression of genes involved in kidney development is altered in conditions of adverse intra-uterine environment such as IUGR. Renin-angiotensin system components, mRNA and protein expression are down-regulated in rats born with intra-uterine growth restriction, further confirming the role of renin as a renal growth factor (45).

Vitamin A deficiency has been shown to alter nephron development in rats, and may be a key factor in nephron mass reduction due to intra-uterine growth restriction (46,47). Indeed, a 50% reduction in maternal retinol circulating concentration leads to a 20% reduction in nephron number in the offspring, while overall fetal development was not affected, a fact confirmed in cultured explanted metanephroi (46). Genes of specific growth-factors, such as midkine, a retinoic-acid responsive gene to a heparin-binding growth-factor, have been shown to interfere with nephron development alteration due to retinoic acid deficiency (48). The regulation cascade of all-trans-retinoic acid control of nephron development involves C-ret, as both C-ret mRNA and protein are significantly altered in conditions of retinoic acid deficiency in vitro (49).

In its early days the thrifty phenotype hypothesis seems to have been largely ignored by the medical profession, possibly due to a lack of a plausible mechanism. The phenomenon was, however, well known to biologists, who refer to it as developmental plasticity to convey the ability to change structure and function in an irreversible fashion, during a critical time window in response to a pre- or postnatal environment (33,50). The environment has great influence on phenotypic expression with the aim of adaptation to the conditions of existence. Adaptation of species follows the line of evolution, which operates over very long periods and many generations, giving rise to genetic variation in populations and ultimately new species driven by mutation, gene flow and genetic drift. Populations adapt on an intermediate scale within one or a few life spans, and individuals adapt in fractions of a life span. Adaptation by mutation cannot parallel short-term environmental alterations and the necessary flexibility comes from regulation of gene expression. This may occur by moment to moment control via transcriptional activators and repressors, which respond through a sequence of signal transduction mechanisms to external stimuli such as nutrients, sunlight, also named labile regulation (51). A second mechanism is by epigenetic regulation (51,52). Epigenetics comprise the stable and heritable (or potentially heritable) changes in gene expression that do not entail a change in DNA sequence.

One molecular background of epigenetic changes is by alteration of chromatin structure through modification of histones by methylation, acetylation, phosphorylation and ubiquitylation, all together giving rise to what is referred to as the epigenotype. But the best characterized epigenetic modifications concern DNA and consist of the methylation of cytosine residues within CpG dinucleotides (53). DNA methylation is of particular importance for gene regulation and is strongly implicated in fetal development. Even minor changes to the degree of gene methylation can have severe consequences. An accurate quantification of the methylation status at any given position within the genome is a powerful diagnostic indicator.

Folate Status, Diet, DNA Methylation, Imprinted Genes and Programming

Folate, a water-soluble B group vitamin, is essential for the transfer of one-carbon units (54). It is indispensable to the methionine cycle and therefore to the synthesis of S-adenosylmethionine, the common methyl donor for DNA methylation. The status of folate and of other substrates and cofactors in one-carbon metabolism may consequently be expected to influence phenotype, an abnormal status or imbalances being able to cause diseases such as neurological disorders, cancer, endocrine and cardiovascular diseases.

Folate deficiency leads to a decrease in S-adenosylmethionine and an increase in homocysteine. Abnormalities in folate metabolism and DNA methylation have been associated with Down's syndrome, and aberrant DNA methylation has been implicated in the pathogenesis of neurological disorders including Alzheimer's, Parkinson's, and Huntington's diseases (55). Altered DNA methylation has been extensively documented in tumorigenesis (54).

Nutritional anomalies, either during the entire pregnancy period, or at critical ontogenetic stages, are likely to have major and persistent effects on the fetal epigenotype and thereby the expression or depression of genes that may cause disease in later life. Nutrition, via nutrient-gene interaction, may in this way at least partially determine phenotypic characteristics and this phenotype may subsequently be transmitted to future generations, given that the epigenome can to some extent be conveyed too. The epigenetic make-up may constitute a link between low birth weight and cardiovascular disease and many other complex diseases at adult age (53).

Several research studies focused on those classes of elements in the genome that are particularly sensitive to nutritional regulation during early life. There is a growing body of evidence from studies of *in vitro* embryo culture that the methylation status of genomically imprinted genes, including IGF2, H19, IGF2R, etc., can be altered with consequences for subsequent organ growth and function (53,56,57). Importantly, the epigenetic lability of imprinted genes is not limited to the preimplantation period and includes the early postnatal period in rodents (58). Recent studies have also demonstrated that retrotransposons are elements within the genome that may also be epigenetically labile to early nutrition (59,60).

Genomic Imprinting and Nutrient Supply to the Fetus

Directional effects on fetal growth of maternally and paternally expressed genes have been documented in a number of mouse knockouts. Paternally expressed genes involved with fetal growth tend to increase fetal size whereas maternally expressed genes decrease fetal size. Imprinted genes are epigenetically regulated and play important roles in development such as fetal growth, placental development and function, and behavior after birth (61,62). The control of fetal growth by imprinted genes can be exerted at the level of cell proliferation, apoptosis and extracellular fluid composition in the fetus.

To prove that such mechanisms are at work in kidney development, asymmetric IUGR was induced through bilateral uterine artery ligation in pregnant rats by Pham et al (63). Uteroplacental insufficiency reduced glomeruli number while increasing TUNEL staining and caspase-3 activity in the IUGR kidney, both indicating increased apoptosis. Furthermore, a significant decrease in Bcl-2 mRNA and a significant increase in Bax and p53 mRNA were observed.

Genomic imprinting is thought to have evolved as a result of genetic conflict between paternal and maternal genomes over the allocation of maternal resources, leading to the prediction that imprinted genes have substantial control over size at birth. This is confirmed by recent studies, from which we have suggested that imprinted genes have central roles in the genetic control of both the fetal demand for, and the placenta supply of, maternal nutrients. Constancia et al have recently provided the demonstration that dys-regulation of an imprinted gene, specifically in the placenta, affects fetal growth by showing that placental-specific Igf2 is an important modulator for fetal growth in the mouse (64). The Ifg2 gene combines and balances the genetic control of supply (through expression in the placenta) with the genetic control of demand (through expression in the fetus) for nutrients. This hypothesis can be extended to other imprinted genes. Paternally expressed genes in the fetus increase the demand for nutrients, and maternally expressed genes in the fetus decrease demand for nutrients. Alterations in demand may create a signal to the placenta to alter supply. Knowledge of how nutrient supply and demand is genetically regulated is crucial for understanding the mechanisms of fetal growth restriction. The role of human imprinted genes in fetal growth restriction, however, remains poorly understood, largely through the difficulties of human experimentation.

CONCLUSION

Increasing, clinical and experimental data support the concept that renal function in adulthood seems partly 'programmed' in utero and/or in the early postnatal period, independently of the eventual occurrence of congenital or acquired kidney disease. Such developmental programming of function and disease in adulthood is related to low birth weight, whether due to intrauterine growth restriction or premature birth and involves a permanent nephron number reduction. The consequent glomerular hyperfiltration contributes to the increased arterial blood pressure in adulthood. The long term influence of postnatal nutrition, especially protein intake, on the development of renal function, especially in conditions of altered perinatal renal development, is still unknown. Knowledge of the molecular mechanisms underlying nephron number reduction and corresponding adaptive changes is in considerable progress. Epigenetic changes are likely to be key molecular factors in the long term memory that characterizes long term consequences of altered perinatal growth and development.

REFERENCES

1. Barker DJ, Winter PD, Osmond C, Margetts B, Simmonds SJ. Weight in infancy and death from ischaemic heart disease. Lancet 2:577–580, 1989.

2. Osmond C, Barker DJ, Winter PD, Fall CH, Simmonds SJ. Early growth and death from cardiovascular disease in women. BMJ 307:1519–1524, 1993.

3. Stein CE, Fall CH, Kumaran K, Osmond C, Cox V, Barker DJ. Fetal growth and coronary heart disease in south India. Lancet 348:1269–1273, 1996.

4. Eriksson JG, Forsen T, Tuomilehto J, Osmond C, Barker DJ. Early growth and coronary heart disease in later life: longitudinal study. BMJ 322:949–953, 2001.

5. Hales CN, Barker DJ, Clark PM, Cox LJ, Fall C, Osmond C, Winter PD. Fetal and infant growth and impaired glucose tolerance at age 64. BMJ 303:1019–1022, 1991.

6. Barker DJ, Hales CN, Fall CH, Osmond C, Phipps K, Clark PM. Type 2 (non-insulin-dependent) diabetes mellitus, hypertension and hyperlipidaemia (syndrome X): relation to reduced fetal growth. Diabetologia 36:62–67, 1993.

7. Huxley RR, Shiell AW, Law CM. The role of size at birth and postnatal catch-up growth in determining systolic blood pressure: a systematic review of the literature. J Hypertens 18:815–831, 2000.

8. Persson E, Jansson T. Low birth weight is associated with elevated adult blood pressure in the chronically catheterized guinea-pig. Acta Physiol Scand 145:195–196, 1992.

9. Moritz K, Butkus A, Hantzis V, Peers A, Wintour EM, Dodic M. Prolonged low-dose dexamethasone, in early gestation, has no long-term deleterious effect on normal ovine fetuses. Endocrinology 143:1159–1165, 2002.

10. Langley-Evans SC, Gardner DS, Welham SJ. Intrauterine programming of cardiovascular disease by maternal nutritional status. Nutrition 14:39–47, 1998.

11. Woodall SM, Johnston BM, Breier BH, Gluckman PD. Chronic maternal undernutrition in the rat leads to delayed postnatal growth and elevated blood pressure of offspring. Pediatr Res 40:438–443, 1996.

12. Ozaki T, Nishina H, Hanson MA, Poston L. Dietary restriction in pregnant rats causes gender-related hypertension and vascular dysfunction in offspring. J Physiol 530:141–152, 2001.

13. Merlet-Benichou C. Influence of fetal environment on kidney development. Int J Dev Biol 43:453–456, 1999.

14. Brenner BM, Garcia DL, Anderson S. Glomeruli and blood pressure. Less of one, more the other? Am J Hypertens 1:335–347, 1988.

15. Keller G, Zimmer G, Mall G, Ritz E, Amann K. Nephron number in patients with primary hypertension. N Engl J Med 348:101–108, 2003.

16. Kistner A, Jacobson L, Jacobson SH, Svensson E, Hellstrom A. Low gestational age associated with abnormal retinal vascularization and increased blood pressure in adult women. Pediatr Res 51:675–680, 2002.

17. Kistner A, Celsi G, Vanpee M, Jacobson SH. Increased systolic daily ambulatory blood pressure in adult women born preterm. Pediatr Nephrol 20:232–233, 2005.

18. Keijzer–Veen MG, Finken MJ, Nauta J, Dekker FW, Hille ET, Frolich M, Wit JM, van der Heijden AJ. Is blood pressure increased 19 years after intrauterine growth restriction and preterm birth? A prospective follow-up study in The Netherlands. Pediatrics 116:725–731, 2005.

19. Irving RJ, Belton NR, Elton RA, Walker BR. Adult cardiovascular risk factors in premature babies. Lancet 355:2135–2136, 2000.

20. Hales CN, Barker DJ. Type 2 (non-insulin-dependent) diabetes mellitus: the thrifty phenotype hypothesis. Diabetologia 35:595–601, 1992.

21. Keijzer-Veen MG, Schrevel M, Finken MJ, Dekker FW, Nauta J, Hille ET, Frolich M, van der Heijden BJ. Microalbuminuria and lower glomerular filtration rate at young adult age in subjects born very premature and after intrauterine growth retardation. J Am Soc Nephrol 16:2762–2768, 2005.

22. Forsdahl A. Are poor living conditions in childhood and adolescence an important risk factor for arteriosclerotic heart disease? Br J Prev Soc Med 31:91–95, 1977.

23. Barker DJ, Osmond C, Forsen TJ, Kajantie E, Eriksson JG. Trajectories of growth among children who have coronary events as adults. N Engl J Med 353:1802–1809, 2005.

24. Law CM, Shiell AW, Newsome CA, Syddall HE, Shinebourne EA, Fayers PM, Martyn CN, de Swiet M. Fetal, infant, and childhood growth and adult blood pressure: a longitudinal study from birth to 22 years of age. Circulation 105:1088–1092, 2002.

25. Adair LS, Cole TJ. Rapid child growth raises blood pressure in adolescent boys who were thin at birth. Hypertension 41:451–456, 2003.

26. Cruickshank JK, Mzayek F, Liu L, Kieltyka L, Sherwin R, Webber LS, Srinavasan SR, Berenson GS. Origins of the 'black/white' difference in blood pressure: roles of birth weight, postnatal growth, early blood pressure, and adolescent body size: the Bogalusa heart study. Circulation 111:1932–1937, 2005.

27. Eriksson J, Forsen T, Tuomilehto J, Osmond C, Barker D. Fetal and childhood growth and hypertension in adult life. Hypertension 36:790–794, 2000.

28. Walker SP, Gaskin P, Powell CA, Bennett FI, Forrester TE, Grantham-McGregor S. The effects of birth weight and postnatal linear growth retardation on blood pressure at age 11–12 years. J Epidemiol Community Health 55:394–398, 2001.

29. Singhal A, Cole TJ, Lucas A. Early nutrition in preterm infants and later blood pressure: two cohorts after randomised trials. Lancet 357:413–419, 2001.

30. Cheung YB, Low L, Osmond C, Barker D, Karlberg J. Fetal growth and early postnatal growth are related to blood pressure in adults. Hypertension 36:795–800, 2000.

31. Vickers MH, Breier BH, Cutfield WS, Hofman PL, Gluckman PD. Fetal origins of hyperphagia, obesity, and hypertension and postnatal amplification by hypercaloric nutrition. Am J Physiol Endocrinol Metab 279:E83–E87, 2000.

32. Plagemann A, Heidrich I, Gotz F, Rohde W, Dorner G. Obesity and enhanced diabetes and cardiovascular risk in adult rats due to early postnatal overfeeding. Exp Clin Endocrinol 99:154–158, 1992.

33. Gluckman PD, Hanson MA. Living with the past: evolution, development, and patterns of disease. Science 305:1733–1736, 2004.

34. Mei-Zahav M, Korzets Z, Cohen I, Kessler O, Rathaus V, Wolach B, Pomeranz A. Ambulatory blood pressure monitoring in children with a solitary kidney—a comparison between unilateral renal agenesis and uninephrectomy. Blood Press Monit 6:263–267, 2001.

35. Woods LL. Neonatal uninephrectomy causes hypertension in adult rats. Am J Physiol 276:R974–R978, 1999.

36. Moritz KM, Wintour EM, Dodic M. Fetal uninephrectomy leads to postnatal hypertension and compromised renal function. Hypertension 39:1071–1076, 2002.

37. Merlet-Benichou C, Gilbert T, Vilar J, Moreau E, Freund N, Lelievre-Pegorier M. Nephron number: variability is the rule. Causes and consequences. Lab Invest 79:515–527, 1999.

38. Hinchliffe SA, Lynch MR, Sargent PH, Howard CV, Van Velzen D. The effect of intrauterine growth retardation on the development of renal nephrons. Br J Obstet Gynaecol 99:296–301, 1992.

39. Hughson M, Farris AB 3rd, Douglas-Denton R, Hoy WE, Bertram JF. Glomerular number and size in autopsy kidneys: the relationship to birth weight. Kidney Int 63:2113–2122, 2003.

40. Rodriguez MM, Gomez AH, Abitbol CL, Chandar JJ, Duara S, Zilleruelo GE. Histomorphometric analysis of postnatal glomerulogenesis in extremely preterm infants. Pediatr Dev Pathol 7:17–25, 2004.

41. Vehaskari VM, Stewart T, Lafont D, Soyez C, Seth D, Manning J. Kidney angiotensin and angiotensin receptor expression in prenatally programmed hypertension. Am J Physiol Renal Physiol 287:F262–F267, 2004.

42. Hammond KA, Janes DN. The effects of increased protein intake on kidney size and function. J Exp Biol 201:2081–2090, 1998.

43. O'Donnell MP, Kasiske BL, Schmitz PG, Keane WF. High protein intake accelerates glomerulosclerosis independent of effects on glomerular hemodynamics. Kidney Int 37:1263–1269, 1990.

44. Lackland DT, Bendall HE, Osmond C, Egan BM, Barker DJ. Low birth weights contribute to high rates of early-onset chronic renal failure in the Southeastern United States. Arch Intern Med 160:1472–1476, 2000.

45. Woods LL, Ingelfinger JR, Nyengaard JR, Rasch R. Maternal protein restriction suppresses the newborn renin-angiotensin system and programs adult hypertension in rats. Pediatr Res 49:460–467, 2001.

46. Lelievre-Pegorier M, Vilar J, Ferrier ML, Moreau E, Freund N, Gilbert T, Merlet-Benichou C. Mild vitamin A deficiency leads to inborn nephron deficit in the rat. Kidney Int 54:1455–1462, 1998.

47. Merlet-Benichou C, Vilar J, Lelievre-Pegorier M, Gilbert T. Role of retinoids in renal development: pathophysiological implication. Curr Opin Nephrol Hypertens 8:39–43, 1999.

48. Vilar J, Lalou C, Duong VH, Charrin S, Hardouin S, Raulais D, Merlet-Benichou C, Lelievre-Pegorier M. Midkine is involved in kidney development and in its regulation by retinoids. J Am Soc Nephrol 13:668–676, 2002.

49. Moreau E, Vilar J, Lelievre-Pegorier M, Merlet-Benichou C, Gilbert T. Regulation of c-ret expression by retinoic acid in rat metanephros: implication in nephron mass control. Am J Physiol 275:F938–F945, 1998.

50. Stewart RJ, Sheppard H, Preece R, Waterlow JC. The effect of rehabilitation at different stages of development of rats marginally malnourished for ten to twelve generations. Br J Nutr 43:403–412, 1980.

51. Jiang YH, Bressler J, Beaudet AL. Epigenetics and human disease. Annu Rev Genomics Hum Genet 5:479–510, 2004.

52. Abdolmaleky HM, Smith CL, Faraone SV, Shafa R, Stone W, Glatt SJ, Tsuang MT. Methylomics in psychiatry: Modulation of gene-environment interactions may be through DNA methylation. Am J Med Genet B Neuropsychiatr Genet 127:51–59, 2004.

53. Waterland RA, Jirtle RL. Early nutrition, epigenetic changes at transposons and imprinted genes, and enhanced susceptibility to adult chronic diseases. Nutrition 20:63–68, 2004.

54. Lucock M. Folic acid: nutritional biochemistry, molecular biology, and role in disease processes. Mol Genet Metab 71:121–138, 2000.

55. Mattson MP. Methylation and acetylation in nervous system development and neurodegenerative disorders. Ageing Res Rev 2:329–342, 2003.

56. Young LE. Imprinting of genes and the Barker hypothesis. Twin Res 4:307–317, 2001.

57. Young LE, Fernandes K, McEvoy TG, Butterwith SC, Gutierrez CG, Carolan C, Broadbent PJ, Robinson JJ, Wilmut I, Sinclair KD. Epigenetic change in IGF2R is associated with fetal overgrowth after sheep embryo culture. Nat Genet 27:153–154, 2001.

58. Waterland RA, Garza C. Early postnatal nutrition determines adult pancreatic glucose-responsive insulin secretion and islet gene expression in rats. J Nutr 132:357–364, 2002.

59. Waterland RA, Jirtle RL. Transposable elements: targets for early nutritional effects on epigenetic gene regulation. Mol Cell Biol 23:5293–5300, 2003.

60. Wolff GL, Kodell RL, Moore SR, Cooney CA. Maternal epigenetics and methyl supplements affect agouti gene expression in Avy/a mice. Faseb J 12:949–957, 1998.

61. Reik W, Walter J. Genomic imprinting: parental influence on the genome. Nat Rev Genet 2:21–32, 2001.

62. Tycko B, Morison IM. Physiological functions of imprinted genes. J Cell Physiol 192:245–258, 2002.

63. Pham TD, MacLennan NK, Chiu CT, Laksana GS, Hsu JL, Lane RH. Uteroplacental insufficiency increases apoptosis and alters p53 gene methylation in the full-term IUGR rat kidney. Am J Physiol Regul Integr Comp Physiol 285:R962–R970, 2003.

64. Constancia M, Hemberger M, Hughes J, Dean W, Ferguson-Smith A, Fundele R, Stewart F, Kelsey G, Fowden A, Sibley C, Reik W. Placental-specific IGF-II is a major modulator of placental and fetal growth. Nature 417:945–948, 2002.

Chapter 7

Renal Modulation: The Renin-Angiotensin-Aldosterone System (RAAS)

Aruna Natarajan, MD, DCh • Pedro A. Jose, MD, PhD

Components of the RAAS
Ontogeny
Current Concepts and Controversies
Summary

The renin-angiotensin-aldosterone system (RAAS) plays a critical role in the maintenance of salt and water homeostasis by the kidney, particularly in hypovolemic or salt-depleted states. The net effect of the unopposed activation of this system results in sodium retention, potassium loss, and an increase in blood pressure (1).

COMPONENTS OF THE RAAS

Angiotensin Generation

Renin is synthesized in the juxtaglomerular (JG) cells (smooth muscle cells in the walls of the afferent arteriole as it enters the glomerulus), and is stored as prorenin (2–5). It is released as renin, and regulated by renal afferent arteriolar baroreceptors and the macula densa of the distal nephron of the kidney. Renin enzymatically causes the formation of angiotensin I (Ang I) from angiotensinogen. Ang I is acted upon by angiotensin converting enzyme (ACE) to form angiotensin II (Ang II). The rate limiting step in this sequence of events in humans is the release of renin, rendering it the most well regulated variable of all constituents of the Renin-Angiotensin System (RAS). Renin secretion/release is increased by three primary pathways: (i) stimulation of renal baroreceptors by a decrease in afferent arterial stretch (pressure) (6,7); (ii) stimulation of renal β_1-adrenergic receptors, in part, through renal sympathetic nerve activity (8–10); and (iii) a decrease in sodium and chloride delivery to, and transport by, the macula densa (11,12). Renin secretion can also be regulated by several endocrine and paracrine hormones.

ACE acts on Ang I (Ang 1-10) to cleave off the active octapeptide, Ang II (Ang 1-8), which is a more potent vasoconstrictor than Ang I (13). Ang II can also be formed by non-ACE enzymes and non-renin enzymes, such as chymase, cathepsin G, cathepsin A and tissue plasminogen activator (t-PA) (14). This assumes greater significance in the organs where not all components of the RAS are expressed, providing alternate means of generation of Ang II, the physiological significance of which is still not well understood, and may be organ specific. For example, mast cells produce renin, and have chymases, which help form Ang II and may play a role in heart failure and generation of arrhythmias (15).

ACE2 is a recently identified human homolog of ACE, sharing about 42% sequence homology. ACE2 converts Ang II to Ang 1-7. Ang 1-7 has vasodilator, antigrowth and antiproliferative properties, and exerts counterregulatory effects on Ang II. ACE 2 also decreases the level of Ang II by converting Ang I to Ang 1-9, an inactive nonapeptide (16,17). Thus, it appears that ACE and ACE2 exert opposing roles on the effects of the RAS. Unlike ACE, ACE2 is unable to inactivate bradykinin, and is insensitive to currently available ACE inhibitors. ACE2 has been identified as the receptor for the SARS-corona virus (SARS-CoV), allowing entry of the SARS-CoV into the cell (18,19). ACE2 may contribute to the localized overproduction of Ang 1-7 in the kidney, observed during pregnancy, which might protect against a rise in blood pressure (20).

Synthesis of the components of the RAAS occurs to a greater extent in certain organs relative to others, such as angiotensinogen in the liver, renin in the kidney, ACE in the lung, and aldosterone in the adrenal glands, which function together as an endocrine system. Some or all of its components are expressed in the brain, heart, vasculature, adipose tissue, pancreas, placenta, and kidney, among others, exerting autocrine, intracrine, and paracrine effects. This adds complexity to our understanding of the modulatory effects of the RAAS in maintaining homeostasis (5). Renin can be produced in the heart, brain, adrenal gland, testes, submaxillary gland, and mast cells, in addition to JG cells. Angiotensinogen is produced in extrahepatic sites such as the kidney, brain, spinal cord, mesentery, adrenal gland, atria, lung, stomach, spleen, large intestine, and ovary, and is also expressed in the ventricle and conduction tissue of the heart (5,21). ACE is ubiquitously expressed; however, the conversion of circulating Ang I to Ang II by ACE occurs mainly in the lung. ACE2 has been identified in the human heart, kidney and testis, and may be present in other tissues as well (21,22).

Ang II stimulates aldosterone synthesis and secretion by zona glomerulosa cells of the adrenal gland (23). Extra-adrenal sites of aldosterone synthesis include brain neurons, where it stimulates thirst, and cardiac myocytes, where it plays a role in the ventricular remodeling associated with salt retention (24). In these areas, the effects of aldosterone oppose those of glucocorticoids (25).

Ang II and its Metabolites

Aminopeptidases cleave Ang II at different sites. Aminopeptidase A acts on Ang II to form the heptapeptide Ang III, which participates, along with Ang II, in the classical effects on body fluid and electrolyte homeostasis, such as drinking behavior, vasopressin release and sodium appetite, in brain centers (5,21,26). Ang IV is a hexapeptide (Ang 3-8), formed by the action of aminopeptidase N on Ang II (27,28). Ang IV negatively regulates aminopeptidase A and thus influences the generation of Ang III.

Gene Targeting of Angiotensin Synthesis

The net impact of the autocrine, endocrine, intracrine, and paracrine effects of the RAAS is understood best in experimental models of controlled hyper-expression or deletion of target genes of the RAAS, such that their effects are enhanced or abolished. Most of these studies have been done in mice. Some have been performed in rats. Mice are different from other species in that they can have one or two renin genes (*Ren-1* and *Ren-2*), depending on the strain (29). *Ren-2* may have arisen from gene duplication during evolution. Thus, C57/BL6 mice express one renin gene while 129 sv mice express two renin genes. Interestingly, the adenosine receptor gene knockout mice, regardless of the strain (30), always express both renin genes. The physiological significance of one versus two genes is unknown thus far: there is no significant difference in plasma renin levels or renal renin mRNA expression between the two.

Deficiency of individual components of the RAAS is associated with low blood pressure while over-expression of individual components of the RAAS increases blood pressure, confirming the essential role of the RAAS in maintaining blood pressure. Angiotensinogen-deficient mice exhibit profound hypotension (31,32). These mice also exhibit delayed glomerular maturation and small papillae and develop nephrosclerosis (33). Transgenic mice, which over-express the human angiotensinogen gene, develop hypertension and renal fibrosis; the latter is ameliorated by the administration of an ACE inhibitor, independent of its blood pressure lowering effects (34).

Tissue-specific targeted ablation helps to elucidate the paracrine and autocrine effects of tissue RAS. In hypertensive mice expressing human renin (hREN) and human angiotensinogen transgenes under the control of their own endogenous promoters, glial-specific deletion of angiotensinogen results in lowered blood pressure (35), indicating that the central nervous system also contributes to the regulation of blood pressure. Introduction of the mouse *Ren-2* gene into normotensive rats creates a transgenic strain that expresses *Ren-2* mRNA in the adrenal gland, and the kidney (36). This transgene provides a monogenic model for a form of sodium dependent malignant hypertension. The *Ren-2* transgenic rat has hyperproreninemia, low plasma and renal renin, high adrenal renin, and increased adrenal corticosteroid production. The hypertension that occurs in this model is responsive to ACE inhibitors. ACE deficient mice have decreased blood pressure and renal disease characterized by perivascular infiltrates and impaired concentration ability, indicating a role of ACE in the development of nephron function (37). ACE2 deficient mice develop dilated cardiomyopathy, and have a hypertensive response to Ang II (38,39).

Angiotensin Receptors

The effects of the angiotensin ligands Ang II, Ang III, and Ang IV are mediated by their interaction with specific angiotensin receptors. Ang II is known to interact mainly with two receptors, AT_1 and AT_2. Ang II and Ang III are full agonists at the AT_1 receptor, while Ang IV binds to the receptor with low affinity (27,28,33,40). Almost all the usual physiological effects of Ang II are mediated by the AT_1 receptor. The human AT_1 receptor gene is located in chromosome 3q21–q25. The human AT_2 receptor is located in chromosome Xq22–q23. AT_1 and AT_2 receptors belong to the seven-transmembrane class of G protein-coupled receptors (27,28,33,41). Adult human renal vasculature, glomeruli, and tubules (proximal, ascending limb of Henle, and collecting duct) express AT_1 receptors; AT_2 receptors are expressed in the vasculature and glomeruli but not in the tubules (42).

Rodents, but not humans, have two AT_1 receptors, AT_{1A} and AT_{1B}. They are 94% homologous, and are located in chromosome 17q12 and chromosome 2q24, respectively (43). These receptor subtypes are differentially expressed: the AT_{1A} receptor is expressed in the hypothalamus while the AT_{1B} receptor mRNA is expressed in the pituitary gland. Both AT_{1A} and AT_{1B} receptors are expressed in the adrenal gland. While aldosterone secretion is mediated by both AT_{1A} and AT_{1B} receptors in the zona glomerulosa, corticosterone secretion is mediated by AT_{1A} in the zona fasciculata (44). Adult rat kidneys express AT_{1A} receptors in blood vessels and glomeruli. More AT_{1A} receptors are expressed in collecting ducts than in other nephron segments (45,46). The AT_{1B} receptor is not expressed in the adult or fetal rat kidney (47). In adult rat kidneys, AT_2 receptors are expressed to a greater extent in glomeruli and to a lesser extent in proximal tubules and blood vessels. Female rats express more AT_2 receptors than male rats (48).

Occupation of the AT_1 receptor by Ang II triggers the generation of various second messengers via heteromeric G-proteins, chiefly $G_{q/11}$. Phospholipase C (PLC) β1 is activated leading to the formation of 1,4,5-inositol trisphosphate (IP_3) and diacylglycerol (DAG) from the hydrolysis of phosphatidylinositol-4,5-bisphosphonate (PIP_2). IP_3 activates IP_3 receptors in the endoplasmic reticulum releasing Ca^{2+}. Ca^{2+} released from the endoplasmic reticulum causes the Ca^{2+}-sensing STIM1 protein to interact with Orai1 in the plasma membrane. This interaction and the activation of IP_3 receptors at the plasma membrane allow the influx of extracellular calcium (49,50). The increase in intracellular calcium and the stimulation of protein kinase C (PKC) by DAG lead to vasoconstriction (51). Activation of the AT_1 receptor stimulates growth factor pathways such as tyrosine phosphorylation and PLCγ activation, leading to activation of downstream proteins, including mitogen-activated protein (MAP) kinases, signal transducers and activators of transcription (STAT protein). These cellular proliferative pathways, mediated by the AT_1 receptor, have been implicated in the proliferative changes seen in cardiovascular and renal diseases (52).

The AT_1 and AT_2 receptors are differentiated based on their affinity for various non-peptide antagonists (51,53). The AT_2 receptor shares 32–34% amino acid homology with the AT_1 receptor, but activates second messenger systems with opposite effects via various signal transduction systems, mainly G_i and G_o proteins (27,28,33,41,49,54). Stimulation of the AT_2 receptor leads to activation of various phosphatases, resulting in inactivation of extracellular signal-regulated kinase (ERK), opening of K^+ channels and inhibition of T-type Ca^{2+} channels. The AT_2 receptor has a higher affinity for Ang III than Ang II. AT_2 receptors may mediate antiproliferative effects, apoptosis, differentiation, and possibly vasodilatation.

Gene Targeting of Angiotensin Receptors

Gene targeting experiments in mice have elucidated the effects of angiotensin receptors. AT_{1A} knockout mice are hypotensive and have a mild reduction in survival, compared to angiotensinogen knockout mice (41,55,56). AT_{1A} receptor knockout mice have minor anomalies in the renal inner medulla and papillary structure (41,55–59). AT_{1B} receptor knockout mice show no specific abnormalities and have normal blood pressure. This indicates that the AT_{1A} receptor can compensate for the absence of the AT_{1B} receptor (60). However, mice lacking both AT_{1A} and AT_{1B} receptors show deficient urinary peristalsis during the perinatal period (61). AT_2 receptor knockout mice have modest elevation of blood pressure, and an enhanced pressor response to Ang II (62–64).

Several proteins interact with the AT_1 and AT_2 receptors. Over-expression of the AT_1 receptor-associated protein (ATRAP) decreases AT_1 receptor number (65). In contrast, the AT_2 receptor-interacting protein (ATIP1) cooperates with the AT_2 receptor in the inactivation of receptor tyrosine kinases, thus playing a role in the initiation of a signaling cascade that inhibits cell growth (66).

Other Ang II Receptors

There are two other receptors for Ang II. The AT_3 receptor represents an angiotensin binding site and is identified in a mouse neuroblastoma cell line (67). The AT_3 receptor has a high affinity for Ang II but a low affinity for Ang III. The AT_4 receptor is an angiotensin binding site, with a high affinity for Ang IV (27,40,68). Unlike the AT_1 and AT_2 receptors, the AT_4 receptor is not coupled to heterotrimeric G proteins, and has been identified as an insulin-regulated transmembrane aminopeptidase (IRAP). A unique binding site for the heptapeptide Ang 1-7 (formed by the action of ACE2 on Ang I) has also been identified (Fig. 7-1).

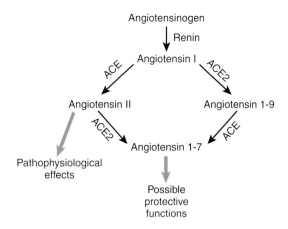

Figure 7-1 Pathways of ANG generation. (After Danilczyk U, Penninger M: Angiotensin-converting enzyme II in the heart and kidney. Circ Res, 98(4): 463–471, 2006.) ACE2-regulated pathways: both ACE and ACE2 are involved in the production of the biologically active peptides Ang II and Ang1-7 from Ang I. Elevated levels of Ang II are known to be detrimental to the function of the heart and kidney. Ang1-7 may function as a key peptide involved in cardioprotection and renoprotection. Genetic experiments suggest that ACE and ACE2 have complementary functions by negatively regulating different RAS products. The fine details of their regulatory function may differ depending on the local RAS environment.

Physiological Effects of Ang II

Ang II exerts most of its physiological effects via the AT_1 receptor. Ang II has pleiotropic actions (69), including direct and indirect vasopressor effects. In response to sodium depletion, hypotension and/or hypovolemia, Ang II is formed, which causes immediate vasoconstriction of arteries and veins, increasing peripheral vascular resistance and venous return respectively, and raising blood pressure. The effect of Ang II on blood pressure secondary to increased ion transport by the renal tubule is more gradual. Ang II increases sodium and chloride reabsorption directly in several segments of the nephron. In the proximal tubule, low concentrations of Ang II play a central role in ion transport by activating luminal Na^+/H^+ exchanger (NHE), Na-glucose cotransporter (70), sodium phosphate cotransporter (NaPi) (71), basolateral $Na^+K^+ATPase$ (72,73) and Na^+-$HCO3^-$ exchanger (74). AT_1 receptors stimulate NHE3 (75–77) but not NHE2 (78). High concentrations of Ang II can inhibit proximal tubule sodium transport via the stimulation of PLA2- and cytochrome P-450-dependent metabolites of arachidonic acid (74,79–82). Ang II also affects ion transport in the medullary thick ascending limb of the loop of Henle in a biphasic manner (83). In this nephron segment, low concentrations of Ang II increase sodium, potassium, and chloride transport by stimulating NHE3 and NaK2Cl cotransporter activities (84). Ang II stimulates NHE1 activity in the macula densa (85). Ang II also stimulates NHE2 in the distal convoluted tubule and amiloride-sensitive Na^+ transport (epithelial sodium channel, ENaC) in the collecting duct (86). All these effects are mediated by the AT_1 receptors.

The role of AT_2 receptors in influencing sodium transport is not well established. AT_2 receptors may inhibit sodium transport. AT_2 receptors are coupled to NHE6 (87), but NHE6 is not involved in sodium reabsorption (88). Ang 1-7 has been reported to inhibit $Na^+K^+ATPase$ in pig outer cortical nephrons (89), and Na^+-HCO_3^- exchanger in mouse renal proximal tubules (90). However, an increase in sodium transport via AT_2 receptors in rat proximal tubules has also been reported (91). These discrepancies may be related to the condition of the animal. For example, AT_2 receptors inhibit $Na^+K^+ATPase$ activity in renal proximal tubules of obese but not lean rats (92), and during AT_1 receptor blockade (93).

Ang II indirectly increases sodium transport by stimulating the synthesis of aldosterone in the zona glomerulosa of the adrenal cortex. Aldosterone increases the density of ENaC in the cortical collecting duct by inducing the transcription of α-ENaC and redistribution of α-ENaC in the early cortical collecting duct from a cytoplasmic to an apical location. However, Ang II can stimulate the expression of α, β, and γ ENaC, independent of aldosterone (94). Aldosterone also activates

Na$^+$K$^+$ATPase in the basolateral membrane of the principal cells of the cortical collecting duct. Aldosterone, like Ang II, can act in an autocrine and paracrine manner. Aldosterone has been reported to be produced by aldosterone producing cells other than the adrenal glomerulosa, such as neuronal glial cells and cardiac myocytes (95).

There is evidence that Ang I and Ang II may act, in ligand-independent ways, to affect cell signaling, cell–cell communication and growth, via their metabolism by the enzyme ACE2, mentioned above. They may also oppose the traditionally accepted effects of the RAAS (96). While AT$_1$ receptors can be stimulated by stretch, independent of Ang II (97), Ang II can have intracellular effects independent of AT$_1$ receptors (98).

Concepts and Controversies in our Current Understanding of the Renal Effects of the RAAS in Maintaining Fluid and Electrolyte Homeostasis and Blood Pressure

Feedback mechanisms in the kidney contribute to the maintenance of renal blood flow and glomerular filtration rate (GFR) in the face of fluctuations in blood pressure. This phenomenon of renal autoregulation was first recognized as early as 1932 (99). In some animals, autoregulation of renal blood flow is negligible at birth (100). In primates, in the immediate neonatal period, autoregulation of renal blood flow is present, but autoregulation of blood flow to other organs, such as

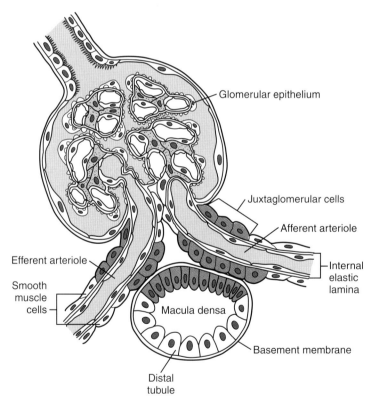

Figure 7-2 The juxtaglomerular apparatus and tubuloglomerular feedback (TGF). (From Guyton AC, Hall JE: The kidneys and body fluids. In Guyton AC, Hall JE (eds): Textbook of Medical Physiology (Fig 26.14, p. 292). Philadelphia, PA: WB Saunders, 2000.) TGF is achieved because of the anatomy of the nephron and juxtaglomerular (JG) apparatus. TGF is a phenomenon that occurs when changes in tubular fluid concentrations of Na+, Cl-, and K+ are sensed by the macula densa, via the luminal Na+-K+-2Cl cotransporter. Increases or decreases in luminal uptake of these ions cause reciprocal changes in GFR by alterations in vascular tone, mainly in the afferent arteriole.

brain, myocardium, and intestines, is not observed (101). Autoregulation of renal blood flow is observed in canine puppies as young as 14 days of age (102). However the set point is lower and the efficiency of autoregulation is less in younger than in older puppies.

Autoregulation is achieved by the interplay of two mechanisms: (i) tubuloglomerular feedback (TGF), which involves a flow-dependent signal from the macula densa and alteration of afferent arteriolar tone, which is mediated by adenosine and/or ATP (103–105); and (ii) myogenic response, which involves direct vasoconstriction of the afferent arteriole in response to increased transmural pressure. These two mechanisms act in concert to prevent acute fluctuations in renal blood flow and GFR in response to changes in blood pressure (Fig. 7-2) (106).

Recent studies challenge pre-existing concepts and merit discussion. Glomerulotubular balance (GTB) is a negative feedback loop that occurs when proximal tubular reabsorption of sodium and water increases in response to increased GFR (107), and vice versa. Thus, GTB affects distal sodium delivery and, consequently, TGF. TGF and GTB may be more critical in the regulation of renal function in the neonate than in the adult as sodium intake is low in the newborn; sodium balance must be tightly regulated to achieve the net positive balance required for growth. Recent advances in our understanding of GTB, specifically in the neonate, will be discussed.

ONTOGENY

Development of the RAAS: Structure of the Kidney and Urinary Tract

Prenatal Changes in RAAS Structure and Function in Rodents and Humans

STUDIES IN HUMANS

In humans, angiotensin-related genes are activated at Stage 11 of the developing embryo (108), which corresponds to 23–24 days of gestation. AT_1 and AT_2 receptors are expressed very early (24 days of gestation), indicating that Ang II may play a role in organogenesis. The AT_1 receptor is expressed in the glomeruli while the AT_2 receptor is found in the undifferentiated mesonephros that surrounds the primitive tubules and glomeruli. AT_2 receptor is maximally expressed at about 8 weeks of gestation, followed by decreasing, but persistent expression until about 20 weeks of gestation (109). At Stage 12–13, which corresponds to 25–29 days of gestation, angiotensinogen is expressed in the proximal part of the primitive tubule, while renin is expressed in glomeruli and JG arterioles. ACE is detected in the mesonephric tubules at stage 14. By 30–35 days, all components of the RAAS are expressed in the human embryonic mesonephros. Expression of these proteins in the future collecting system occurs later, at about 8 weeks of gestation.

ACE has a role in fetal growth and development. ACE inhibitor-induced fetopathy, consisting of oligohydramnios, intrauterine growth retardation, hypocalvaria, renal dysplasia, anuria, and death, has been described in mothers exposed to ACE inhibitors during the second and third trimesters of pregnancy (110). These effects were initially believed to arise from a decrease in organ perfusion (111). More recent evidence indicates that ACE inhibition has teratogenic effects during development. Fetuses exposed to ACE inhibitors during the first trimester have an increased risk of congenital malformations, with an incidence of 7.1%, compared to those with no maternal exposure to antihypertensive medications during the same time period. The congenital anomalies are major and include cardiovascular defects such as atrial septal defect, patent ductus arteriosus, ventricular septal defects and pulmonic stenosis; skeletal malformations, including polydactyly, upper limb defects and craniofacial anomalies; gastrointestinal malformations such as pyloric stenosis and intestinal atresia; central nervous system malformations such as hydrocephalus, spina bifida and microcephaly; and genitourinary malformations including renal malformations (112). Angiotensin receptor blockers (ARB) have also been reported to be fetotoxic (113). Inhibition of the activity of the RAAS in pregnancy may have effects on the fetus that manifest later on in life, such as hypertension, which are addressed later.

STUDIES IN RODENTS

The expression patterns of the RAS components in the embryonic kidney are similar in rodents and humans (108,114). Angiotensinogen is expressed in the proximal part of the primitive tubule in the mouse at embryonic day 12.5 (30 days' gestation in humans) (115). Renin is widely expressed initially in the renal vasculature in the embryonic rat, but its expression becomes localized to the afferent arteriole with development. Renin secretion is greater during the early embryonic period and decreases gradually. Circulating renin levels are higher in the neonatal rodent than in the adult, and appear to be due to increased production (115). Rodent ACE follows a similar expression pattern as in humans. Ang II and AT_1 receptors are important in nephron development and afferent arterial growth. AT_1 receptors may guide Ang II to its target sites to induce cell growth and differentiation (116–118). AT_1 receptor mRNA is strongly expressed during the early embryonic period (E17 to E20 in the rat), with increased expression in mature nephron segments by E17, persisting until adulthood (119). AT_2 expression is seen in both the undifferentiated mesenchyme in the maturing kidney and the mature nephron, including the proximal tubule. Collectrin, a novel homolog of ACE2 (120) shares about 47% homology with ACE2 in humans, but lacks the carboxypeptidase function. Collectrin mRNA is expressed in the mouse embryo at day 13, is localized to the ureteric bud, the progenitor of the collecting duct, increases throughout development, and decreases after birth.

Mutations of genes encoding renin, angiotensinogen, ACE, or AT_1 receptor are associated with skull ossification defects (121), as well as autosomal recessive renal tubular dysgenesis (122–124). AT_1 receptor deficient mice do not develop a renal pelvis (122). AT_2 receptor deficient mice have congenital abnormalities of the kidney and urinary tract (CAKUT), such as multicystic dysplastic, and aplastic kidneys (124). The more dramatic phenotypes seen in mice with deficient AT_2 receptor, as compared to humans with similar defects, is attributed to the fact that human nephrogenesis is completed in utero, while maturation of rodent nephrons occurs for up to 10 days after birth. However, AT_1 receptor gene deficient phenotypes are similar in rodents and humans. As indicated earlier, mutations in angiotensin-related genes in humans are associated with renal tubular dysgenesis (123). These studies demonstrate the importance of the RAAS in development and maturation of the kidney and collecting systems (115).

Postnatal Changes in RAAS Structure and Function in Rodents and Humans

STUDIES IN RODENTS

In rats, angiotensionogen mRNA expression is negligible immediately after birth, but increases dramatically by day 5, only to decrease again over the next few days, followed by a gradual increase to adult levels by 2 months of life. The newborn rat kidney can generate Ang II directly from angiotensinogen via a serine-protease that is induced in the newborn (125). Renin levels are higher in the neonatal than the adult rodent, and appear to be due to increased production (107). Ang II levels are high in the early neonatal period, and decrease with age.

The RAAS is more highly activated in the neonatal period and infancy compared to later in childhood (126). Plasma renin activity and plasma aldosterone levels are markedly increased in preterm human infants in the first 3 weeks of life (127). While fetal ACE levels remain stable during gestation in rats (128), serum ACE activity has been reported by some to be higher in late fetal than in neonatal life in humans (128–130), lambs and guinea pigs (131,132). In contrast, renal ACE activity may increase with age, at least in pigs and horses (133,134). A similar pattern may be found in humans based on measurement of urine ACE isoforms (135). Recent studies measuring plasma Ang II levels in 46 normal and low birth weight human infants have shown increased Ang II levels at 7 days of life in very low birth weight infants (136). Maximum serum aldosterone levels are seen at 2 h of age, and gradually decrease over the first year of life (137).

Sodium Homeostasis in the Neonatal Period

Sodium intake is low in infants compared to adults, as milk is a poor source of sodium. However, a positive balance of sodium in the neonate is needed to sustain growth, in contrast to normal adults who are in sodium balance. The kidney of a full term infant filters 4–5% of the volume of plasma filtered by an adult (120 mL/min/1.73M^2). Despite the relative paucity of sodium transporters, the full-term neonate does retain sodium, in part because of the low GFR (3). Although renal sodium transporters are reduced, neonates cannot excrete a sodium load compared to adults. This has been attributed to the increased activity of agents that increase sodium reabsorption in the neonatal period, including the RAAS and α-adrenergic receptors (117,138). Endogenous Ang II inhibits the natriuresis of acute expansion in the neonatal rat (139). The decreased effects of natriuretic factors (e.g., atrial natriuretic peptide, dopamine, nitric oxide) in the term neonate compared to the adult may also impair its ability to excrete a sodium load (140–142). Water transport across the proximal tubule also differs in adults and neonates. The adult tubule transports water by the water channels called aquaporins, which belong to the category of non-solute carrier-related genes. These are present in very low concentrations in the neonatal nephron. However, water is transported effectively in the neonatal nephron by paracellular and transmembrane mechanisms and by passage through non-aquaporin channels to maintain GTB (see below) (143). Aquaporin expression increased with age, an effect that is mediated by glucocorticoids (144).

Development of TGF

Growth and maturation affect the influence of distal ion delivery on the sensors of the macula densa in producing a vascular response. TGF responses are operative in neonatal rats, as early as 3.5 weeks of age (145,146). The inflection point for TGF may also be different between younger and older rats. Extracellular fluid volume and dietary protein affect the TGF response profoundly. The effect of dietary protein on the TGF response varies in different studies, with high protein diets stimulating or blunting the TGF response.

Despite a lower GFR, urinary sodium losses are highest in the most premature babies but fractional sodium excretion (FE_{Na}) is exponentially related to gestational age. The renal sodium loss in prematurity appears, in part, to result from the immaturity of the TGF mechanism. Postnatal age has been shown to have an independent effect on FE_{Na} but not on GFR. These findings indicate that in infants of greater than 33 weeks' gestation, sodium conservation is possible because of adequate TGF. The rapid increase in sodium reabsorption in the first few postnatal days seems to be due to maturation of distal tubular function. Although this was initially attributed to aldosterone (147), the decreased amount of transporters that are targets of aldosterone makes this mechanism unlikely. An increase in maturity of the $Na^+K^+ATPase$ in the distal tubule and a decrease in extracellular fluid volume may be contributory factors to postnatal maturation of sodium transport in the distal tubule.

Development of GTB

The essential regulatory mechanisms of tubule transport include GTB and neural and hormonal factors such as sympathetic innervation, Ang II, endothelin, parathormone, and other mediators. As defined earlier, GTB is the capacity of each segment of the nephron to reabsorb a constant fraction of the GFR, fluid and solute delivered to it, and is influenced by peritubular and intratubular capillary pressures and GFR (148). The capacity of the proximal tubule to reabsorb sodium, chloride and water, bicarbonate, glucose and organic substances is adjusted to GFR: the higher the GFR, the greater the reabsorption. The underlying physical mechanism of GTB is a flow-dependent reabsorption of ions and water across the renal proximal tubular luminal membrane in response to changes in GFR, which is independent of neural and hormonal systems. Maintenance of GTB is influenced by flow rate, substrate delivery and other unknown systems. It is signaled by the hydrodynamic torque (bending movement) on epithelial microvilli (149). Increases in luminal diameter have the effect of blunting the impact of flow velocity on microvillous shear stress and, thus, on microvillous torque. Variations in microvillous torque produce nearly identical fractional changes in sodium reabsorption. Furthermore, the flow-dependent sodium transport is enhanced by increasing luminal fluid viscosity, diminished in NHE3 knockout mice, and abolished by nontoxic disruption of the actin cytoskeleton. These data suggest that the 'brush-border' microvilli serve a mechanosensory function wherein fluid dynamic torque is transmitted to the actin cytoskeleton to modulate sodium absorption in renal proximal tubules.

Clinical studies have been conducted to study GTB in term and preterm human infants, which suggest that GTB is operational from about 33 weeks of gestational age (147). In a study of 70 infants of gestational ages 27–40 weeks and postnatal ages 3–68 days, 24-h sodium balance studies and creatinine clearance measurements showed that intrauterine age and extrauterine existence independently increased the maturation of this function. The incidence of hyponatremia was associated with a negative sodium balance, which varied directly with the degree of prematurity. Indeed, no babies born after 36 weeks had a negative sodium balance. Studies in rats also show that GTB is present in 4.5 month old rats. Thus, it appears that GTB is maintained during development by proportional maturation of GFR and tubular reabsorptive mechanisms (150).

CURRENT CONCEPTS AND CONTROVERSIES

The changes in preglomerular resistance that regulate renal blood flow and GFR in the face of changing blood pressure is attributed to TGF and the renal myogenic response, acting in concert, as mentioned earlier. This is the classic paradigm. However, over the last 20 years, the importance of TGF and renal autoregulation has been challenged, and the role of the myogenic response as a renoprotective mechanism to prevent renal damage due to increased blood pressure has been demonstrated in several studies.

There is evidence that renal protection is lost when autoregulation fails (151,152). The changes in glomerular capillary pressure to maintain GFR at a relatively constant level in the face of increasing or decreasing blood pressure is different from the vascular response needed to reduce GFR to limit pressure-induced increases, which cause renal injury. Thus, TGF and the myogenic response occur at different levels and may have different goals in the balance between renal autoregulation and renal protection. Classic studies in the two kidney, one clip model of hypertension (153,154) were followed by studies in the uninephrectomized deoxycorticosterone acetate (DOCA)/salt model of malignant nephrosclerosis (155), confirming the damage engendered by a dilated renal vascular bed in the face of hypertension. In a 5/6 ablation model of chronic kidney disease, the loss of autoregulation increases susceptibility to hypertensive renal injury.

There are different requirements for protection versus regulation. The myogenic response, which constricts the afferent arteriole, occurs after every 3–4 s in response to a blood pressure change. A TGF response takes up to 20 s, as it involves the sequence of increased distal delivery, sensing by the macula densa, release of mediator (now presumed to be adenosine/ATP) and generation of arteriolar afferent response (156). Thus, very brief perturbations of blood pressure have insignificant effects on renal blood flow and GFR. Such brief episodes should alter the myogenic response, but there are no convincing in vivo data available that support this. Similarly, there are no studies on the effects of spikes in systolic versus spikes in mean arterial blood pressure in generating a renal myogenic response. A delay in the onset of pressure-induced vasoconstriction has been reported in the intact kidney (157), with a longer delay in vasodilatation induced by decreasing blood pressure in the intact kidney and an even longer delay in a hydronephrotic kidney.

The advocates for TGF as the dominant mechanism argue that as GFR is influenced by several factors, including plasma colloid pressure, proximal tubular pressure and the filtration coefficient (158), a vascular response to changes in pressure alone may not be adequate for regulation. TGF, with its response to alteration in distal sodium delivery, may thus play the stronger autoregulatory role, while its immediate renoprotective role may be less important.

Differentiating these two closely aligned mechanisms is difficult. In the Fawn-Hooded rat, the Brown-Norway rat, and the Dahl salt-sensitive rat, the genetic defect in autoregulation seems to involve the myogenic response, with an intact or even enhanced TGF (159–161). Studies of renal injury in these models may shed more light on this issue. We do know that humans with uncomplicated, essential hypertension and intact renal autoregulation do not exhibit renal injury (151,152).

If autoregulation is essential for volume homeostasis, one would expect an unequivocal relationship between the two. However, there is little evidence that impaired autoregulation leads to impaired volume homeostasis. Hypertension is not clearly linked to loss of autoregulation. In the Brown-Norway rat, blood pressure is reduced and administration of DOCA or NaCl has little effect (162). In genetic knockout mice without the TGF mechanism, no overt volume disturbances are noted (163). Similarly, if distal delivery is manipulated, such as by the chronic use of loop diuretics, the effects should be catastrophic, since these also suppress TGF. However after an initial loss of volume, steady state adaptations occur within 3–4 days. GTB helps in this adjustment.

Mediators and Modulators of TGF

There are several recent studies aimed at identifying the mediator of the TGF mechanism, which is critical to autoregulation. As defined earlier, TGF is a phenomenon that occurs when changes in tubular ion transport by the macula densa cause reciprocal changes in GFR by alterations in vascular tone, mainly in the afferent arteriole (106). The initial step in the TGF mechanism is the sensing of the luminal signal by the Na^+K^+2Cl cotransporter at the macula densa. The activation of the Na^+K^+2Cl cotransporter generates adenosine, which stimulates A_1

adenosine (A_1) receptors, resulting in increased cytosolic calcium. Some investigators have suggested that ATP, activating P2X1 receptors, triggers the increase in cytosolic calcium. The calcium signal is propagated to extraglomerular mesangial cells, constricting vascular smooth muscle cells of the afferent arteriole and decreasing GFR. Renin secretion is also inhibited, which allows recovery of arteriolar flow and GFR. TGF is absent in A_1 receptor knockout mice. In contrast, TGF response persists in mice in which the ACE, AT_1 receptor, NOS1, or thromboxane receptor genes are disrupted (164). Vasoconstrictors, such as Ang II, increase the sensitivity of the TGF response, while vasodilators, such as nitric oxide, blunt the response (106). These studies indicate that TGF is modulated by Ang II, arachidonic acid metabolites, and nitric oxide, while the primary mediators are adenosine and/or ATP.

Adenosine

A recent study of cd73-/- mice, which cannot generate ATP/adenosine, suggests that a humoral factor, adenosine, may mediate TGF response. Thus, a lack of adenosine abrogates the change in GFR engendered by TGF, but does not affect distal reabsorption of sodium and water along the tubule, likely mediated by aldosterone (165). The cells of the macula densa display a role in regulation, by sensing increased NaCl delivery to the distal tubule, and activation of Na^+K^+2Cl cotransporter activity to reduce GFR, with adenosine most likely being the mediator of this response. Indeed, TGF is absent in A_1 receptor knockout, mice (165). In anesthetized wild type, and A_1 receptor knockout mice, GFR and renal blood flow were measured before and after reducing renal perfusion pressure by a suprarenal aortic clamp. A reduction in blood pressure produced a significantly greater fall in A_1 receptor knockout mice compared to the wild type, indicating reduced regulatory responses in the knockout mice. This suggests that deficient autoregulation in the absence of the effector adenosine or A_1 receptor is mediated by abrogation of the TGF response.

The administration of highly selective adenosine 1 receptor antagonist, CVT-124, results in marked diuresis and natriuresis, indicating failure of autoregulation (148). The diuresis and natriuresis are associated with a reduction in absolute proximal tubular reabsorption and its uncoupling from glomerular filtration. In addition, the response of the macula densa to increased distal delivery of sodium chloride and water is blunted, as there is no corresponding decrease in GFR. This indicates inhibition of the TGF mechanisms, and provides additional support for adenosine being the mediator of the TGF response. The lack of proximal tubular regulation in GTB could be indicative of adenosine being a player in GTB, in addition to the known and accepted peritubular, luminal and oncotic controls that regulate it. However, the mechanism underlying the increased formation of adenosine in response to an increase in Na^+K^+2Cl cotransporter activity remains to be determined.

ATP

Navar et al (166) make the case for ATP being the mediator of the TGF response based on their finding that ATP selectively affects renal afferent arteriolar tone, the demonstration of the presence of ATP-specific receptors P2X1 in the renal afferent arteriole, the absence of the TGF response in mice lacking the P2X1 receptor, and evidence that ATP directly stimulates the L-type voltage gated calcium channel, leading to calcium influx and vascular smooth muscle cell contraction (167,168).

Nitric Oxide (NO)

NO, derived from arginine, modulates TGF. Type I NO synthase (NOS) is expressed in the macula densa (169). Other NOS isoforms may be expressed in the mesangium and glomerular microvessels. These enzymes are strategically positioned to influence each step of the TGF process (170). However, micropuncture experiments using NOS antagonists have shown that NO does not mediate TGF. Instead, local NOS blockade causes the curve that represents TGF to shift leftward and become steeper. Changes in NO production in the macula densa may underlie the resetting of TGF, which is needed to maintain the TGF curve so that it adapts to different conditions of ambient tubular flow to accommodate physiologic circumstances and maintain homeostasis (171). Also, macula densa NO production may be substrate limited and dissociated from NOS protein content. The importance of NO to TGF resetting and the substrate dependence of NO production have both been found during changes in dietary salt. Changes in neuronal NOS (nNOS or NOS1) function have been shown to occur in the JGA of the spontaneously hypertensive rat (SHR) (172). NOS inhibition has been demonstrated to have a reduced effect on TGF in the SHR (173).

Reactive Oxygen Species

Reactive oxygen species and ongoing oxidative stress are increasingly implicated in the pathophysiology of vascular changes in many diseases, including hypertension. AT_1 receptors increase the sensitivity of the TGF response, which could also be related to reactive oxygen species. While the superoxide anion may lead to vaso-constriction and an increase in myogenic tone, directly, and via many signaling pathways, it also influences vasoconstriction and vasodilatation as a consequence of TGF. These effects occur due to changes in macula densa cell function in response to changes in sodium chloride delivery to the distal tubule. The macula densa expresses nNOS (171), which is activated during sodium chloride reabsorption and has a vasodilatory effect; this blunts the vasoconstriction caused by the TGF in response to increased sodium chloride transport. Oxygen radicals enhance the TGF response and limit NO signaling from the macula densa (174). Reactive oxygen species react with NO, producing peroxynitrate, which impairs vasorelax-ation and promotes hypertrophy (175–177): thus reactive oxygen species effectively counteract the effects of NO.

The interaction between NO and superoxide anion has been studied in micro-perfusion experiments. The infusion of a nitric oxide precursor into the macula densa caused a graded reduction in the TGF-mediated afferent arteriolar vasocon-striction; this response was more pronounced in the Wistar Kyoto (WKY) rat compared to the (SHR) (171). The thick ascending limb of the loop of Henle also produces NO, as it expresses endothelial NOS (eNOS or NOS III) (170,173). Here, studies have shown that NO decreases net absorption of chloride and bicar-bonate in the isolated thick ascending limb (178), thus indirectly decreasing the TGF response by increasing delivery of these to the distal tubule. Superoxide anion activates 5′-nucleotidase, thereby increasing adenosine generation in the kidney (which we know to be a mediator of TGF). These studies implicate reactive oxygen species in the enhancement of TGF (106).

Calcium Wave

Intracellular calcium modulates vascular smooth muscle tone and is the mediator for stimulation of renin release. There is evidence for a calcium wave that spreads through the mesangial cell field and constricts the afferent arteriolar smooth muscle cells. It appears that both gap junctional communication and extracellular ATP are integral components of the TGF calcium wave. The finding that the calcium wave is generated by ATP, but not by adenosine, offers a new model for a direct effect of ATP, not necessarily mediated by adenosine, as the final common pathway of changes in vascular tone in response to signals from the JGA and macula densa. A recent study demonstrates this using ratiometric calcium imaging of the in vitro microperfused isolated JGA-glomerular complex dissected rabbits (179).

New Directions

Fetal Programming for Hypertension: Failure of renoprotection?

The association of low birth weight with the development of hypertension later in life has been validated epidemiologically (180) and, more recently, has been demonstrated experimentally in animal models (181). A suboptimal fetal environment may lead to maladaptive responses, including failure of renal autoregulation and the development of hypertension. A reduction in nephron number during development may contribute to a reduction in GFR, but this is not always borne out in experimental studies. Multiple factors may contribute to the development of hypertension, but we will restrict ourselves to the role of renal hemodynamics. The RAAS may play a more important role as it is expressed early and associated with nephrogenesis. Blockade of the AT_1 receptor during the nephrogenic period after birth in the rat led to a decrease in nephron number, a reduction in renal function and hypertension (182). Protein restricted diets have also shown a rise in ACE levels in pregnant ewes (183) and a general stimulation of all components of the systemic RAS in other studies in response to protein restriction, which is blocked by treatment with an ACE inhibitor or an AT_1 receptor blocker. Thus, the adverse environment in utero, which programs the fetus to develop hypertension could be critically linked to abnormalities in the RAS (182).

Unconventional Behavior of RAS Components

While the canonical scheme of activation of the RAS components, from renin to Ang II and its effects on AT receptors is well recognized, recent evidence of other effects merit discussion. Both Ang I and Ang II may lead to effects that are independent of, or even antagonistic to, the accepted effects of the RAS (96). ACE may also function as a 'receptor' that initiates intracellular signaling and influences gene expression (184). AT_1 and AT_2 receptors have been shown to form heterodimers with other 7-transmembrane receptors, and influence signal transduction pathways (185–188). Intracellular Ang II exerts effects on cell communication, cell growth and gene expression via the AT_1 receptor, but also has independent effects (189,190).

Clinical Aspects

As discussed earlier, the development of the kidney occurs during the first 35 days postconception in humans. The integrity of the RAAS is essential for normal development, and Ang II is essential for normal structural development of the kidney and collecting system. The complex interplay of GTB and TGF increases with gestational age. The excretory function of the kidney begins soon after clamping of the umbilical cord at birth and continues through the first year of life. It follows that the neonate is exquisitely sensitive to stressors, which activate the RAAS, and lead to profound oligoanuric states.

Ischemia and Asphyxia Generate Renin by Sympathetic Stimulation

Drugs such as furosemide increase distal delivery of sodium and water, but reduce Na^+K^+2Cl activity, which should decrease renin release. However, decreased cotransporter activity impairs the TGF and, in the face of continued ion and water excretion, may result in hypovolemia, activation of the RAS and may lead to anuria. Indomethacin, used to treat patent ductus arteriosus in the neonate, could lead to altered renal vasoregulation (191). Congenital abnormalities in steroid synthesis could lead to deficiencies in aldosterone production, and cause profound salt-wasting states (192). In pseudohypoaldosteronism Type 1, mutations in the sodium channel may cause profound neonatal salt wasting (193). To counter the heightened awareness of the RAAS in neonates, adenosine receptor antagonists may offer new avenues of therapy.

SUMMARY

In summary, the RAAS is an important developmental and physiological system that contributes to renal blood flow and GFR autoregulation. Together with the myogenic response, the RAAS serves to maintain volume homeostasis in sodium and volume depleted states, and renoprotection in hypertensive states. The relative contributions of these two systems continue to be an area of controversy and debate. We also know that central and peripheral sympathetic input influences all aspects of renal autoregulation. More studies in transplanted or denervated kidneys in animal models and humans will elucidate these areas of controversy. A better understanding of these mechanisms would translate to better care for premature and full term newborns with renal dysregulation, hyponatremia and oligoanuric renal failure.

REFERENCES

1. Guyton AC, Hall JE. Dominant role of the kidney in long-term regulation of arterial pressure and in hypertension: The integrated system for pressure control. In Textbook of Medical Physiology, 10th edn (pp. 201–203), Philadelphia, PA: W.B. Saunders, 2001.
2. Gomez RA, McReddie TA, Everett AD, et al. Ontogeny of renin and AT1 receptor in the rat. Pediatr Nephrol 5:635–638, 1993.
3. Chevalier RL. The moth and the aspen tree: sodium in early postnatal development. Kidney Int 59(5):1617–1625, 2001.
4. Persson AE, Ollerstam A, Liu R, et al. Mechanisms for macula densa cell release of renin. Acta Physiol Scand 181:471–474, 2004.
5. Lavoie JL, Sigmund CD. Minireview: overview of the renin-angiotensin system—an endocrine and paracrine system. Endocrinology 144(6):2179–2183, 2003.
6. Krieger MH, Moreira ED, Oliveira EM, et al. Dissociation of blood pressure and sympathetic activation of renin release in sinoaortic-denervated rats. Clin Exp Pharmacol Physiol 33(5–6):471–476, 2006.
7. Schweda F, Segerer F, Castrop H, et al. Blood pressure-dependent inhibition of renin secretion requires A1 adenosine receptors. Hypertension 46(4):780–786, 2005.
8. Milavec-Krizman M, Evenou JP, Wagner H, et al. Characterization of beta-adrenoceptor subtypes in rat kidney with new highly selective beta 1 blockers and their role in renin release. Biochem Pharmacol 34(22):3951–3957, 1985.
9. DiBona GF. Neural regulation of renal tubular sodium reabsorption and renin secretion. Fed Proc 44(13):2816–2822, 1985.
10. Goldsmith SR. Interactions between the sympathetic nervous system and the RAAS in heart failure. Curr Heart Fail Rep 1(2):45–50, 2004.
11. Bell PD, Lapointe JY, Peti-Peterdi J. Macula densa signaling. Annu Rev Physiol 65:481–500, 2003.
12. Lorenz JN, Greenberg SG, Briggs JP. The macula densa mechanism for control of renin secretion (1993). Semin Nephrol 13(6):531–542, 1993.
13. Erdos EG. Conversion of angiotensin I to angiotensin II. Am J Med 60:749–759, 1976.
14. Urata H, Nishimura H, Ganten D. Mechanisms of angiotensin II formation in humans. Eur Heart J 16 (Suppl N):79–85, 1995.
15. Le TH, Coffman TM. A new cardiac MASTer switch for the renin-angiotensin system. J Clin Invest 116(4):866–869, 2006.
16. Chappel MC, Ferrario CM. ACE and ACE2: their role to balance the expression of angiotensin II and angiotensin-(1-7). Kidney Int 70:8–10, 2006.
17. Donoghue M, Hsieh F, Baronas E, et al. A novel angiotensin-converting enzyme-related carboxy-peptidase (ACE2) converts angiotensin I to angiotensin 1-9. Circ Res 87(5):E1–E9, 2000.
18. Li W, Moore MJ, Vasilieva N, et al. Angiotensin-converting enzyme 2 is a functional receptor for the SARS coronavirus. Nature 426(6965):450–454, 2003.
19. Han DP, Penn-Nicholson A, Cho MW, et al. Identification of critical determinants on ACE2 for SARS-CoV entry and development of a potent entry inhibitor. Virology 350(1):15–25, 2006.
20. Brosnihan KB, Neves LA, Joyner J, et al. Enhanced renal immunocytochemical expression of ANG-(1-7) and ACE2 during pregnancy. Hypertension 42(4):749–753, 2003.
21. Gavras I, Gavras H. Angiotensin II as a cardiovascular risk factor. J Hum Hypertens 16 (Suppl 2):S2–S6, 2002.
22. Danilczyk U, Penninger JM. Angiotensin-converting enzyme II in the heart and kidney. Circ Res 98(4):463–471, 2006.
23. Romero DG, Plonczynski M, Vergara GR, et al. Angiotensin II early regulated genes in H295R human adrenocortical cells. Physiol Genomics 19:106–116, 2004.
24. Declayre C, Swynghedauw B. Molecular mechanisms of myocardial remodeling. The role of aldostorone. J Mol Cell Cardiol 34:1577–1584, 2002.

25. Colombo L, Dala Valle L, Fiore C, et al. Aldosterone and the conquest of land. J Endocrinol Invest 29(4):373–379, 2006.

26. Veerasingham SJ, Raizada MK. Brain renin-angiotensin system dysfunction in hypertension: recent advances and perspectives. Br J Pharmacol 139:191–202, 2003.

27. Chai SY, Fernando R, Peck G, et al. The angiotension IV/AT4 receptor. Cell Mol Life Sci 61:2728–2737, 2004.

28. Saavedra JM, Ando H, Armando I, et al. Brain angiotensin II, an important stress hormone: regulatory sites and therapeutic opportunities. Ann N Y Acad Sci 1018:76–84, 2004.

29. Pan L, Gross KW. Transcriptional regulation of renin: an update. Hypertension 45:3–8, 2005.

30. Schweda F, Wagner C, Kremer BK, et al. Preserved macula densa dependent renin secretion in A1 adenosine receptor knockout mice. Am J Physiol Renal Physiol 284(4):F770–F777, 2003.

31. Kim HS, Krege JH, Kluckman KD, et al. Genetic control of blood pressure and the angiotensinogen locus. Proc Natl Acad Sci USA 92(7):2735–2739, 1995.

32. Tanimoto K, Sugiyama F, Goto Y, et al. Angiotensinogen deficient mice with hypotension. J Biol Chem 269(50):31334–31337, 1994.

33. Niimura F, Labosky PA, Kakuchi J, et al. Gene targeting in mice reveals a requirement for angiotensin in the development and maintenance of kidney morphology and growth factor regulation. J Clin Invest 96(6):2947–2954, 1995.

34. Fern RJ, Yesko CM, Thornhill BA, et al. Reduced angiotensinogen expression attenuates renal interstitial fibrosis in obstructive nephropathy in mice. J Clin Invest 103(1):39–46, 1999.

35. Sherrod M, David DR, Zhou X, et al. Glial-specific ablation of angiotensinogen lowers arterial pressure in renin and angiotensin transgenic mice. Am J Physiol Regul Integr Comp Physiol 289(6):R1763–R1769, 2005.

36. Wagner J, Thiele F, Ganten D. The renin-angiotensin system in transgenic rats. Pediatr Nephrol 10(1):108–112, 1996.

37. Bernstein KE. Views of the renin-angiotensin system: brilling, mimsy and slithy tove. Hypertension 47(3):509–514, 2006.

38. Yamamoto K, Ohishi M, Katsuya T, et al. Deletion of angiotensin-converting enzyme 2 accelerates pressure overload-induced cardiac dysfunction by increasing local angiotensin II. Hypertension 47(4):718–726, 2006.

39. Crackower MA, Sarao R, Oudit GY, et al. Angiotensin-converting enzyme 2 is an essential regulator of heart functionfunction. Nature 417(6891):822–828, 2002.

40. Davis CJ, Kramar EA, De A, et al. AT4 receptor activation increases intracellular calcium influx and induces a non-N-methyl-D-aspartate dependent form of long-term potentiation. Neuroscience 37:1369–1379, 2006.

41. Crowley SD, Tharaux PL, Audoly LP, et al. Exploring type I angiotensin (AT1) receptor functions through gene targeting. Acta Physiol Scand 181:561–567, 2004.

42. Mifune M, Sasamura H, Nakazato Y, et al. Examination of Ang II type 1 and type 2 receptor expression in human kidneys by immunohistochemistry. Clin Exp Hypertens 23(3):257–266, 2001.

43. Iwai N, Inagamii T. Identification of two subtypes in the rat type 1 angiotensin II receptor. FEBS Lett 8(2–3):257–260, 1992.

44. Naruse M, Tanabe A, Sugaya T, et al. Deferential roles of angiotensin receptor subtypes in adrenocortical function in mice. Life Sci 63(18):1593–1598, 1998.

45. Bonnet F, Candida R, Carey RM, et al. Renal expression of angiotensin receptors in long-term diabetes and the effects of angiotensin typ. 1 receptor blockade. J Hypertens 20(8):1615–1624, 2002.

46. Imanishi K, Nonoguchi H, Nakayama Y, et al. Type IA Ang II receptor is regulated differently in proximal and distal nephron segments. Hypertens Res 267:E260–E267, 2003.

47. Burson JM, Aguilera G, Gross KW, et al. Differential expression of angiotensin receptor 1A and 1B in mouse. Am J Physiol 267:E260–E267, 1994.

48. Baiardi G, Macova M, Armando I, et al. Estrogen upregulates Ang II AT1 and AT2 receptors in the rat. Regul Pept 124(1–3):7–17, 2005.

49. Dellis O, Dedos SG, Tovey SC, et al. Ca^{2+} entry through plasma membrane IP3 receptors. Science 313:229–233, 2006.

50. Gill DL, Spassova MA, Soboloff J. Signal transduction. Calcium entry signals—trickles and torrents. Science 313:183–184, 2006.

51. Sandberg K, Ji H. Comparative analysis of amphibian and mammalian angiotensin receptors. Comp Biochem Physiol A Mol Integr Physiol 128:53–57, 2001.

52. Kalantarinia K, Okusa MD: The renin-angiotensin system and its blockade in diabetic renal and cardiovascular disease. Curr Diab Rep (1):8–16, 2006.

53. De Gasparo M, Catt KJ, Inagami T, et al. International union of pharmacology XXIII. The angiotensin II receptors. Pharmacol Rev 52:415–472, 2000.

54. Zhang J, Pratt RE. The AT2 receptor selectively associates with Gia2 and Gia3 in the rat fetus. J Biol Chem 271:15026–15033, 1996.

55. Ito M, Oliviero P, Mannon C, et al. Regulation of blood pressure by the type 1A receptor for angiotensin II. Proc Natl Acad Sci USA 92:3521–3525, 1995.

56. Schnermann J, Travnor T, Yang Y, et al. Absence of tubuloglomerular feedback responses in AT1A receptor-deficient mice. Am J Physiol 273:F315–F320, 1997.

57. Matsusaka T, Nishimura H, Utsonomiya H, et al. Chimeric mice carrying 'regional' targeted deletion of the angiotensin type 1A receptor gene. Evidence against the role for local angiotensin in the in vivo feedback regulation of renin synthesis in juxtaglomerular cells. J Clin Invest 98(8):1867–1877, 1996.

58. Oliverio MI, Madsen K, Best CF, et al. Renal growth and development in mice lacking the AT1A receptors for Angiotensin II. Am J Physiol 274:F43–F50, 1998.

59. Sugaya T, Nishimatsu S, Tanimoto K, et al. Angiotensin II type 1a receptor-deficient mice with hypotension and hyperreninemia. J Biol Chem 270(32):18719–18722, 1995.

60. Chen XW, Li H, Yoshida S, et al. Targeting deletion of angiotensin type 1B receptor gene in the mouse. Am J Physiol 272:F299–F304, 1997.

61. Miyazaki Y, Tsuchida S, Nishimura H, et al. Angiotensin induces the urinary peristaltic machinery during the perinatal period. J Clin Invest 102(8):1489–1497, 1998.

62. Hein LG, Barsh R, Pratt V, et al. Behavioral and cardiovascular effects of disrupting the angiotensin II type-2 receptor gene in mice. Nature 377:744–747, 1995.

63. Siragy HM, Inagami T, Ichiki T, et al. sustained hypersensitivity to Ang II and its mechanism in mice lacking the subtype 2 (AT2) angiotensin receptor. Proc Natl Acad Sci USA 96(11):6506–6510, 1996.

64. Ichiki T, Labosky PA, Shiota C, et al. Effects on blood pressure and exploratory behaviour of mice lacking Ang II type-2 receptor. Nature 377(6551):748–750, 1995.

65. Tanaka Y, Tamura K, Kkoide Y, et al. The novel angiotensin II type 1 receptor (AT1R)-associated protein ATRAP downregulates AT1R and ameliorates cardiomyocyte hypertrophy. FEBS Lett 579(7):1579–1586, 2005.

66. Nouet S, Amzallag N, Li JM. Transactivation of receptor tyrosine kinases by novel angiotensin II receptor-interacting protein, ATIP. J Biol Chem 279(28):28989–28997, 2005.

67. Chaki S, Inagami T. Identification and characterization of a new binding site for angiotensin II in mouse neuroblastoma neuro-2A cells. Biochem Biophys Res Commun 182(1):388–394, 1992.

68. Albiston AL, McDowall SG, Matsacos D, et al. Evidence that the angiotensin IV (AT4) receptor is the enzyme insulin-regulated aminopeptidase. J Biol Chem 276(52):48623–48626, 2001.

69. Hunyadi L, Catt KJ. Pleiotropic AT1 receptor signaling pathways mediating physiological and pathogenic actions of Ang II. Mol Endocrinol 20(5):953–970, 2006.

70. Garvin JL. Angiotensin stimulates glucose and fluid absorption by rat proximal straight tubules. J Am Soc Nephrol 1(3):272–277, 1990.

71. Xu L, Dixit MP, Chen R, et al. Effects of angiotensin II on NaPi-II a co-transporter expression and activity in rat renal cortex. Biochim Biophys Acta 1667(2):114–121, 2004.

72. Yingst DR, Massey KJ, Rossi NF, et al. Angiotensin II directly stimulates the activity and alters the phosphorylation of Na-K-ATPase in rat proximal tubule with a rapid time course. Am J Physiol Renal Physiol 287(4):F713–F721, 2004.

73. Shah S, Hussain T. Enhanced angiotensin II-induced activation of Na$^+$- K$^+$- ATPase in the proximal tubules of obese Zucker rats. Clin Exp Hypertens 28:29–40, 2006.

74. Horita S, Zheng Y, Hara C. Biphasic regulation of Na$^+$ HCO3$^-$ cotransporter by angiotensin II type 1A receptor. Hypertension 40(5):707–712, 2002.

75. Noonan WT, Woo AL, Nieman ML, et al. Blood pressure maintenance in NHE3-deficient mice with transgenic expression of NHE3 in small intestine. Am J Physiol Regul Integr Comp Physio 288(3):R685–R691, 2005.

76. Kolb RJ, Woost PG, Hopfer U, et al. Membrane trafficking of angiotensin receptor type-1 and mechanochemical signal transduction in proximal tubule cells. Hypertension 44(3):352–359, 2004.

77. Quan A, Chakravarty S, Chen JK, et al. Androgens augment proximal tubule transport. Am J Physiol Renal Physiol 287(3):F452–F459, 2004.

78. Dixit MP, Xu L, Xu H, et al. Effect of angiotensin II on renal Na+/H+ exchanger-NHE3 and NHE2. Biochim Biophys Acta 1664(1):38–44, 2004.

79. Han HJ, Park SH, Kob HJ, et al. Mechanism of regulation of Na$^+$ transport by angiotensin II in primary renal cells. Kidney International 57:2457–2467, 2000.

80. Romero MF, Hopfer U, Madhun ZT et al. Angiotensin II actions in the rabbit proximal tubule: angiotensin II mediated signaling mechanisms and electrolyte transport in the rabbit proximal tubule. Ren Physiol Biochem 14(4–5):199–207, 1991.

81. Houillier P, Chambrey R, Achard JM, et al. Signaling pathways in the biphasic effect of angiotensin II on apical Na/H antiport activity in proximal tubule. Kidney Int 50(5):1496–1505, 1996.

82. Romero MF, Madhun ZT, Hopfer U, et al. An epoxygenase metabolite of arachidonic acid, 5, 6 epoxy-eicosatetranoic acid mediates angiotensin-induced natriuresis in proximal tubular epithelium. Adv Prostaglandin Thromboxane Leukot Res 21A:205–208, 1991.

83. Good DW, George T, Wang DH, et al. Angiotensin II inhibits HCO3 absorption via a cytochrome P450 dependent pathway in MTAL. Am J Physiol 276:F726–F736, 1999.

84. Kwon TH, Nielsen J, Kim H, et al. Regulation of sodium transporters in the thick ascending limb of rat kidney: response to angiotensin II. Am J Physiol Renal Physiol 285(1):F152–F165, 2003.

85. Bell PD, Peti-Peterdi J. Angiotensin II stimulates macula densa basolateral sodium/hydrogen exchange via type 1 angiotensin II receptors. J Am Soc Nephrol Suppl 11:S225–S229, 1999.

86. Wang T, Geibisch G. Eeffects of angiotensin II on electrolyte transport in the early and late distal tubule in rat kidney. Am J Physiol 271:F143–F149, 1996.

87. Pulakat L, Cooper S, Knowle D, et al. Ligand-dependent complex formation between the Angiotensin II receptor subtype AT2 and Na$^+$/H$^+$ exchanger NHE6 in mammalian cells. Peptides 26(5):863–873, 2005.

88. Bobulescu IA, Di Sole F, Moe OW. Na+/H+ exchangers; physiology and link to hypertension and organ ischemia. Curr Opin Nephrol Hypertens 14(5):485–494, 2005.

89. Lara LS, Cavalcante F, Axelband F, et al. Involvement of Gi/o/cGMP/PKG pathway in the AT2-mediated inhibition of outer cortex proximal tubule Na$^+$K$^+$ATPase by Ang (1-7). Bichem J 395(1):183–190, 2006.

90. Haithcock D, Jiao H, Cui XL, et al. Renal proximal tubular AT2 receptor: Signaling and transport. J Am Soc Nephrol Suppl 11:S69–S74, 1999.

91. Quan A, Baum M. Effect of luminal angiotensin II receptor antagonists on proximal tubule transport. Am J Hypertens 12(5):499–503, 1999.

92. Hakam AC, Hussain T. Angiotensin II type 2 receptor agonist directly inhibits proximal tubule sodium pump activity in obese but not in lean Zucker rats. Hypertension 47(6):1117–1124, 2006.

93. Padia SH, Howell NL, Siragy HM, et al. Renal angiotensin type 2 receptors mediate natriuresis via angiotensin III in the angiotensin II type 1 receptor-blocked rat. Hypertension 47(3):537–544, 2006.

94. Beutler KT, Masilamani S, Turban S, et al. Long-term regulation of ENaC expression in kidney by angiotensin II. Hypertension 41(5):1143–1150, 2003.

95. Davies E, McKenzie SM. Extra adrenal production of corticosteroids. Clin Exp Pharmacol Physiol 30(7):437–445, 2003.

96. Kurdi M, De Mello WC, et al. Working outside the system: an update on the unconventional behavior of the renin-angiotensin system components. Int J Biochem Cell Biol 37:1357–1367, 2005.

97. Zou Y, Akazawa H, Qin Y, et al. Mechanical stress activates angiotensin II type 1 receptor without the involvement of angiotensin II. Nat Cell Biol 6(6):499–506, 2004.

98. Baker KM, Kumar R: Intracellular Ang II induces cell proliferation independent of AT1 receptor. Am J Physiol Cell Physiol 291(5):C995–1001, 2006.

99. Rein H. Vasomotorische regulationen. Ergebn de Physiol 32:28–72, 1932.

100. Buckley NM, Brazeau P, Frasier ID. Renal blood flow autoregulation in developing swine. Am J Physiol 245(1):H1–H6, 1983.

101. Paton JB, Fisher DE. Organ blood flows of fetal and infant baboons. Early Hum Dev 10(1–2):137–144, 1984.

102. Jose PA, Slotkoff LM, Montgomery S, et al. Autoregulation of renal blood flow in the puppy. Am J Physiol 229(4):983–988, 1975.

103. Castrop H, Schnermann J. Impairment of tubuloglomerular feedback regulation of GFR in ecto-5'-nucleotidase/CD73-deficient mice. J Clin Invest 114:634–642, 2004.

104. Inscho EW, Cook AK, Imig JD, et al. Physiological role for P2X1 receptors in renal microvascular autoregulatory behavior. JCI 112(12):1895–1905, 2003.

105. Sun D, Samuelson LC, Yang T, et al. Mediation of tubuloglomerular feedback by adenosine: evidence from mice lacking adenosine 1 receptors. Proc Natl Acad Sci USA 98(17):9938–9989, 2001.

106. Wilcox CS. Redox regulation of the afferent arteriole and tubuloglomerular feedback. Acta Physiol Scand 179(3):217–223, 2003.

107. Bank N. Physical factors in glomerular tubular balance. Renal Physiol 2:289–294, 1979–1980.

108. Schutz S, Le Moullec JM, Corvoll P, et al. Early expression of all the components of the renin-angiotensin system in human development. Am J Pathol 149:2067–2079, 1996.

109. Niimura F, Kon V, Ichikawa I. The renin-angiotensin system in the development of congenital anomalies of the kidney and urinary tract. Curr Opin Pediatr 18(2):161–166, 2006.

110. Tabacova S, Little R, Tsong Y, et al. Adverse pregnancy outcomes associated with maternal enalapril antihypertensive treatment. Pharmacoepidemiol Drug Saf 12:633–646, 2003.

111. Buttar HS. An overview of the influence of ACE inhibitors on fetal-placental circulation and perinatal development. Mol Cell Biochem 176(1–2):61–67, 1997.

112. Cooper WO, Harnandez-Diaz S, Arbogast PG, et al. Major congenital malformations after first-trimester exposure to ACE inhibitors. N Engl J Med 354:2443–2451, 2006.

113. Schaefer C. Angiotensin II receptor antagonists: further evidence of fetotoxicity but not terratogenicity. Birth Defect Res 67:591–594, 2003.

114. Niimura F, Okubo S, Togo A, et al. Temporal and spatial expression of the angiotensinogen gene in mice and rats. Am J Physiol 272:142–147, 1997.

115. Gomez RA, Lynch KR, Sturgill BC, et al. Distribution of renin mRNA and its distribution in the developing kidney. Am J Physiol 257:F850–F858, 1989.

116. Schieffer B, Bernstein KE, Marrero MB, et al. The role of tyrosine phosphorylation in angiotensin II mediated intracellular signalling and cell growth. J Mol Med 74(2):85–95, 1996.

117. Marrero MB, Schieffer B, Paxton WG, et al. The role of tyrosine phosphorylation in angiotensinII-mediated intracellular signaling. Cardiovasc Res 30(4):530–536, 1995.

118. Sadoshima J, Izumo S. Molecular characterization of angiotensin II-induced hypertrophy of cardiac myocytes and hyperplasia of cardiac fibroblasts. Critical role of the AT1 receptor subtype. Circ Res 73(3):413–423, 1993.

119. Norwood VF, Craig MR, Harris JM, et al. Differential expression of angiotensin II receptors during early renal morphogenesis. Am J Physiol 272:R662–R668, 1997.

120. Zhang H, Wada J, Hida K, et al. Collectrin, a collecting duct-specific transmembrane glycoprotein, is a novel homolog of ACE2 and is developmentally regulated in embryonic kidneys. J Biol Chem 276(20):17132–17139, 2001.

121. Kumar D, Moss G, Primhak R, et al. Congenital renal tubular dysplasia and skull ossification defects similar to teratogenic effects of angiotensin converting enzyme (ACE) inhibitors. J Med Genet 34:541–545, 1997.

122. Gribouval O, Gonzales M, Neuhaus T, et al. Mutations in genes in the renin-angiotensin system are associated with autosomal recessive renal tubular dysgenesis. Nat Genet 37:964–968, 2005.
123. Lacoste M, Cai Y, Guicharnaud L, et al. Renal tubular dysgenesis, a not uncommon autosomal recessive disorder leading to oligohydramnios: role of the renin-angiotensin system. J Am Soc Nephrol 17(8):2253–2263, 2006.
124. Nishimura H, Yerkes E, Hohenfellner K, et al. Role of the angiotensin type 2 receptor l gene in congenital anomalies of the kidney and urinary tract, CAKUT, of mice and men. Mol Cell 3:1–10, 1999.
125. Yosypiv IV, El-Dahr SS. Role of the renin-angiotensin system in the development of the ureteric bud and renal collecting system. Pediatr Nephrol 20:1219–1229, 2005.
126. Fiselier T, Monnens L, van Munster P, et al. The renin-angiotensin-aldosterone system in infancy and childhood in basal conditions and after stimulation. Eur J Pediatr 143(1):18–24, 1984.
127. Sulyok E, Nemeth M, Tenyi I, et al. Relationship between the postnatal development of the renin-angiotensin-aldosterone system and electrolyte and acid-base status of the NaCl-supplemented premature infants. In: Spizer A, (ed.): The Kidney during Development Morphogenesis and Function. New York: Masson; 1982: 273.
128. Peleg E, Peleg D, Yaron A, et al. Perinatal development of angiotensin-converting enzyme in the rat's blood. Gynecol Obstet Invest 25(1):12–15, 1988.
129. Walther T, Faber R, Maul B, et al. Fetal, neonatal cord and maternal plasma concentrations of angiotensin converting enzyme (ACE). Prenat Diagn 22(2):111–113, 2002.
130. Bender JW, Davitt MK, Jose P. Angiotensin-1-converting enzyme activity in term and premature infants. Biol Neonate 34(1–2):19–23, 1978.
131. Forhead AJ, Melvin R, Balouzet V, et al. Developmental changes in plasma angiotensin-converting enzyme concentration in fetal and neonatal lambs. Reprod Fertil Dev 10(5):393–398, 1998.
132. Raimbach SJ, Thomas AL. Renin and angiotensin converting enzyme concentrations in the fetal and neonatal guinea-pig. J Physiol 423:441–451, 1990.
133. Forhead AJ, Gulati V, Poore KR, et al. Ontogeny of pulmonary and renal angiotensin-converting enzyme in pigs. Mol Cell Endocrinol 185(1–2):127–133, 2001.
134. O'Connor SJ, Fowden AL, Holdstock N, et al. Developmental changes in pulmonary and renal angiotensin-converting enzyme concentration in fetal and neonatal horses. Reprod Fertil Dev 14(7–8):413–417, 2002.
135. Hattori MA, Del Ben GL, Carmona AK, et al. Angiotensin I-converting enzyme isoforms (high and low molecular weight) in urine of premature and full-term infants. Hypertension 35(6):1284–1290, 2000.
136. Miyawaki M, Okutani T, Higuchi R et al: Plasma angiotensin II levels in the early neonatal period. Arch Dis Child Fetal Neonatal 91(5):F359–F362.
137. Sippell WG, Dorr HG, Bidlingmaier F, et al. Plasma levels of aldosterone, corticosterone, 11-deoxycorticosterone, progesterone, 17-hydroxyprogesterone, cortisol, and cortisone during infancy and childhood. Pediatr Res 14:39–46, 1980.
138. Felder RA, Pelayo JC, Calcagno PL, et al. Alpha adrenoreceptors in the developing kidney. Pediatr Res 17(2):177–180, 1983.
139. Chevalier RL, Thornhill BA, Belmonte DC, et al. Endogenous angiotensin II inhibits natriuresis after acute volume expansion in the neonatal rat. Am J Physiol 270:R393–R397, 1996.
140. Pelayo JC, Fildes RD, Jose PA. Age-dependent renal effects of intrarenal infusion dopamine infusion. Am J Physiol 247:R212–R216, 1984.
141. Muchant DG, Thornhill BA, Belmonte DC, et al. Chronic sodium loading augments natriuretic response to acute volume expansion in the preweaned rat. Am J Physiol 269:R15–R22, 1995.
142. Solhaug MJ, Dong XO, Adelman RD, et al. Ontogeny of neuronal nitric oxide synthase NOS1, in the developing porcine kidney. Am J Physiol Regul Integr Comp Physiol 278(6):R1453–R1459, 2000.
143. Mulder J, Baum M, Quigley R. Diffusional water permeability (PDW) of adult and neonatal rabbit renal brush border membrane vesicles. J Membr Biol 187:167–174, 2002.
144. Mulder J, Chakravarty S, Haddad MN, et al. Glucocorticoids increase osmotic water permeability (Pf) of neonatal rabbit renal brush border membrane vesicles. Am J Physiol Regul Integr Comp Physiol 288:R1417–R1421, 2005.
145. Boberg U, Persson AE. Increased tubuloglomerular feedback activity in Milan hypertensive rats. Am J Physiol 250:F967–F974, 1986.
146. Dilley JR, Arendshorst WJ. Enhanced tubuloglomerular feedback activity in rats developing spontaneous hypertension. Am J Physiol 274:F672–F679, 1984.
147. Al-Dahhan J, Haycock GB, Chantler C, et al. Sodium Homeostasis in term and preterm neonates. I. Renal aspects. Arch Dis Child 58(5):335–342, 1983.
148. Wilcox CS, Welch WJ, Schreiner GF, et al. Natriuretic and diuretic actions of a highly-selective adenosine A1 receptor antagonist. J Am Soc Nephrol 10:714–720, 1990.
149. Du Z, Duan Y, Yan Q, et al. Mechanosensory function of microvilli of the kidney proximal tubule. Proc Natl Acad Sci USA 101(35):13068–13073, 2004.
150. Kon V, Highes ML, Ichikawa I. Physiological basis for the maintenance of glomerulotubular balance in young growing rats. Kidney Int 25(2):391–396, 1984.
151. Bidani AK, Griffin KA. Long-term renal consequences of hypertension for normal and diseased kidneys. Curr Opin Nephrol Hypertens 11:73–80, 2002.
152. Bidani AK, Griffin KA. Pathophysiology of hypertensive renal damage: implications for therapy. Hypertension 44:1–7, 2004.

153. Wilson C, Byrom FB. Renal changes in malignant hypertension. Lancet 1:136–139, 1939.
154. Wilson C, Byrom FB. The vicious circle in chronic Bright's disease. Experimental evidence from the hypertensive rat. Q J Med 10:65–93, 1941.
155. Hill GS, Heptinstall RH. Steroid-induced hypertension in the rat. A microangiopathic and histologic study on the pathogenesis of hypertensive vascular and glomerular lesions. Am J Pathol 52:1–39, 1968.
156. Loutzenhiser R, Griffin K, Williamson G, et al. Renal Autoregulation: new perspectives: the protective and regulatory roles of the underlying mechanisms. Am J Physiol Regul Integr Comp Physiol 290:1153–1167, 2006.
157. Just A, Arendshorst WJ. Dynamics and contribution of mechanisms mediating renal blood flow autoregulation. Am J Physiol Regul Integr Comp Physiol 285:R619–R631, 2003.
158. Navar LG. Renal autoregulation; perspectives from whole kidney and single nephron studies. Am J Physiol Renal Fluid Electrolyte Physiol 234:F357–F370, 1978.
159. Karlsen FM, Anderson PP, Holstein-Rathlou NH. Dynamic autoregulation and renal injury in Dahl rats. Hypertension 30:975–983, 1997.
160. Takemaka T, Forster H, De Micheli A, et al. Impaired myogenic responsiveness of renal microvessels in Dahl salt-sensitive rats. Circ Res 71:471–480, 1992.
161. Karlsen FM, Leysacc PP, Holstein Rathlou NH. Tubuloglomerular feedback in Dahl rats. Am J Physiol Renal Physiol 274:F1561–F1569, 1998.
162. Churchill PC, Churchill MC, Bidani AK, et al. Genetic susceptibility to hypertension-induced renal damage in the rat: evidence based on kidney specific genome transfer. J Clin Invest 100:1373–1382, 1997.
163. Castrop H, Huang Y, Hashimoto S, et al. Impairment of tubuloglomerular feedback regulation of GFR in ecto-5' nucleotidase/CD73-deficient mice. J Clin Invest 114:634–642, 2004.
164. Vallon V. Tubuloglomerular feedback in the kidney: insights from gene-targeted mice. Pflugers Arch-Eur J Physiol 445:470–476, 2003.
165. Hashimoto S, Huang Y, Briggs J, et al. Reduced autoregulatory effectiveness in adenosine 1 receptor-deficient mice. Am J Physiol Renal Physiol 290:888–891, 2006.
166. Nishayama A, Navar LG. ATP mediates tubuloglomerular feedback. Am J Physiol Regulatory Integrative Comp Physiol 283:R273–R275, 2002.
167. Inscho EW. PX2 receptors in regulation of renal microvascular function. Am J Physiol Renal Physiol 280:F927–F944, 2001.
168. Inscho EW, Belott TP, Mason MJ, et al. Extracellular ATP increases cytosolic calcium in cultured rat renal arterial smooth muscle cells. Clin Exp Pharmacol Physiol 23:503–507, 1996.
169. Tojo A, Madsen KM, Wilcox CS, et al. Expression of immunoreactive nitric oxide synthase isoforms in rat kidney: effects of dietary salt and losartan. Jpn Heart J 36:389–398, 1995.
170. Wilcox CS, Welch WJ, Murad F, et al. Nitric oxide synthase in macula densa regulates glomerular capillary pressure. Proc Natl Acad Sci USA 89:11993–11997, 1992.
171. Welch WJ, Wilcox CS, Thomson SC. Nitric oxide and tubuloglomerular feedback. Semin Nephrol 19(3):251–62, 1999.
172. Welch WJ, Tojo A, Lee Ju, et al. Nitric oxide synthase in the JGA of the SHR: expression and role in tubuloglomerular feedback. Am J Physiol 277:F1301–F1308, 1999.
173. Thorup C, Persson AE. Impaired effect of nitric oxide synthesis inhibition on tubuloglomerular feedback in hypertensive rats. Am J Physiol 271:F246–F252, 1996.
174. Welch JW, Tojo A, Wilcox CS. Roles of NO and oxygen radicals in tubuloglomerular feedback in SHR. Am J Physiol Renal Physiol 278(5):F769–F776, 2000.
175. Chen YF, Li PL, Zuo AP. Oxidative stress enhances the production and actions of adenosine in the kidney. Am J Physiol Regul Integr Comp Physiol 281(6):R1808–R1816, 2001.
176. McIntyre M, Bohr DF, Dominiczak AF. Endothelial function in hypertension: the role of superoxide anion. Hypertension 34:539–545, 1999.
177. Yang ZZ, Zhang AY, Yi FX et al: Redox regulation of HIF-1alpha levels and HO-1 expression in renal medullary interstitial cells. Am J Physiol Renal Physiol 284(6):F1207–15, 2003.
178. Ortiz PA, Garvin JL. Role of nitric oxide in the regulation of nephron transport. Am J Physiol Renal Physiol 282(5):F777–F784, 2002.
179. Peti-Peterdi et al. Calcium wave of tubuloglomerular feedback. Am J Physiol Renal Physiol 291(2):F473–802, 2006.
180. Barker DJ, Osmond C, Golding J, et al. Growth in utero, blood pressure in childhood and adult life, and mortality from cardiovascular disease. BMJ 298:564–567, 1989.
181. Alexander BT. Fetal programming of hypertension. Am J Physiol Regul Integr Comp Physiol 290:1–10, 2006.
182. Woods LL, Rasch R. Perinatal Ang II programs adult blood pressure, glomerular number and renal function in rats. Am J Physiol Regul Integr Comp Physiol 275:R1593–R1599, 1998.
183. Gilbert JS, Lang AL, Grant AR, et al. Maternal nutrient restriction in sheep: hypertension and decreased nephron number in offspring at 9 months of age. J Physiol 565:137–147, 2005.
184. Kohlstedt K, Brandis RP, Muller-Esterl W, et al. Angiotensin-converting enzyme is involved in outside-in signaling in endothelial cells. Circ Res 94:60–67, 2002.
185. Zeng C, Wang Z, Hopfer U, et al. Rat strain effects of AT1 receptor activation on D1 dopamine receptors in immortalized renal proximal tubule cells. Hypertension 46:799–805, 2005.
186. Zeng C, Hopfer U, Asico LD, et al. Altered AT1 receptor regulation of ETB receptors in renal proximal tubule cells of spontaneously hypertensive rats. Hypertension 46:926–931, 2005.

187. AbdAlla S, Lother H, Quitterer U. AT1-receptor heterodimers show enhanced G-protein activation and altered receptor sequestration. Nature 407:94–98, 2000.
188. Abadir PM, Periasamy A, Carey RM, et al. Angiotensin II type 2 receptor-bradykinin B2 receptor functional heterodimerization. Hypertension 48:316–322, 2006.
189. Zhuo JL. Intracrine renin and angiotensin II: a novel role in cardiovascular and renal cellular regulation. J Hypertens 24:1017–1020, 2006.
190. Zou Y, Akazawa H, Qin Y, Sano M, et al. Mechanical stress activates angiotensin II type 1 receptor without the involvement of angiotensin II. Nat Cell Biol 6:499–506, 2004.
191. Drukker A, Guignard JP. Renal aspects of the term and preterm infant: a selective update. Current Opin Pediatr 14:175–182, 2002.
192. Menke DR, Bornstein SR. Congenital adrenal hyperplasia. Lancet 365:2125–2136, 2005.
193. Chang SS, Grunder S, Hanukoglu A, et al. Mutations in subunits of the epithelial sodium channel cause salt wasting with hyperkalemic acidosis, pseudohypoaldosteronism type 1. Nat Genet 53:248–533, 1996.

Chapter 8

Renal Modulation: Arginine Vasopressin and Atrial Natriuretic Peptide

Marco Zaffanello, MD, PhD • Maria Antonietta Procaccino, MD • Gilda Stringini, MD • Francesco Emma, MD

Arginine Vasopressin
Atrial Natriuretic Peptide

Total body water (TBW) is distributed in compartments divided by semi-permeable membranes. In postnatal life, approximately two thirds of TBW is located in the intracellular space and one third is located in the extracellular space. The latter is further divided with a 3:1 ratio in the interstitial and plasma compartments.

Passive equilibration of solutes between body compartments is driven by electrochemical gradients and is mediated by a complex system of transport mechanisms that includes pumps, channels, facilitated carriers and selective paracellular pathways. With few exceptions, water diffuses rapidly across epithelia and cell membranes, following osmotic gradients. High transcellular water transport cannot occur through pure lipid bilayers, as these have low osmotic water permeability ($\sim$0.002 cm/s) (1). Water diffusion through cell membranes is therefore mediated by specific water channels, termed aquaporins (AQPs), which enhance osmotic water permeability by 10–1000 fold. Because solutes diffuse less rapidly than their solvent, the relative water content of body compartments is primarily regulated by their solute distribution. This allows the organism to adjust its TBW distribution by regulating the activity of solute transporters located in biological membranes that separate body compartments.

During early fetal life, TBW represents approximately 90% of body mass. As pregnancy progresses, TBW decreases progressively, to reach 75–80% of body mass at the end of gestation. These changes are primarily due to a decline in extracellular water, while intracellular water increases. In the first 24–48 h after birth, the extracellular compartment further decreases, as a result of a negative fluid balance in the immediate postnatal period (2).

The fetus constantly regulates its TBW by salt and water exchanges through the placenta membrane. After birth, uptake of water and solutes is limited to gastrointestinal intakes, while insensible fluid losses increase dramatically. The newborn needs therefore to activate mechanisms that are aimed at controlling water and salt losses. Most of these mechanisms involve the secretion of hormones, which act directly on the kidney. To be efficient, these mechanisms require that sensors, hormone secretion pathways and target organs have reached an appropriate level of maturity.

Water excretion or retention is primarily modulated through the regulation of arginine vasopressin (AVP) secretion. Stimulation of thirst has only limited value in newborns, because of their restricted access to free water and immaturity of the central nervous system.

Salt retention by the kidney is predominantly achieved by activation of the renin-angiotensin-aldosterone system, which is potentiated by endotelins and adrenergic renal nerve activity. Conversely renal salt losses are stimulated by natriuretic peptides (NPs), prostaglandins, kinins, nitric oxide (NO) and adrenomedullin.

In this review, the roles of AVP and NPs in the regulation of body fluid composition during the prenatal and perinatal periods are briefly reviewed. It is important to notice however, that their action is part of a complex network in which all of the above mentioned pathways are synergistically activated or inhibited to maintain body homeostasis.

ARGININE VASOPRESSIN

Normal AVP Physiology

AVP Synthesis

AVP is a cyclic nonapeptide that constitutes the principal antidiuretic hormone for regulation of free water excretion by the kidney. It is composed of an intra-chain disulfide bridge and has a structure similar to oxytocin, which acts primarily as a vasoconstrictor hormone with marginal antidiuretic effects (3). AVP-induced vasoconstriction, on the other hand, is elicited only at non-physiological plasma concentrations in humans (3).

AVP is encoded by the pre-pro-vasopressin gene (PPV), which is translated into protein as a pro-hormone. The PPV peptide undergoes two post-translational modifications, which generate equimolar quantities of AVP and neurophysin II peptides (3). Both AVP and oxytocin are synthesized in cell bodies of neurosecretory axons located in the neurohypophysis. Once synthesized, they are packaged in granules, together with their neurophysin carrier protein, and stored in nerve terminals (4). Neurons containing AVP originate primarily from the supraoptic and paraventricular nuclei of the hypothalamus and are surrounded by a rich network of capillaries scattered throughout the neurohypophysis (5).

Sensor Mechanisms for AVP Secretion

AVP secretion can be stimulated by several mechanisms. The two prominent stimuli are changes in plasma osmolality and changes in blood pressure or volume (6). Other triggers for AVP secretion include emetic stimuli, hypoglycemia, pain, thermic stresses, hypoxia, hypercapnia, acidosis and angiotensin II (ATII) stimulation (7).

Under physiological conditions, serum AVP levels are chiefly dependent on plasma osmolality, which is detected by osmoresponsive cells located near the supraoptic nuclei. These cells act as set-point receptors that inhibit AVP secretion below a given plasma osmolality and gradually stimulate AVP secretion above this set-point (3). Normal subjects differ considerably on a genetic basis, in their osmoreceptor sensitivity and in their set-point for AVP secretion (8). Some subjects respond to changes in plasma osmolality as small as 0.5 mOsm/kg/H_2O, while other subjects require changes as high as 5 mOsm/kg/H_2O (9). The set point for AVP secretion can range from 275 mOsm/kg/H_2O to 290 mOsm/kg/H_2O (9). Additionally to the genetic background, other factors such as age, sex, blood volume, serum calcium levels, can also modify the set point (9). To date, there is very little information on the ontogenicity of osmoreceptors. In particular, it has not been clearly established if the sensitivity of osmoreceptors is fully mature at birth.

The second most important stimuli for AVP secretion are blood pressure and blood volume. Changes lower then 10% in blood volume or blood pressure have little effect on serum AVP levels (10). Above these values, AVP secretion increases rapidly (11). Because these changes are not physiological, AVP levels are primarily regulated by osmoreceptors under normal conditions. Blood volume and pressure changes do not override osmoreceptors, but produce a shift in the set-point for AVP secretion (8). Hemodynamic sensors that mediate AVP secretion are chiefly located in baroreceptor cells of the cardiac atria, carotid sinus and aorta (11).

In adults, the ability to regulate water intake and excretion exceeds by far physiological needs, which allows the maintenance of serum sodium and plasma osmolality within a very narrow range. In contrast, renal immaturity limits the ability of the neonatal kidney to dilute or concentrate the urine and water intake is poorly regulated by activation of thrust in newborns. Consequently, serum sodium levels and plasma osmolality are less stable in neonates, particularly in premature infants.

AVP Receptors and Signal Transduction

AVP receptors are members of the rhodopsin subfamily of G protein-coupled receptors (12). Classically, two types of AVP receptors, V1 and V2, have been identified. The V2 receptor is the primary target of AVP in the kidney and is primarily expressed on the basolateral membranes of collecting duct tubular cells. The V2 receptor is composed of seven transmembrane domains that come together to form a groove for ADH binding in the extracellular region, and contains a binding site for a G_S protein in its intracellular domain (13).

V1 receptors are mainly located in vascular endothelial cells and are sub-divided in V1a and V1b sub-types, according to their location and genetic sequence (14). In addition, it is now well established that V1 receptors are also expressed in renal tubular cells, where they modulate AVP action (15). Unlike V2 receptors, V1 receptors are generally coupled to the inositol tri-phosphate pathway, which causes a vasoconstrictive response induced by increased cytosolic calcium levels (16).

Renal AVP Action and Aquaporin 2 (AQP2) Water Channels

Basolateral binding of AVP to V2 receptors in collecting duct cells activates cytosolic adenylate cyclase, leading to increased intracellular cAMP concentrations. This stimulates protein kinase A (PKA), which in turn promotes phosphorylation of AQP2 proteins and their translocation into the apical membrane (17). In vitro, membrane insertion of AQP2 increases cell water permeability from $\sim$0.005 cm/s to $\sim$0.1 cm/s (18). AQP2 is a member of the AQP superfamily, which to date contains 12 different human water channels (19). AQPs are 26–34 kD glycosylated proteins sharing 50–85% homology. They contain 6 transmembrane spanning domains and are organized in homotetramers. AQPs differ between them by their water transport properties, solute selectivity and tissue expression.

In the kidney, AQP1 is mostly expressed in water permeable proximal tubular cells and capillaries, whereas water transport in the collecting duct is mediated basolaterally by AQP3 and AQP4 and by AVP-dependent insertion of AQP2 on the apical aspects of cells.

AVP stimulation also decreases glomerular capillary ultrafiltration and renal medulla blood flow, increases sodium reabsorption in cortical collecting ducts and in the thick ascending limb of Henle, promotes urea reabsorption in medullary collecting ducts and stimulates prostaglandin synthesis in medullary interstitial cells (20). Most of these actions increase the osmotic gradient for renal water reabsorption.

Extra-renal actions of AVP include limited vasoconstrictive action, platelet activation (release of Von Willebrand factor) and regulation of several central nervous system functions including learning and memory abilities, neuro-endocrine reactions, social behaviors, circadian rhythm, thermoregulation and autonomic functions (20). The clinical relevance of these effects remains uncertain.

Modulation of AVP Action

Renal responses of AVP can be blunted in several conditions. These conditions may have significant clinical relevance as they may interfere with normal mechanisms of body water regulation.

Chronic water-loading in animals, for example, produces vasopressin-independent inhibition of V2 receptor mRNA transcription (21,22). This phenomenon is referred to as 'ADH-escape.' Similarly, ADH escape can be induced by hypercalciuria secondary to inhibition of cAMP production through activation of the calcium-sensing receptor (23), by chronic hypokalemia (24) or acute water loading (21). AQP2 and AQP3 expression are also down-regulated in experimental nephrotic syndrome (25). Conversely, prolonged fasting increases AVP-independent collecting duct renal water reabsorption (26).

Several hormones and molecules modulate AVP action. Oestrogens, for example, can directly increase renal fluid reabsorption (27), while endothelin-1 decreases the sensitivity to AVP of collecting ducts (28). Lithium also produces water diuresis by inhibiting AVP-stimulated translocation of AQP2 through inhibition of adenylate cyclase, while prolonged indomethacin treatment can induce AVP escape, by modulating the intrarenal synthesis of prostaglandins (29,30).

Developmental Differences between the Fetus and the Newborn Infant

Role of AVP in the Placenta

Normal fetal growth is dependent on constant exchanges of fluids at the level of the placenta. V1a receptors are expressed in the placenta, particularly during the first half of the pregnancy (31). In sheep, the time of maximal placental expression of V1a receptor correlates with the time of maximal placental growth, suggesting that AVP stimulation through V1a receptors may play a role in placental growth and differentiation (31). The expression of V1a receptors in the placenta also suggests that AVP may exert a vasoconstrictor effect on the placental circulation, although no definitive evidence has been produced to date.

Low levels of placenta V2 receptor expression are also found throughout gestation. Fetal infusion of AVP in sheep, however, produces no changes in placenta adenylate cyclase activity, questioning the physiologic relevance of V2 receptor expression in this organ (32). No evidence indicating a physiological role of maternal AVP on placenta water permeability or solute transport has been reported (33,34). In particular, maternal or fetal infusion of AVP, at least in experimental ovine models, has no effect on placental fluid exchanges (34).

Several water channels are expressed in human and ovine placenta. AQP1 is primarily expressed in the placental vasculature and fetal membranes, AQP3 and AQP8 in trophoblast epithelial cells and AQP9 in the amnion and allantoid (35–38). No expression of AQP2 has been documented to date.

The relationship between maternal AVP levels and maternal plasma osmolality or maternal renal water clearance is not significantly modified in pregnant animals (39).

In humans, maternal serum AVP levels decrease progressively in the third trimester of pregnancy as total body water increases (40). Despite decreased plasma AVP concentrations, maternal urinary AQP2 excretion increases during pregnancy, indicating a AVP-independent mechanism of renal AQP2 stimulation (40). Because maternal AVP does not cross the placenta membrane, maternal AVP levels do not influence fetal plasma osmolality (41,42).

Amniotic fluid contains AVP of fetal origin (43). Assays using reverse-transcription PCR have shown no evidence of AVP gene expression in the placenta, which reasonably excludes that amniotic AVP is produced by the placenta membranes (44). Intra-amniotic infusion of AVP, on the other hand, produces a sharp increase in fetal serum AVP levels, indicating fast equilibration of AVP concentrations across the amniotic membranes, and that amniotic AVP levels reflect fetal concentrations (45).

Increased concentrations of AVP in the amniotic fluid have been shown to correlate with fetal growth retardation in rats and with fetal stress, particularly fetal acidosis, in humans (46).

AVP in Fetal Life

In humans, AVP and V1b receptors are detectable in the fetal pituitary gland at 11–12 weeks of gestation (44,47). AVP concentrations increase rapidly thereafter until the second trimester of pregnancy (44). In sheep, expression of pituitary V1b receptors decreases progressively during pregnancy, despite increased AVP responsiveness to glucocorticoid, indicating maturation of the feedback mechanisms that regulate AVP secretion throughout gestation (47).

Maternal infusion of mannitol to early pregnant ewes (<120 days) increases fetal AVP secretion in response to increased fetal plasma osmolality (32,34). AVP secretion can also be stimulated in ovine fetuses by angiotensin II (ATII), while inhibition of V1 receptors inhibits ATII-induced pressure changes, suggesting that AVP may play a role in blood pressure regulation during fetal life (48).

Although renal V1a and V2 receptors in rats have been shown to be already significantly expressed at 16 days of gestation (49), AVP has probably little involvement in modulating urine concentration during fetal life, because of renal unresponsiveness to this hormone.

Fetal serum AVP concentrations are relatively stable during normal pregnancy but correlate poorly with fetal urine production (32). Only limited correlation has been reported between amniotic fluid volume and fetal AVP levels (50). These clinical evidences are also substantiated by experimental data, showing that AVP infusion in different fetal animal models produces marginal changes in urine osmolarity or plasma osmolarity, although a certain degree of maturation of these responses during gestation has been documented (32,34,51).

AVP in the Newborn

AVP is released during labour in term newborns, as demonstrated by high levels of the hormone in the umbilical cord (52). Nonetheless, AVP concentrations are similar in infants born by cesarean section or natural delivery, questioning the physiologic relevance of AVP during labor and the exact mechanisms that stimulate AVP secretion (53).

In humans, the urine concentration ability develops progressively during the first year of life and reaches full maturity around 18 months of age (54,55).

Functional impairment of the neonatal kidney to respond to AVP has been established by several investigators in the 1950s–1979s, by direct injection of ADH or pituitary extracts to neonates (56,57). Renal AVP unresponsiveness does not appear to be related to lack of receptors. Murine V2 receptor expression, for example, increases rapidly after the first weeks of life, reaching adult levels by the fifth week (58), demonstrating an adequate number of binding sites for AVP during renal development.

Several investigators have dissected the mechanisms involved in the maturation of cortical collecting ducts' water permeability (reviewed in (49)). Overall, these data show that transduction pathways for AVP are limited by PGE2-mediated inhibition of cAMP synthesis and by increased degradation of cAMP secondary to high phosphodiesterase activity (59–62). Water movement across collecting ducts is also limited by low medullary tonicity, which is caused primarily by the immaturity of the salt reabsorption machinery in the thick ascending limb of Henle and of the urea recycling mechanisms (59). Low dietary protein intake may also play a limiting role in urea generation. In addition, the performance of the countercurrent system is limited by the physical length of the loop of Henle, which increases progressively with renal growth after birth (63).

Finally, it has been proposed that renal concentration ability is limited during the first year of life by expression of AQPs, as AQP2 expression increases progressively after birth in humans and animal models (59). Several investigators have failed, however, to demonstrate alterations in AQP2 expression at birth, both in preterm and term infants (64) and in animal models (65). Urinary AQP-2 excretion decreases postnatally from day 1 to 4, then remains stable during the first 4 weeks of life and increases rapidly between weeks 4 to 6 (64), but the correlation between urinary AQP-2 excretion, AVP levels and renal water concentration ability in the early postnatal period is relatively poor (66).

Experimental studies have also shown that AQP2 synthesis in immature kidneys can be efficiently stimulated by intravenous AVP or dehydration, which is not followed by an increase in urine osmolality (67).

Altogether, this data indicates that AQP2 expression is probably not a limiting factor for the urinary concentration ability of neonates and that low levels of AQP2 expression are related to low stimulation of their synthesis in collecting duct cells. Similarly, the expression of AQP1, AQP3 and AQP4 increases progressively during fetal and early postnatal life, and does not limit water reabsorption in the kidney (49,68,69).

Role of AVP in Pathological Conditions of the Neonate

Diabetes Insipidus

Genetic forms of diabetes insipidus are caused by lack of AVP secretion (central diabetes insipidus, CDI) or by insensibility of the kidney to AVP (nephrogenic diabetes insipidus, NDI). CDI is caused by autosomal dominant mutations of the pre-pro-vasopressin gene (PPV) (70), whereas NDI is caused by X-linked mutations of the V2 receptor gene or autosomal recessive mutations of the AQP2 gene (71). Exceptionally, these later mutations can be transmitted following an autosomal dominant pattern (72). In addition to genetic forms, CDI develops in association with malformations of the central nervous system, particularly midline defects, or is caused by tumor processes that disrupt the neurohypophysis and its connections (73). Acquired forms of NDI are generally secondary to the renal toxic effects of drugs such as lithium, antibiotics, antifungals, antineoplastic agents and antivirals (74). Maternal lithium treatment for bipolar disorders aggravates neonatal unresponsiveness to AVP (29).

Because AVP has a limited role in prenatal and neonatal fluid balance, CDI and NDI do not cause polyhydramnios and newborns are generally asymptomatic. Although genetic defects are present at birth, infants do not develop classic symptoms, including failure to thrive, polyuria, dehydration and hypernatremia, because human milk has relatively low salt and protein content and therefore generates low urine osmolar load. Symptoms usually begin after the first months of life when infants are switched to formulas, which generate twice the osmolar load of breast milk, and are nearly always present when cow's milk and solid foods are introduced (71).

Syndrome of Inappropriate Secretion of ADH (SIADH)

Inappropriate secretion of ADH causes hyponatremia with extracellular volume expansion. In older children, SIADH is caused by neurological lesions, pulmonary diseases or tumors, or treatment with drugs that increase ADH release such as barbiturates, clofibrate, isoproterenol or vincristine (75).

In SIADH, the urine is inappropriately concentrated in comparison to plasma osmolality. Because newborns cannot efficiently concentrate their urine, excessive AVP secretion is generally asymptomatic in the neonatal period and SIADH does not develop. Therefore, the association of hyponatremia with extracellular volume expansion in newborns is nearly invariably caused by excessive intravenous infusion of dextrose solutions or, less frequently, by decreased renal clearance of free water caused by congenital or acquired renal diseases.

AVP Secretion in Neonatal Pathological Conditions

AVP is a hormone released during conditions of stress. Increased AVP secretion has been reported in numerous clinical conditions, including cardiomyopathy, intra-cardiac shunts, congestive heart failure, respiratory distress, mechanical ventilation, systemic infections, meningitis, gastroenteritis, pneumonia, botulism (76–80). Here again, the relative unresponsiveness of the neonatal kidney to AVP questions the clinical relevance of this secretion.

ATRIAL NATRIURETIC PEPTIDE

Normal Physiology of Atrial Natriuretic Peptide (ANP) and Related NPs

Introduction to NPs

The existence of NPs has been suspected since the mid 1950s after the observation that saline infusion released circulating factors that increased natriuresis (81). It was not until the 1980s that De Bold et al demonstrated for the first time that extracts of rat atrial cells contained peptides, which inhibited renal sodium reabsorption (82).

NPs are a family of peptides encoded by three different genes. Type A natriuretic peptide or ANP was first isolated in 1984 from cardiac atrial cells (83). Soon after, two other NPs were isolated from brain cells, namely BNP and CNP (84,85). Although initially isolated from brain tissue, BNP is primarily expressed by cardiac myocytes and CNP by endothelial cells (86,87).

Synthesis of NPs

Similarly to other hormones such as AVP and ACTH, NPs are synthesized as pro-hormones that undergo a series of post-translational modifications. The major site of synthesis of NPs is the heart. NPs' mRNA has also been documented in several tissues, including aorta, brain, lungs, kidneys, adrenal glands, intestine and adipose tissue (87,88). Gene expression in these tissues, however, is far lower than in the heart (87). Therefore, the majority of circulating NPs acting on the cardiovascular and renal systems is of cardiac origin. Nonetheless, extra-cardiac synthesis of NPs has important local effects. In hypothalamic neurons, for example, regional ANP production is thought to regulate AVP secretion and sympathic nerve activity (89), whereas in the kidney the locally secreted urodilatin regulates sodium and water tubular reabsorption (87). CNP also has important functions of regulating chondrocyte proliferation and differentiation, as demonstrated by CNP knock-out mice that suffer from severe dwarfism (90).

Similarly to AVP and oxytocin, NPs are short peptides (28-32 AA) that differ in few residues within a 17 aminoacid ring, closed by a disulfide bridge.

Unlike its BNP and CNP analogues, post-translational processing of the pre-pro-ANP gene generates three additional peptides, namely the long acting natri-uretic peptide (LANP), the vessel dilator peptide and the kaliuretic peptide, which are released into the circulation and enhance ANP activity (88). Additionally, post-translational processing of the ANP gene in the kidney results in a 4 aminoacid longer ANP molecule, termed urodilatin (91).

Sensor Mechanisms for ANP Secretion

Both ANP and BNP are stored in secretory granules of atrial and to a lesser degree ventricular myocytes (86). The major triggers for ANP release are increased cardiac wall stretch and increased blood pressure (82,86,91). In the first case, ANP release is triggered by changes in the central venous return and dilatation of the atrial chambers. The second type of stimulation is brought about by sustained hemodynamic and neuroendocrine stimuli and involves, at least in part, a separate pertussis toxin-sensitive pathway (92). Various hormones, including glucocorticoids, AVP, ATII and catecholamines modulate the rate of ANP release (89).

NP Receptors and Signal Transduction

To date, three different membrane receptors for NPs have been identified. ANP and BNP bind to a specific guanyl cyclase receptor type A, termed NPR-A, and increase intracellular cGMP levels, similar to NO and endothelium derived relaxing factor (93,94). cGMP in turn, activates cGMP-gated channels, cGMP-dependent phosphodiesterases and the cGMP-dependent protein kinases cGKI and cGKII (87,94,95). CNP binds to another guanyl cyclase receptor, named NPR-B, which activates similar pathways (87,94,95). The third receptor, NPR-C, is expressed in target organs in similar or even greater amounts than receptors A and B (8). Unlike its other two homologues, NPR-C has no guanyl cyclase activity and has been reported to decrease cAMP levels (96). Its most major role is to internalize and degrade NPs in order to modulate their activity in various tissues (8). The predominant clearance function of NPR-C is well documented in the NPR-C knockout mouse, which exhibits hypotension, reduced urinary concentration ability and hypotension, as a result of increased bio-availability of both ANP and BNP (97).

Biological Action of NPs

ANP and BNP are potent natriuretic, diuretic and vasodilator hormones, which act primarily on the cardiovascular and renal system. In the kidney, the type A receptors are expressed throughout the nephron. The highest levels of ANP-stimulated accumulation of cGMP are found in the inner medulla collecting ducts and, at higher concentrations of the hormone, in the glomerulus (98,99). Both ANP and BNP increase the glomerular filtration rate by promoting vasodilatation of the afferent arteriole and vasoconstriction of the efferent arteriole, an effect opposed to the action of ATII (100). Glomerular podocytes also express NP receptors and respond to ANP stimulation similarly to NO, by upregulating their cGMP synthesis. The podocyte foot processes contractile apparatus seems to be an obvious target for this signaling cascade (101).

In collecting duct cells, low concentrations of ANP can reduce Na reabsorption by as much as 50%, even in the presence of AVP (97,102–106). Additionally, ANP has been shown to inhibit water permeability by 40–50% in non AVP-stimulated renal collecting ducts (107). In other tubular segments, the action of AVP is more controversial. Decreased ATII-stimulated sodium reabsorption, in the presence of ANP, has been reported in proximal tubular cells and in the thick ascending limb of Henle (106,108), but these data have not been confirmed by other authors (109–111).

Urodilatin, which is locally synthesized in the kidney, is secreted directly in the renal tubules, where it has similar actions to the cardiac-derived ANP (112).

The above-mentioned ATII antagonist effect of ANP is further reinforced by direct inhibition of renin secretion and aldosterone secretion (113–115). At the cardiovascular level, stimulation of type A receptors induces vessel dilatation, increased endothelial permeability and inhibition of the sympathetic system, which adds to the inhibition of the renin-ATII-aldosterone axis (8,90).

The essential role of NPs in blood pressure regulation is best demonstrated by experiments in transgenic animals, where targeted deletion of the ANP gene, or of the type A receptor gene, leads to severe arterial hypertension, while overexpression of the same genes induces hypotension (86). Deletion of the NPR-A gene limited to vascular smooth muscle cells, on the other hand, does not cause hypotension under normal conditions, but abolishes the vasodilatatory response after acute volume loading, demonstrating the complexity of the biological activities that are mediated by NPs (116).

In conditions of chronic volume expansion or hypertension, ANP also exerts an antihypertrophic effect and BNP exerts an antifibrotic effect by inhibiting myocyte and fibroblast proliferation, respectively (87,117–119).

Modulation of ANP Action

The above-discussed data shows that NPs counteract the renal and cardiovascular effects of a combined secretion of ATII and AVP. These various systems are heavily interdependent and can influence each other significantly. ATII receptor blockade during heart failure, for example, mitigates renal hyporesponsiveness to ANP (120). These interactions occur at different levels, including reciprocal modulation of gene transcription, of sensor mechanisms that trigger hormone secretion, of receptor expression and activity on second messengers (121). Inhibition of PKA, for example, increases NPR-A activity, which results in increased generation of cGMP after ANP stimulation (122). Conversely, activation of cGMP-coupled phosphodiesterases by ANP decreases intracellular cAMP levels (87,95), which is the second messenger for AVP activity in the kidney, where it activates PKA (see above).

These various levels of interaction have a critical role in creating a dynamic balance between different hormonal pathways, allowing the preservation of TBW and blood pressure control. Other hormones also modulate the activity of NPs at different levels. The neutral endopeptidase (NEP) for example, is a zinc-metallopeptidase that degrades biologically active peptides. In the kidney, NEP is heavily expressed in the brush border of renal proximal epithelial cells (123) and in mesangial cells, where it is thought to have an important role in modulating renal hemodynamics, in part by inactivation of NPs (124). Endothelin 1, on the other hand, promotes gene expression of NP in ventricular myocytes (125), while bradykinin counteracts the ANP-stimulated sodium and water excretion, by acting directly on the kidney (126,127).

Developmental Differences between the Fetus and the Newborn Infant

Role of ANP in the Placenta

Maternal ANP levels increase steadily during pregnancy and decline significantly in the postpartum period (128). There is no evidence suggesting that ANP or other NPs cross the placenta. In 20-days pregnant rats for example, no active or passive transport of intact radiolabeled ANP across the placenta has been documented (129). Since ANP plays a major role in the regulation of vascular tone, several investigators have studied the role of ANP in regulating placenta hemodynamics. In particular, because the placenta lacks an autonomic innervation, it has been hypothesized that locally produced vasoactive factors, such as NPs, contribute to placental vascular tone control (130). This hypothesis has now been confirmed by several studies showing that NPs and their receptors are expressed in the placenta.

Placental synthesis of ANP has been documented by immunocytochemistry and RT-PCR in human extravillous trophoblasts and to a lesser degree in decidual cells, whereas villous trophoblasts do not appear to express significant amounts of ANP (130). ANP and BNP synthesis has also been documented in vitro, in cultured human umbilical vein endothelial cells and human amnion cells, respectively (131,132). In mice, strong expression of CNP and, to a lesser degree, of BNP, has been shown early during gestation in the decidua, whereas placental synthesis of ANP remains controversial (133–135).

The presence of NP receptors was demonstrated using binding assays, in non villous microsomal placental extracts, even before their isolation and molecular characterization (136). Subsequently, the expression of NPR-A and NPR-B was confirmed in human uterine tissues, including decidua, chorion, myometrium and in the placenta itself (132). ANP receptors in the human placenta have been found to be significantly more expressed in its fetal components than in the maternal microvillous membranes (137). The human placental artery has also been found to be the site of expression of large amounts of ANP and BNP receptors and expresses the clearance receptor (NPR-C) (138).

Clearance receptors are downregulated in fetoplacental artery endothelial cells towards the end of gestation, which increases the local concentrations of ANP and corresponds to increased generation of cGMP (139). This is thought to be, at least in part, secondary to increased placental secretion of basic fibroblast growth factor during the last trimester of the pregnancy (139). On this basis, it has been postulated that ANP and other NPs are critical for maintaining adequate blood flow in the placental and uterine tissues and that in pathological conditions, such as preeclampsia, these hormones play an important role.

In fact, the number of guanyl cyclase-coupled receptors in the placental vasculature, maternal ANP plasma levels and fetal ANP plasma levels, are increased during preeclampsia (140–145). Increased ANP and ANP receptor expression in this condition may represent a local defense mechanism to prevent further increases in maternal blood pressure, by promoting arterial vasodilatation and natriuresis (141). Accordingly, infusion of ANP in human placenta inhibits arterial vasoconstriction induced by L-arginine, ATII and to a lesser extent endothelin-1 (140,146–148). These effects are not mediated by NO and may also extend to thromboxane-induced vasoconstriction at higher, non-physiological, ANP concentrations (147,148).

Intravenous infusion of low doses of ANP (10 ng/kg/min) to women with preeclampsia has been shown to induce a mean uteroplacental blood flow increase of 28% (149). An individual increase in placental blood flow correlates with increased cGMP synthesis and with a decrease in maternal blood pressure, indicating effective uteroplacental vasodilatation (149).

ANP in Fetal Life

Several studies indicate that ANP levels in fetal blood are not related to maternal ANP concentrations. In the rat embryo, gene expression of ANP mRNA is detectable at 8.5 days of gestation (150). Fetal ANP levels during pregnancy are higher then maternal levels, in murine and ovine experimental models (151,152). Higher fetal ANP levels do not result from slower removal rates by the developing kidney or by transfer from maternal circulation (153,154). In fact, ANP secretion is markedly increased in rats during mid-gestation, although the major site of synthesis is in the ventricles rather then the atria (151,155). Similarly, in 17–19 weeks' gestation human fetuses, ANP expression is higher in the ventricles (133). In ovine fetuses on the other hand, ANP is mainly synthesized in the atria (156). These differences may be relevant when translating animal data to humans, as the mechanisms stimulating NP release may not be entirely comparable.

A number of experimental data, mostly obtained in murine and ovine fetal models, have shown that mid- and late-gestation animals can readily release NPs in response to various stimuli, including ATII infusion, AVP infusion, indomethacin treatment, acute fetal volume expansion, hypertonicity and fetal hypoxia (151,154,157,158). Nonetheless, NPs have probably little role in renal homeostasis and fluid balance during intrauterine life, which is chiefly insured by the placenta. In general, ANP infusion at supra-physiological doses in fetal animals decreases arterial blood pressure, has a moderate diuretic effect, but does not increase natriuresis significantly (155,158).

ANP in the Newborn

At birth, loss of the placenta circulation produces dramatic hemodynamic changes that significantly modify the atria sizes and pressures, and stimulate NP secretion. Increased perinatal secretion of ANP and BNP has been well established in both preterm and term newborns. This secretion starts at birth and peaks at days 1–2 of life to decrease thereafter, reaching a plateau after 1–2 weeks (159). Because of their known natriuretic and diuretic action, it has been logically proposed that NPs play a predominant role in promoting the transition from fetal to postnatal circulation and stimulate the postnatal natriuretic phase that causes the contraction of the extracellular space (160).

Plasma ANP levels and the onset of the postnatal diuretic phase in human newborns, have been found, however, to be relatively poorly correlated, both in preterm and term infants (161,162). This probably highlights the complexity of interactions between the cardiovascular and renal system after birth, where NPs are only part of a complex hormonal and hemodynamic system that is activated after birth.

Several experimental data also indicate that the renal response to NPs is still, in large, immature at birth. ANP infusion, for example, induces a blunted natriuretic and diuretic response in newborn rabbits, which has been attributed to immaturity of ANP receptors and signal transduction pathways and to overriding interactions with other hormonal systems (163). Similarly, the natriuretic and diuretic response to ANP in sheep has been shown to undergo a maturation phase that extends well into the first postnatal weeks (153). In rats, expression of renal ANP receptors is low at birth and increases thereafter to reach adult levels only at the end of the 5th week of life (163). This correlates with a parallel maturation of their signal transduction pathways, as demonstrated by a progressive increase in ANP-induced renal cGMP synthesis during the first weeks of life (164).

In humans, a similar pattern of postnatal increase in cGMP urinary excretion has also been documented, although it is highly variable (165).

In summary, these data indicate that the sensor and synthesis mechanisms leading to ANP and BNP secretion are mature at birth. The vasodilatatory response to NPs is also satisfactory in utero, but the renal responses require a phase of postnatal maturation (166). Increased ANP levels in neonates, therefore, indicate primarily a state of volume expansion or disturbances of the pulmonary circulation related to cardiovascular and respiratory diseases (160,167), but do not necessarily anticipate a phase of negative fluid balance related to increased renal fluid losses.

Role of ANP in Pathological Conditions of the Newborn

Fetal Distress

Levels of ANP have been found to be elevated during fetal distress and fetal hypoxia (168–171). On these bases, it has been postulated that increased cord levels of NPs may predict the development of periventricular leukomalesia lesions. One study has prospectively addressed this hypothesis (172). No significant association was found between brain lesions and cord ANP or BNP levels in four patients that later developed periventricular leukomalacia, when compared to control infants (172).

Postnatal Diseases

After birth, ANP levels often remain elevated in infants with respiratory distress. Most likely, high ANP levels indicate increased atrial wall stretch secondary to volume expansion, pulmonary hypertension, mechanical ventilation or patent ductus arteriosus (PDA). In the hypothesis that ANP and/or BNP levels could be predictive of the clinical outcome or may anticipate a phase of increased diuresis coinciding with clinical improvement, several investigators have studied NPs in sick neonates. Increased interest in NPs has also been stimulated by the recent availability of whole blood assays, allowing on-site BNP measurements within 10 min, from as little as 250 mcl of blood samples (173).

The available data however has generated controversial results. Discrepancies between studies are probably related to differences in the studied populations, in particular to the co-existence of a PDA, to differences in policies for fluid and respiratory management between centers and may reflect changes over time in these policies. In addition, ANP secretion is often variable in infants within a 24-h period. This may be related to sudden changes in atrial filling pressures, secondary for example to small fluid boluses, variations in PDA shunting or in the mean airway pressure when infants are mechanically ventilated.

In this respect, the study by Modi et al is extremely illustrative (174). These authors have measured ANP levels every 4 h in 18 preterm infants with respiratory distress. A clear period of respiratory improvement was observed in 15 babies, which was preceded by a peak in circulating ANP in 8 babies and was concomitant with the same peak in 7 babies, demonstrating a temporal relationship between circulating ANP and improvement in respiratory function (174). The same study, however, has also documented in several infants peaks of ANP that were not followed by immediate respiratory improvement (174). This observation illustrates the problem of assessing the clinical usefulness of NP dosage in neonates, and probably explains a significant part of the large variance that has been reported by several authors when correlating NP levels with respiratory improvement (167,175–179). A similar variability has also been reported when NP levels have been correlated with the timing of onset of the postnatal diuretic phase. Overall, a majority of studies report nonetheless a temporal relationship between increased ANP or BNP levels and a phase of negative sodium and water balance (162,174,175,177,180,181).

The persistence of a PDA is probably the most confounding factors in neonatal ANP and BNP studies. In fact, left-to-right shunting resulting from a PDA, by its dramatic hemodynamic effects on atrial filling pressures, is one of the most potent triggers for ANP and BNP secretion in the neonatal period. Infants with PDA have high levels of circulating NPs (173,182–184). A recent study by Choi et al has shown very significant correlations between BNP levels and PDA (173). Non-symptomatic infants with PDA had a five fold increase in their BNP levels when compared with controls, and infants with symptomatic PDA had five times higher levels than infants with asymptomatic PDA. BNP levels returned to normal concentrations after duct closure with indomethacin (173). Other authors have also reported similar results, although their data were considerably less significant (182–186). Similarly, increased levels of BNP have also been documented in infants with persistent pulmonary hypertension of the newborn, in comparison with healthy infants or with infants with respiratory disease but no evidence of pulmonary hypertension (187).

Congestive Heart Failure and Congenital Heart Diseases

ANP and BNP levels are increased during congestive heart failure and in most congenital heart diseases, including septal and atrial defects, transposition of great arteries, tetralogy of Fallot, pulmonary stenosis, tricuspid valve atresia, mitral valve stenosis or regurgitation (188–191). In general, reported data indicate higher NP levels in conditions with marked atrial distension, left ventricle overload, left-to-right shunt and pulmonary hypertension. Cardiopulmonary bypass has been shown to cause in these conditions a dramatic decrease in NP levels (189).

REFERENCES

1. Goodman BE. Transport of small molecules across cell membranes: water channels and urea transporters. Adv Physiol Educ 26:146, 2002.
2. Shaffer SG, Weisman DN. Fluid requirements in the preterm infant. Clin Perinatol 19:233, 1992.
3. Robertson GL, Berl T. Pathophysiology of water metabolism. In Brenner BM (ed.): The Kidney, 5th edn (Philadelphia, PA: Saunders), pp. 873–928, 1996.
4. Miyata S, Takamatsu H, Maekawa S, et al. Plasticity of neurohypophysial terminals with increased hormonal release during dehydration: ultrastructural and biochemical analyses. J Comp Neurol 434:413, 2001.
5. Hoffman GE, McDonald T, Figueroa JP, Nathanielsz PW. Neuropeptide cells and fibers in the hypothalamus and pituitary of the fetal sheep: comparison of oxytocin and arginine vasopressin. Neuroendocrinology 50:633, 1989.
6. Hammer M, Olgaard K, Schapira A, et al. Hypovolemic stimuli and vasopressin secretion in man. Acta Endocrinol 118:465, 1988.
7. Engelmann M, Ludwig M. The activity of the hypothalamo-neurohypophysial system in response to acute stressor exposure: neuroendocrine and electrophysiological observations. Stress 7:91, 2004.
8. Brenner BM, Ballermann BJ, Gunning ME, Zeidel ML. Diverse biological actions of atrial natriuretic peptide. Physiol Rev 70:665, 1990.
9. Toto KH. Regulation of plasma osmolality: thirst and vasopressin. Crit Care Nurs Clin North Am 6:661, 1994.
10. Mannix ET, Farber MO, Aronoff GR, et al. Hemodynamic, renal, and hormonal responses to lower body positive pressure in human subjects. J Lab Clin Med 128:585, 1996.
11. Schrier RW, Berl T, Anderson RJ. Osmotic and nonosmotic control of vasopressin release. Am J Physiol 236:F321, 1979.
12. Czaplewski C, Kazmierkiewicz R, Ciarkowski J. Molecular modeling of the human vasopressin V2 receptor/agonist complex. J Comput Aided Mol Des 12:275, 1998.
13. Ruiz-Opazo N, Akimoto K, Herrera VL. Identification of a novel dual angiotensin II/vasopressin receptor on the basis of molecular recognition theory. Nat Med 1:1074, 1995.
14. Thibonnier M, Conarty DM, Preston JA, et al. Human vascular endothelial cells express oxytocin receptors. Endocrinology 140:1301, 1999.
15. Bankir L. Antidiuretic action of vasopressin: quantitative aspects and interaction between V1a and V2 receptor-mediated effects. Cardiovasc Res 51:372, 2001.
16. Son MC, Brinton RD. Vasopressin-induced calcium signaling in cultured cortical neurons. Brain Res 793:244, 1998.
17. Valenti G, Procino G, Tamma G, et al. Minireview: aquaporin 2 trafficking. Endocrinology 146:5063, 2005.
18. Kuwahara M, Fushimi K, Terada Y, et al. cAMP-dependent phosphorylation stimulates water permeability of aquaporin-collecting duct water channel protein expressed in Xenopus oocytes. J Biol Chem 270:10384, 1995.
19. Itoh T, Rai T, Kuwahara M, et al. Identification of a novel aquaporin, AQP12, expressed in pancreatic acinar cells. Biochem Biophys Res Commun 330:832, 2005.
20. Harris HW, Zeidel ML. Cell biology of vasopressin. In Brenner BM (ed.): The Kidney, 5th edn (Philadelphia, PA: Saunders), pp 516–531, 1996.
21. Ecelbarger CA, Nielsen S, Olson BR, et al. Role of renal aquaporins in escape from vasopressin-induced antidiuresis in rat. J Clin Invest 99:1852, 1997.
22. Tian Y, Sandberg K, Murase T, et al. Vasopressin V2 receptor binding is down-regulated during renal escape from vasopressin-induced antidiuresis. Endocrinology 141:307, 2000.
23. Hebert SC, Brown EM, Harris HW. Role of the Ca2+-sensing receptor in divalent mineral ion homeostasis. J Exp Biol 200:295, 1997.
24. Marples D, Frokiaer J, Dorup J, et al. Hypokalemia-induced downregulation of aquaporin-2 water channel expression in rat kidney medulla and cortex. J Clin Invest 97:1960, 1996.
25. Apostol E, Ecelbarger CA, Terris J, et al. Reduced renal medullary water channel expression in puromycin aminonucleoside-induced nephrotic syndrome. J Am Soc Nephrol 8:15, 1997.
26. Wilke C, Sheriff S, Soleimani M, Amlal H. Vasopressin-independent regulation of collecting duct aquaporin-2 in food deprivation. Kidney Int 67:201, 2005.

27. Stachenfeld NS, Taylor HS, Leone CA, Keefe DL. Estrogen effects on urine concentrating response in young women. J Physiol 552:869, 2003.

28. Ge Y, Stricklett PK, Hughes AK, et al. Collecting duct-specific knockout of the endothelin A receptor alters renal vasopressin responsiveness, but not sodium excretion or blood pressure. Am J Physiol Renal Physiol 289:F692, 2005.

29. Walker RJ, Weggery S, Bedford JJ, et al. Lithium-induced reduction in urinary concentrating ability and urinary aquaporin 2 (AQP2) excretion in healthy volunteers. Kidney Int 67:291, 2005.

30. Agnoli GC, Borgatti R, Cacciari M, et al. Low-dose desmopressin infusion: renal action in healthy women in moderate salt retention and depletion, and interactions with prostanoids. Prostaglandins Leukot Essent Fatty Acids 67:263, 2002.

31. Koukoulas I, Risvanis J, Douglas-Denton R, et al. Vasopressin receptor expression in the placenta. Biol Reprod 69:679, 2003.

32. Herin P, Kim JK, Schrier RW, et al. Ovine fetal response to water deprivation: aspects on the role of vasopressin. Q J Exp Physiol 73:931, 1988.

33. Irion GL, Mack CE, Clark KE. Fetal hemodynamic and fetoplacental vascular response to exogenous arginine vasopressin. Am J Obstet Gynecol 162:1115, 1990.

34. Towstoless MK, Congiu M, Coghlan JP, Wintour EM. Placental and renal control of plasma osmolality in chronically cannulated ovine fetus. Am J Physiol 253:R389, 1987.

35. Liu H, Koukoulas I, Ross MC, et al. Quantitative comparison of placental expression of three aquaporin genes. Placenta 25:475, 2004.

36. Wang S, Chen J, Beall M, et al. Expression of aquaporin 9 in human chorioamniotic membranes and placenta. Am J Obstet Gynecol 191:2160, 2004.

37. Ishibashi K, Morinaga T, Kuwahara M, et al. Cloning and identification of a new member of water channel (AQP10) as an aquaglyceroporin. Biochim Biophys Acta 1576:335, 2002.

38. Mobasheri A, Wray S, Marples D. Distribution of AQP2 and AQP3 water channels in human tissue microarrays. J Mol Histol 36:1, 2005.

39. Bell RJ, Laurence BM, Meehan PJ, et al. Regulation and function of arginine vasopressin in pregnant sheep. Am J Physiol 250:F777, 1986.

40. Buemi M, D'Anna R, Di Pasquale G, et al. Urinary excretion of aquaporin-2 water channel during pregnancy. Cell Physiol Biochem 11:203, 2001.

41. Stegner H, Leake RD, Palmer SM, Fisher DA. Permeability of the sheep placenta to 125I-arginine vasopressin. Dev Pharmacol Ther 7:140, 1984.

42. Desai M, Guerra C, Wang S, Ross MG. Programming of hypertonicity in neonatal lambs: resetting of the threshold for vasopressin secretion. Endocrinology 144:4332, 2003.

43. Oosterbaan HP, Swaab DF, Boer GJ. Oxytocin and vasopressin in the rat do not readily pass from the mother to the amniotic fluid in late pregnancy. J Dev Physiol 7:55, 1985.

44. Mastorakos G, Ilias I. Maternal and fetal hypothalamic-pituitary-adrenal axes during pregnancy and postpartum. Ann N Y Acad Sci 997:136, 2003.

45. Gilbert WM, Cheung CY, Brace RA. Rapid intramembranous absorption into the fetal circulation of arginine vasopressin injected intraamniotically. Am J Obstet Gynecol 164:1013, 1991.

46. Oosterbaan HP, Swaab DF. Amniotic oxytocin and vasopressin in relation to human fetal development and labour. Early Hum Dev 19:253, 1989.

47. Young SF, Smith JL, Figueroa JP, Rose JC. Ontogeny and effect of cortisol on vasopressin-1b receptor expression in anterior pituitaries of fetal sheep. Am J Physiol Regul Integr Comp Physiol 284:R51, 2003.

48. Shi L, Guerra C, Yao J, Xu Z. Vasopressin mechanism-mediated pressor responses caused by central angiotensin II in the ovine fetus. Pediatr Res 56:756, 2004.

49. Bonilla-Felix M. Development of water transport in the collecting duct. Am J Physiol Renal Physiol 287:F1093, 2004.

50. Bajoria R, Ward S, Sooranna SR. Influence of vasopressin in the pathogenesis of oligohydramnios-polyhydramnios in monochorionic twins. Eur J Obstet Gynecol Reprod Biol 113:49, 2004.

51. Robillard JE, Weitzman RE. Developmental aspects of the fetal renal response to exogenous arginine vasopressin. Am J Physiol 238:F407, 1980.

52. Ramin SM, Porter JC, Gilstrap LC 3rd, Rosenfeld CR. Stress hormones and acid-base status of human fetuses at delivery. J Clin Endocrinol Metab 73:182, 1991.

53. Pochard JL, Lutz-Bucher B. Vasopressin and oxytocin levels in human neonates. Relationships with the evolution of labour and beta-endorphins. Acta Paediatr Scand 75:774, 1986.

54. Zelenina M, Zelenin S, Aperia A. Water channels (aquaporins) and their role for postnatal adaptation. Pediatr Res 57:47R, 2005.

55. Polacek E, Vocel J, Neugebauerova L, et al. The osmotic concentrating ability in healthy infants and children. Arch Dis Child 40:291, 1965.

56. Svenningsen NW, Aronson AS. Postnatal development of renal concentration capacity as estimated by DDAVP-test in normal and asphyxiated neonates. Biol Neonate 25:230, 1974.

57. Winberg J. Renal function in water-losing syndrome due to lower urinary tract obstruction before and after treatment. Acta Paediatr 48:149, 1959.

58. Ammar A, Roseau S, Butlen D. Pharmacological characterization of V1a vasopressin receptors in the rat cortical collecting duct. Am J Physiol 262:F546, 1992.

59. Bonilla-Felix M, Vehaskari VM, Hamm LL. Water transport in the immature rabbit collecting duct. Pediatr Nephrol 13:103, 1999.

60. Gengler WR, Forte LR. Neonatal development of rat kidney adenyl cyclase and phosphodiesterase. Biochim Biophys Acta 279:367, 1972.

61. Quigley R, Chakravarty S, Baum M. Antidiuretic hormone resistance in the neonatal cortical collecting tubule is mediated in part by elevated phosphodiesterase activity. Am J Physiol Renal Physiol 286:F317, 2004.

62. Sulyok E. Renal response to vasopressin in premature infants: what is new? Biol Neonate 53:212, 1988.

63. Celsi G, Jakobsson B, Aperia A. Influence of age on compensatory renal growth in rats. Pediatr Res 20:347, 1986.

64. Tsukahara H, Hata I, Sekine K, et al. Renal water channel expression in newborns: measurement of urinary excretion of aquaporin-2. Metabolism 47:1344, 1998.

65. Devuyst O, Burrow CR, Smith BL, et al. Expression of aquaporins-1 and -2 during nephrogenesis and in autosomal dominant polycystic kidney disease. Am J Physiol 271:F169, 1996.

66. Nyul Z, Vajda Z, Vida G, Sulyok E, et al. Urinary aquaporin-2 excretion in preterm and full-term neonates. Biol Neonate 82:17, 2002.

67. Bonilla-Felix M, Jiang W. Aquaporin-2 in the immature rat: expression, regulation, and trafficking. J Am Soc Nephrol 8:1502, 1997.

68. Yasui M, Serlachius E, Lofgren M, et al. Perinatal changes in expression of aquaporin-4 and other water and ion transporters in rat lung. J Physiol 505:3, 1997.

69. Yamamoto T, Sasaki S, Fushimi K, et al. Expression of AQP family in rat kidneys during development and maturation. Am J Physiol 272:F198, 1997.

70. Rutishauser J, Boni-Schnetzler M, Boni J, et al. A novel point mutation in the translation initiation codon of the pre-pro-vasopressin-neurophysin II gene: cosegregation with morphological abnormalities and clinical symptoms in autosomal dominant neurohypophyseal diabetes insipidus. J Clin Endocrinol Metab 81:192, 1996.

71. Knoers NVAM, Monnens LAH: Nephrogenic diabetes insipidus. In Avner ED, Harmon WE, Niaudet P (Eds), Pediatric Nephrology 5th edn (pp. 777–787). Philadelphia, PA: Lippincott Williams and Wilkins, 2004.

72. Knoers NV, Deen PM. Molecular and cellular defects in nephrogenic diabetes insipidus. Pediatr Nephrol 16:1146, 2001.

73. Abernethy LJ, Qunibi MA, Smith CS. Normal MR appearances of the posterior pituitary in central diabetes insipidus associated with septo-optic dysplasia. Pediatr Radiol 27:45, 1997.

74. Garofeanu CG, Weir M, Rosas-Arellano MP, et al. Causes of reversible nephrogenic diabetes insipidus: a systematic review. Am J Kidney Dis 45:626, 2005.

75. Baylis PH. The syndrome of inappropriate antidiuretic hormone secretion. Int J Biochem Cell Biol 35:1495, 2003.

76. Price JF, Towbin JA, Denfield SW, et al. Arginine vasopressin levels are elevated and correlate with functional status in infants and children with congestive heart failure. Circulation 109:2550, 2004.

77. Rocha JL, Friedman E, Boson W, et al. Molecular analyses of the vasopressin type 2 receptor and aquaporin-2 genes in Brazilian kindreds with nephrogenic diabetes insipidus. Hum Mutat 14:233, 1999.

78. Kavvadia V, Greenough A, Dimitriou G, et al. A comparison of arginine vasopressin levels and fluid balance in the perinatal period in infants who did and did not develop chronic oxygen dependency. Biol Neonate 78:86, 2000.

79. Kobayashi R, Iguchi A, Nakajima M, et al. Hyponatremia and syndrome of inappropriate antidiuretic hormone secretion complicating stem cell transplantation. Bone Marrow Transplant 34:975, 2004.

80. Papadimitriou A, Kipourou K, Manta C, et al. Adipsic hypernatremia syndrome in infancy. J Pediatr Endocrinol Metab 10:547, 1997.

81. Henry JP, Gauer OH, Sieker HO. The effect of moderate changes in blood volume on left and right atrial pressures. Circ Res 4:91, 1956.

82. de Bold AJ, Borenstein HB, Veress AT, Sonnenberg H. A rapid and potent natriuretic response to intravenous injection of atrial myocardial extract in rats. Life Sci 28:89, 1981.

83. Kangawa K, Matsuo H. Purification and complete amino acid sequence of alpha-human atrial natriuretic polypeptide (alpha-hANP). Biochem Biophys Res Commun 118:131, 1984.

84. Sudoh T, Kangawa K, Minamino N, Matsuo H. A new natriuretic peptide in porcine brain. Nature 332:78, 1988.

85. Sudoh T, Minamino N, Kangawa K, Matsuo H. C-type natriuretic peptide (CNP): a new member of natriuretic peptide family identified in porcine brain. Biochem Biophys Res Commun 168:863, 1990.

86. de Bold AJ, Ma KK, Zhang Y, et al. The physiological and pathophysiological modulation of the endocrine function of the heart. Can J Physiol Pharmacol 79:705, 2001.

87. Kuhn M. Cardiac and intestinal natriuretic peptides: insights from genetically modified mice. Peptides 26:1078, 2005.

88. Vesely DL. Natriuretic peptides and acute renal failure. Am J Physiol Renal Physiol 285:F167, 2003.

89. Ruskoaho H. Atrial natriuretic peptide: synthesis, release, and metabolism. Pharmacol Rev 44:479, 1992.

90. Chusho H, Tamura N, Ogawa Y, et al. Dwarfism and early death in mice lacking C-type natriuretic peptide. Proc Natl Acad Sci USA 98:4016, 2001.

91. Levin ER, Gardner DG, Samson WK. Natriuretic peptides. N Engl J Med 339:321, 1998.

92. McGrath MF, de Bold AJ. Determinants of natriuretic peptide gene expression. Peptides 26:933, 2005.

93. Joubert S, Jossart C, McNicoll N, De Lean A. Atrial natriuretic peptide-dependent photolabeling of a regulatory ATP-binding site on the natriuretic peptide receptor-A. FEBS J 272:5572, 2005.

94. Inoue T, Nonoguchi H, Tomita K. Physiological effects of vasopressin and atrial natriuretic peptide in the collecting duct. Cardiovasc Res 51:470, 2001.

95. Garbers DL, Lowe DG. Guanylyl cyclase receptors. J Biol Chem 269:30741, 1994.

96. Fuller F, Porter JG, Arfsten AE, et al. Atrial natriuretic peptide clearance receptor. Complete sequence and functional expression of cDNA clones. J Biol Chem 263:9395, 1988.

97. Matsukawa N, Grzesik WJ, Takahashi N, et al. The natriuretic peptide clearance receptor locally modulates the physiological effects of the natriuretic peptide system. Proc Natl Acad Sci USA 96:7403, 1999.

98. Nonoguchi H, Knepper MA, Manganiello VC. Effects of atrial natriuretic factor on cyclic guanosine monophosphate and cyclic adenosine monophosphate accumulation in microdissected nephron segments from rats. J Clin Invest 79:500, 1987.

99. Terada Y, Moriyama T, Martin BM, et al. RT-PCR microlocalization of mRNA for guanylyl cyclase-coupled ANF receptor in rat kidney. Am J Physiol Renal Physiol 261:1080, 1991.

100. Gunning ME, Brenner BM. Natriuretic peptides and the kidney: current concepts. Kidney Int Suppl 38:S127, 1992.

101. Lewko B. [Interaction between guanylate cyclases in the kidney glomerulus]. Postepy Hig Med Dosw 53:225, 1999.

102. Nonoguchi H, Sands JM, Knepper MA. ANF inhibits NaCl and fluid absorption in cortical collecting duct of rat kidney. Am J Physiol 256:F179, 1989.

103. Zeidel ML, Silva P, Brenner BM, Seifter JL. cGMP mediates effects of atrial peptides on medullary collecting duct cells. Am J Physiol 252:F551, 1987.

104. Zeidel ML, Kikeri D, Silva P, et al. Atrial natriuretic peptides inhibit conductive sodium uptake by rabbit inner medullary collecting duct cells. J Clin Invest 82:1067, 1988.

105. Sonnenberg H, Honrath U, Chong CK, Wilson DR. Atrial natriuretic factor inhibits sodium transport in medullary collecting duct. Am J Physiol 250:F963, 1986.

106. Harris PJ, Thomas D, Morgan TO. Atrial natriuretic peptide inhibits angiotensin-stimulated proximal tubular sodium and water reabsorption. Nature 326:697, 1987.

107. Nonoguchi H, Sands JM, Knepper MA. Atrial natriuretic factor inhibits vasopressin-stimulated osmotic water permeability in rat inner medullary collecting duct. J Clin Invest 82:1383, 1988.

108. Nonoguchi H, Tomita K, Marumo F. Effects of atrial natriuretic peptide and vasopressin on chloride transport in long- and short-looped medullary thick ascending limbs. J Clin Invest 90:349, 1992.

109. Baum M, Toto RD. Lack of a direct effect of atrial natriuretic factor in the rabbit proximal tubule. Am J Physiol 250:F66, 1986.

110. Capasso G, Rosati C, Giordano DR, De Santo NG. Atrial natriuretic peptide has no direct effect on proximal tubule sodium and water reabsorption. Pflugers Arch 415:336, 1989.

111. Kondo Y, Imai M, Kangawa K, Matsuo H. Lack of direct action of alpha-human atrial natriuretic polypeptide on the in vitro perfused segments of Henle's loop isolated from rabbit kidney. Pflugers Arch 406:273, 1986.

112. Herten M, Lenz W, Gerzer R, Drummer C. The renal natriuretic peptide urodilatin is present in human kidney. Nephrol Dial Transplant 13:2529, 1998.

113. Villarreal D, Freeman RH, Taraben A, Reams GP. Modulation of renin secretion by atrial natriuretic factor prohormone fragment 31-67. Am J Med Sci 318:330, 1999.

114. Burnett JC Jr, Granger JP, Opgenorth TJ. Effects of synthetic atrial natriuretic factor on renal function and renin release. Am J Physiol 247:F863, 1984.

115. Aguilera G. Differential effects of atrial natriuretic factor on angiotensin II- and adrenocorticotropin-stimulated aldosterone secretion. Endocrinology 120:299, 1987.

116. Holtwick R, Gotthardt M, Skryabin B, et al. Smooth muscle-selective deletion of guanylyl cyclase-A prevents the acute but not chronic effects of ANP on blood pressure. Proc Natl Acad Sci USA 99:7142, 2002.

117. Nakayama T. The genetic contribution of the natriuretic peptide system to cardiovascular diseases. Endocr J 52:11, 2005.

118. Calderone A, Thaik CM, Takahashi N, et al. Nitric oxide, atrial natriuretic peptide, and cyclic GMP inhibit the growth-promoting effects of norepinephrine in cardiac myocytes and fibroblasts. J Clin Invest 101:812, 1998.

119. Cao L, Gardner DG. Natriuretic peptides inhibit DNA synthesis in cardiac fibroblasts. Hypertension 25:227, 1995.

120. Charloux A, Piquard F, Doutreleau S, et al. Mechanisms of renal hyporesponsiveness to ANP in heart failure. Eur J Clin Invest 33:769, 2003.

121. Stevens TL, Wei CM, Aahrus LL, et al. Modulation of exogenous and endogenous atrial natriuretic peptide by a receptor inhibitor. Hypertension 23:613, 1994.

122. Ledoux S, Dussaule JC, Chatziantoniou C, et al. Protein kinase A activity modulates natriuretic peptide-dependent cGMP accumulation in renal cells. Am J Physiol 272:C82, 1997.

123. Aviv R, Gurbanov K, Hoffman A, et al. Urinary neutral endopeptidase 24.11 activity: modulation by chronic salt loading. Kidney Int 47:855, 1995.

124. Ebihara F, Di Marco GS, Juliano MA, Casarini DE. Neutral endopeptidase expression in mesangial cells. J Renin Angiotensin Aldosterone Syst 4:228, 2003.

125. Bianciotti LG, de Bold AJ. Modulation of cardiac natriuretic peptide gene expression following endothelin type A receptor blockade in renovascular hypertension. Cardiovasc Res 49:808, 2001.

126. Boric MP, Bravo JA, Corbalan M, et al. Interactions between bradykinin and ANP in rat kidney in vitro: inhibition of natriuresis and modulation of medullary cyclic GMP. Biol Res 31:281, 1998.

127. McDougall JG, Yates NA. Natriuresis and inhibition of Na+/K(+)-ATPase: modulation of response by physiological manipulation. Clin Exp Pharmacol Physiol Suppl 25:S57, 1998.

128. Yoshimura T, Yoshimura M, Yasue H, et al. Plasma concentration of atrial natriuretic peptide and brain natriuretic peptide during normal human pregnancy and the postpartum period. J Endocrinol 140:393, 1994.

129. Mulay S, Varna DR. Placental barrier to atrial natriuretic peptide in rats. Can J Physiol Pharmacol 67:1, 1989.

130. Graham CH, Watson JD, Blumenfeld AJ, Pang SC. Expression of atrial natriuretic peptide by third-trimester placental cytotrophoblasts in women. Biol Reprod 54:834, 1996.

131. Cai WQ, Terenghi G, Bodin P, et al. In situ hybridization of atrial natriuretic peptide mRNA in the endothelial cells of human umbilical vessels. Histochemistry 100:277, 1993.

132. Itoh H, Sagawa N, Hasegawa M, et al. Transforming growth factor-beta stimulates, and glucocorticoids and epidermal growth factor inhibit brain natriuretic peptide secretion from cultured human amnion cells. J Clin Endocrinol Metab 79:176, 1994.

133. Cameron VA, Aitken GD, Ellmers LJ, et al. The sites of gene expression of atrial, brain, and C-type natriuretic peptides in mouse fetal development: temporal changes in embryos and placenta. Endocrinology 137:817, 1996.

134. Huang W, Lee D, Yang Z, et al. Evidence for atrial natriuretic peptide-(5-28) production by rat placental cytotrophoblasts. Endocrinology 131:919, 1992.

135. Inglis GC, Kingdom JC, Nelson DM, et al. Atrial natriuretic hormone: a paracrine or endocrine role within the human placenta? J Clin Endocrinol Metab 76:1014, 1993.

136. Hatjis CG, Grogan DM. Atrial natriuretic peptide receptors in normal human placentas. Am J Obstet Gynecol 159:587, 1988.

137. Zhang LC, Liang GD, Zhang YH, et al. Distribution and characteristics of placental ANP receptors in normal and hypertensive pregnancy. Chin Med J 105:39, 1992.

138. McQueen J, Kingdom JC, Whittle MJ, Connell JM. Characterization of atrial natriuretic peptide receptors in human fetoplacental vasculature. Am J Physiol 264:H798, 1993.

139. Itoh H, Zheng J, Bird IM, et al. Basic FGF decreases clearance receptor of natriuretic peptides in fetoplacental artery endothelium. Am J Physiol 277:R541, 1999.

140. Szukiewicz D, Szukiewicz A, Maslinska D, Markowski M. In vitro effect of bioactive natriuretic peptides on perfusion pressure in placentas from normal and pre-eclamptic pregnancies. Arch Gynecol Obstet 263:37, 1999.

141. Thomsen JK, Storm TL, Thamsborg G, et al. Atrial natriuretic peptide concentrations in pre-eclampsia. Br Med J (Clin Res Ed) 294:1508, 1987.

142. Fievet P, Fournier A, de Bold A, et al. Atrial natriuretic factor in pregnancy-induced hypertension and preeclampsia: increased plasma concentrations possibly explaining these hypovolemic states with paradoxical hyporeninism. Am J Hypertens 1:16, 1988.

143. Miyamoto S, Shimokawa H, Sumioki H, Nakano H. Physiologic role of endogenous human atrial natriuretic peptide in preeclamptic pregnancies. Am J Obstet Gynecol 160:155, 1989.

144. Hatjis CG, Greelish JP, Kofinas AD, et al. Atrial natriuretic factor maternal and fetal concentrations in severe preeclampsia. Am J Obstet Gynecol 161:1015, 1989.

145. Bond AL, August P, Druzin ML, et al. Atrial natriuretic factor in normal and hypertensive pregnancy. Am J Obstet Gynecol 160:1112, 1989.

146. McQueen J, Jardine J, Kingdom J, et al. Interaction of angiotensin II and atrial natriuretic peptide in the human fetoplacental unit. Am J Hypertens 3:641, 1990.

147. Holcberg G, Kossenjans W, Brewer A, et al. Selective vasodilator effects of atrial natriuretic peptide in the human placental vasculature. J Soc Gynecol Investig 2:1, 1995.

148. Stebbing PN, Gude NM, King RG, Brennecke SP. Alpha-atrial natriuretic peptide-induced attenuation of vasoconstriction in the fetal circulation of the human isolated perfused placenta. J Perinat Med 24:253, 1996.

149. Grunewald C, Nisell H, Jansson T, et al. Possible improvement in uteroplacental blood flow during atrial natriuretic peptide infusion in preeclampsia. Obstet Gynecol 84:235, 1994.

150. Zeller R, Bloch KD, Williams BS, et al. Localized expression of the atrial natriuretic factor gene during cardiac embryogenesis. Genes Dev 1:693, 1987.

151. Wei YF, Rodi CP, Day ML, et al. Developmental changes in the rat atriopeptin hormonal system. J Clin Invest 79:1325, 1987.

152. Cheung CY, Gibbs DM, Brace RA. Atrial natriuretic factor in maternal and fetal sheep. Am J Physiol 252:E279, 1987.

153. Robillard JE, Nakamura KT, Varille VA, et al. Ontogeny of the renal response to natriuretic peptide in sheep. Am J Physiol 254:F634, 1988.

154. Deloof S, Chatelain A. Effect of blood volume expansion on basal plasma atrial natriuretic factor and adrenocorticotropic hormone secretions in the fetal rat at term. Biol Neonate 65:390, 1994.

155. Cameron VA, Ellmers LJ. Minireview: natriuretic peptides during development of the fetal heart and circulation. Endocrinology 144:2191, 2003.

156. Cheung CY, Roberts VJ. Developmental changes in atrial natriuretic factor content and localization of its messenger ribonucleic acid in ovine fetal heart. Am J Obstet Gynecol 169:1345, 1993.

157. Rosenfeld CR, Samson WK, Roy TA, et al. Vasoconstrictor-induced secretion of ANP in fetal sheep. Am J Physiol 263:E526, 1992.

158. Cheung CY. Regulation of atrial natriuretic factor secretion and expression in the ovine fetus. Neurosci Biobehav Rev 19:159, 1995.

159. Mir TS, Laux R, Hellwege HH, et al. Plasma concentrations of aminoterminal pro atrial natriuretic peptide and aminoterminal pro brain natriuretic peptide in healthy neonates: marked and rapid increase after birth. Pediatrics 112:896, 2003.

160. Bierd TM, Kattwinkel J, Chevalier RL, et al. Interrelationship of atrial natriuretic peptide, atrial volume, and renal function in premature infants. J Pediatr 116:753, 1990.

161. Ekblad H, Kero P, Vuolteenaho O, et al. Atrial natriuretic peptide in the preterm infant. Lack of correlation with natriuresis and diuresis. Acta Paediatr 81:978, 1992.

162. Shaffer SG, Geer PG, Goetz KL. Elevated atrial natriuretic factor in neonates with respiratory distress syndrome. J Pediatr 109:1028, 1986.

163. Semmekrot B, Roseau S, Vassent G, Butlen D. Developmental patterns of renal atrial natriuretic peptide receptors: [125I]alpha-rat atrial natriuretic peptide binding in glomeruli and inner medullary collecting tubules microdissected from kidneys of young rats. Mol Cell Endocrinol 68:35, 1990.

164. Chevalier RL, Fern RJ, Garmey M, et al. Localization of cGMP after infusion of ANP or nitroprusside in the maturing rat. Am J Physiol 262:F417, 1992.

165. Midgley J, Modi N, Littleton P, et al. Atrial natriuretic peptide, cyclic guanosine monophosphate and sodium excretion during postnatal adaptation in male infants below 34 weeks gestation with severe respiratory distress syndrome. Early Hum Dev 28:145, 1992.

166. Norling LL, Vaughan CA, Chevalier RL. Maturation of cGMP response to ANP by isolated glomeruli. Am J Physiol 262:F138, 1992.

167. Stephenson TJ, Broughton Pipkin F, Hetmanski D, Yoxall B. Atrial natriuretic peptide in the preterm newborn. Biol Neonate 66:22, 1994.

168. Itoh H, Sagawa N, Hasegawa M, et al. Brain natriuretic peptide levels in the umbilical venous plasma are elevated in fetal distress. Biol Neonate 64:18, 1993.

169. Andersson S, Hallman M, Tikkanen I, Fyhrquist F. Birth stress increase fetal atrial natriuretic factor. Am J Obstet Gynecol 162:872, 1990.

170. Itoh H, Sagawa N, Hasegawa M, et al. Umbilical venous guanosine 3′,5′-cyclic phosphate (cGMP) concentration increases in asphyxiated newborns. Reprod Fertil Dev 7:1515, 1995.

171. Yamada J, Fujimori K, Ispida T, et al. Plasma endothelin-1 and atrial natriuretic peptide levels during prolonged (24-h) non-acidemic hypoxemia in fetal goats. J Matern Fetal Med 10:409, 2001.

172. Okumura A, Toyota N, Hayakawa F, et al. Cerebral hemodynamics during early neonatal period in preterm infants with periventricular leukomalacia. Brain Dev 24:693, 2002.

173. Choi BM, Lee KH, Eun BL, et al. Utility of rapid B-type natriuretic peptide assay for diagnosis of symptomatic patent ductus arteriosus in preterm infants. Pediatrics 115:e255, 2005.

174. Modi N, Betremieux P, Midgley J, Hartnoll G. Postnatal weight loss and contraction of the extracellular compartment is triggered by atrial natriuretic peptide. Early Hum Dev 59:201, 2000.

175. Rozycki HJ, Baumgart S. Atrial natriuretic factor and postnatal diuresis in respiratory distress syndrome. Arch Dis Child 66:43, 1991.

176. Bauer K, Buschkamp S, Marcinkowski M, et al. Postnatal changes of extracellular volume, atrial natriuretic factor, and diuresis in a randomized controlled trial of high-frequency oscillatory ventilation versus intermittent positive-pressure ventilation in premature infants <30 weeks gestation. Crit Care Med 28:2064, 2000.

177. Kojima T, Hirata Y, Fukuda Y, et al. Plasma atrial natriuretic peptide and spontaneous diuresis in sick neonates. Arch Dis Child 62:667, 1987.

178. Ronconi M, Fortunato A, Soffiati G, et al. Vasopressin, atrial natriuretic factor and renal water homeostasis in premature newborn infants with respiratory distress syndrome. J Perinat Med 23:307, 1995.

179. Onal EE, Dilmen U, Adam B, et al. Serum atrial natriuretic peptide levels in infants with transient tachypnea of the newborn. J Matern Fetal Neonatal Med 17:145, 2005.

180. Tulassay T, Rascher W, Seyberth HW, et al. Role of atrial natriuretic peptide in sodium homeostasis in premature infants. J Pediatr 109:1023, 1986.

181. Kojima T, Fukuda Y, Hirata Y, et al. Effects of aldosterone and atrial natriuretic peptide on water and electrolyte homeostasis of sick neonates. Pediatr Res 25:591, 1989.

182. Holmstrom H, Hall C, Thaulow E. Plasma levels of natriuretic peptides and hemodynamic assessment of patent ductus arteriosus in preterm infants. Acta Paediatr 90:184, 2001.

183. Holmstrom H, Omland T. Editorial Board: Natriuretic peptides as markers of patent ductus arteriosus in preterm infants. Clin Sci 103:79, 2002.

184. Puddy VF, Amirmansour C, Williams AF, Singer DR. Plasma brain natriuretic peptide as a predictor of haemodynamically significant patent ductus arteriosus in preterm infants. Clin Sci 3:75, 2002.

185. Kaapa P, Seppanen M, Kero P, et al. Hemodynamic control of atrial natriuretic peptide plasma levels in neonatal respiratory distress syndrome. Am J Perinatol 12:235, 1995.

186. Pesonen E. Role of natriuretic hormones in the diagnosis of patent ductus arteriosus in newborn infants. Acta Paediatr 90:363, 2001.

187. Reynolds EW, Ellington JG, Vranicar M, Bada HS. Brain-type natriuretic peptide in the diagnosis and management of persistent pulmonary hypertension of the newborn. Pediatrics 114:1297, 2004.

188. Holmgren D, Westerlind A, Lundberg PA, Wahlander H. Increased plasma levels of natriuretic peptide type B and A in children with congenital heart defects with left compared with right ventricular volume overload or pressure overload. Clin Physiol Funct Imaging 25:263, 2005.

189. Costello JM, Backer CL, Checchia PA, et al. Alterations in the natriuretic hormone system related to cardiopulmonary bypass in infants with congestive heart failure. Pediatr Cardiol 25:347, 2004.
190. Ootaki Y, Yamaguchi M, Yoshimura N, et al. Secretion of A-type and B-type natriuretic peptides into the bloodstream and pericardial space in children with congenital heart disease. J Thorac Cardiovasc Surg 126:1411, 2003.
191. Oberhansli I, Mermillod B, Favre H, et al. Atrial natriuretic factor in patients with congenital heart disease: correlation with hemodynamic variables. J Am Coll Cardiol 15:1438, 1990.

Section IV

Special Pathology

Chapter 9

Body Fluid Compartments in the Fetus and Newborn Infant with Growth Aberration

Karl Bauer, MD[†]

Methods for Measuring Body Fluid Compartments in Neonates

Fetal Body Fluid Compartments (TBW, ECV, ICV) in Intrauterine Growth Restriction

Adaptation of Body Fluid Compartments in SGA Neonates in the Immediate Postnatal Period

Fluid Therapy in SGA Preterm Neonates in the Immediate Postnatal Period

Body Fluid Compartments in LGA Neonates

Summary

Neonates with aberrations in growth—small for gestational age (SGA) or large for gestational age (LGA)—have an increased perinatal mortality, more neonatal complications and more health problems in later life (1). The type and severity of the growth aberration can be characterized more precisely by the analysis of body composition than by body weight alone. Therefore, fetal and neonatal body composition has received considerable attention (2,3).

Water is the most abundant substance in the body, accounting for about two thirds of body weight in the adult. Growth not only increases the absolute volume of body water but also influences the proportion of water in the body as well as the relative size of the different body fluid compartments. The most dramatic changes in body fluid compartments occur during intrauterine growth when approximately 4000 mL of water accumulate in the human uterus, 2800 mL in the fetus, 800 mL in the amniotic fluid, and 400 mL in the placenta, and during the postnatal adaptation of the neonate from the 'aquatic' intrauterine to the 'terrestrial' extrauterine environment.

In this chapter the effects of fetal growth aberrations on body water will be reviewed. First, a short overview about methods used to measure body fluid compartments in neonates will be presented. With this background, the alterations of body composition in neonates born after intrauterine growth retardation will be discussed. We will then highlight differences in the postnatal adaptation of fluid homeostasis between SGA neonates and appropriate for gestational age (AGA) neonates to answer the question if SGA neonates need a different postnatal fluid

---

†Deceased.

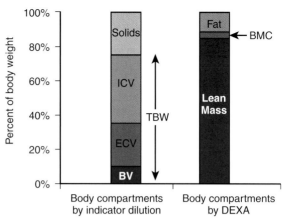

Figure 9-1 Body compartments defined by indicator dilution (TBW = total body water, ICV = intracellular volume, ECV = extracellular volume, BV = blood volume) or by dual X-ray absorptiometry (BMC = bone mineral content) studies.

therapy. Finally, the limited available information about body fluid compartments in LGA neonates will be summarized.

METHODS FOR MEASURING BODY FLUID COMPARTMENTS IN NEONATES

There are various methods for studying human body composition in vivo (4). Indicator dilution is the most widely used method for in vivo measurements of body fluid compartments in perinatal medicine (5). More recently, since validation studies for measurements in neonates have become available, dual X-ray absorptiometry (DEXA) has become another tool for body composition studies during growth (Fig. 9-1).

The basic principle of indicator dilution is to calculate the distribution volume of an indicator from the amount of indicator given and the indicator concentration after an equal distribution and equilibrium has been achieved. Indicators used for the measurement of total body water (TBW) are antipyrine or stable isotopes of water (D_2O or $H_2{}^{18}O$); indicators used for the measurement of extracellular volume (ECV) are bromide or sucrose, and plasma volume (PV) can be measured with Evan's blue. Body solids can than be calculated as body weight−TBW, intracellular volume as TBW−ECV, and blood volume as PV × Hct.

Dual X-ray absorptiometry utilizes the different absorption of X-rays by different body tissues to measure the three body compartments: bone mineral content, lean tissue mass and fat mass. Accuracy of results critically depends on the method of calibration. DEXA has been validated for neonates (6).

In vivo measurements of body fluid compartments are usually confined to relatively small groups of subjects because they are either invasive or require expensive equipment.

FETAL BODY FLUID COMPARTMENTS (TBW, ECV, ICV) IN INTRAUTERINE GROWTH RESTRICTION

Intrauterine growth restriction can result from a variety of factors that can be broadly grouped into three categories: (i) maternal factors such as maternal under nutrition, maternal disease (e.g., pre-eclampsia, toxemia of pregnancy) or maternal exposure to adverse environmental factors, (ii) placental factors such as placental vascular disease, placental anomalies, and (iii) fetal factors such as genetic abnormalities or fetal infection (1).

Impaired growth in the neonate is clinically diagnosed when the birth weight is lower than a predetermined cut-off value, for example a birth weight below the third percentile for gestational age. This clinical diagnosis of a SGA infant, which is also used in most body composition studies, does not differentiate between the different etiologies for impaired growth, includes small infants with normal intrauterine growth, and is a categorical rather than a continuous description of growth impairment. All these limitations complicate the interpretation of body composition measurements.

Total Body Water and Body Solids

The measurement of TBW allows the analysis of growth in a two-compartment model of TBW and body solids, which are calculated as body weight−TBW. Total body water decreases from 75% of body weight at birth to 60% in adulthood (7). Body solids encompass protein (approximately 12% of body weight), minerals (approximately 3% of body weight) and body fat (15–30% of body weight). Body fat is the most variable body solid compartment throughout life. In healthy term neonates 10–15% of body weight is body fat, yet there are considerable inter-individual differences, so that the variation in fat mass explains 46% of the observed variance in birth weight (8). There are physiologic changes during infant growth, when body fat increases markedly from 10–15% of body weight at birth to 25–30% at 2 years of age (9). Females have more body fat than males at birth (10), and the gender difference widens with sexual maturation during adolescence. Throughout life, body fat varies considerably with nutritional status.

During normal intrauterine growth TBW content decreases from 94% of body weight in the first trimester of pregnancy to 76% at term caused by the accumulation of body solids during growth (7). In the first two-thirds of gestation body solids increase due to the accretion of protein and minerals, whereas there is little fat deposition. We know from postmortem chemical analyses that at 27 weeks' gestation 86% of body weight is water, 12% is fat-free dry solids, and only 2% is fat (11). In vivo measurements in AGA preterm infants with a birth weight below 1500 g showed a TBW content of 83% (12) and no fat was detectable by dual photon absorptiometry using ^{153}Gd magnetic resonance tomography (MRT) in preterm infants (13). During the last trimester of gestation the proportion of body solids increases from 14% to 24% of body weight due to the deposition of body fat, which is 2% of body weight at 27 weeks' gestation and 10–15% of body weight at birth (11).

Normal intrauterine growth critically depends on the delivery of sufficient nutrients to the fetus via the placenta. When nutrient delivery was reduced by uterine artery ligation during experimental intrauterine growth restriction in rats, TBW was increased, reflecting the reduced deposition of body fat and protein (14). In human neonates born after intrauterine growth restriction the TBW content of the body was also increased compared to normal intrauterine growth. In SGA preterm neonates mean TBW content was 62 mL/kg higher than in AGA preterm neonates (15) and in SGA term neonates mean TBW content was increased by 76 mL/kg (16) or by 102 mL/kg (17), respectively. No reduction in total body water was found in only one study of a small group of SGA neonates with a wide range of gestational ages (18) (Table 9-1).

The relative increase in TBW in SGA neonates is caused by the reduction in body solids and not by an accumulation of excess water due to a disturbed fluid homeostasis. In preterm SGA neonates the higher body water content reflects the reduced deposition of protein and minerals because, during the first two thirds of gestation, the fetal body consists of water and fat-free dry solids, whereas

Table 9-1   Total Body Water (TBW) and Extracellular Volume (ECV) in Appropriate for Gestational Age (AGA) and Small for Gestational Age (SGA) Human Neonates

Author	Subjects		N	TBW (mL/kg)	Significance	Method
Cassady & Milstead 1971	Term (37–43 weeks)	AGA	12	688±16	p<0.001	Indicator dilution (Antipyrine)
		SGA	23	790±13		
Hartnoll et al 2000	Preterm (25–30 weeks)	AGA	35	906 (833–954)	p=0.019	Indicator dilution (H2 18O)
		SGA	7	844 (637–958)		
Cheek et al 1984	Term (≥ 37 weeks)	AGA	7	749	not reported	Indicator dilution (D2O)
		SGA	6	825		
vdWagen et al 1986	GA (34–40 weeks)	AGA	11	780±38	NS	Indicator dilution (D2O)
		SGA	10	776±13		

Author	Subjects		N	ECV (mL/kg)	Significance	Method
Cassady 1970	Term (≥37 weeks)	AGA	13	376±20	p=0.025	Indicator dilution (bromide)
		SGA	20	419±45		
Cheek et al 1984	Term (≥37 weeks)	AGA	7	361±16	not reported	Indicator dilution (bromide)
		SGA	6	395±35		
vd Wagen et al 1986	GA (34–40 weeks)	AGA	11	355±55	NS	Indicator dilution (sucrose)
		SGA	10	344±35		

Cassady G, Milstead RR: Antipyrine space studies and cell water estimates in infants of low birth weight. Pediatr Res 5:673–682, 1971.

Hartnoll G, Betremieux P, Modi N: Body water content of extremely preterm infants at birth. Arch Dis Child Fetal Neonatal Ed 83:F56–F59, 2000.

Cheek DB, Wishart J, MacLennan A, Haslam R: Cell hydration in the normally grown, the premature, and the low weight for gestational age infant. Early Hum Dev 10:75–84, 1984.

vd Wagen A, Okken A, Zweens J, Zijlstra WG: Body composition at birth of growth-retarded newborn infants demonstrating catch-up growth in the first year of life. Biol Neonate 49:121–125, 1986.

Cassady G: Body composition in intrauterine growth retardation. Pediatr Clin North Am 17:79–99, 1970.

there is little deposition of fat. A reduction in fetal lean mass during intrauterine growth restriction has been demonstrated by ultrasound measurements of the cross-sectional lean body area of the fetal thigh (19). A reduced protein and mineral deposition early in gestation is likely to disrupt organ development. In fact, preterm SGA neonates have a higher mortality and more chronic lung disease than preterm AGA neonates (20) and SGA preterm neonates are still smaller and lighter at three years of age than AGA preterm neonates (21). Different from preterm SGA neonates, the increase in body water content in term SGA neonates reflects primarily the reduced deposition of fat. The accumulation of fat is the primary cause of the physiologic reduction in TBW during normal growth throughout the third trimester of gestation. Aside from body water measurements there are several lines of evidence indicating that adipose tissue is indeed reduced in SGA term neonates. Reduced abdominal wall fat thickness measured by ultrasound in a late gestation fetus was found during intrauterine growth restriction (22). The percentage of adipose tissue estimated from dual photon absorptiometry using ^{153}Gd MRT was 2% in SGA term neonates compared to 13% in AGA term neonates (13) and thinner skin folds in SGA term neonates indicated a thinner subcutaneous fat layer (23). One recent study using DEXA analysis also found a reduced fat content in SGA near-term and term infant, though the difference did not reach statistical significance due to the small sample size (24).

No conclusions about the effect of altered body composition of SGA neonates on the risk for neonatal complications or long term outcome can be drawn from body fluid compartment measurements because studies including body composition measurements are usually small and no clinical outcomes are reported. Yet, from anthropometric studies that include large numbers of neonates, the prognostic utility of body composition estimated from anthropometry can be analyzed. Body weight below a certain cut-off point is the parameter most often used to diagnose impaired fetal growth. In future studies of impaired fetal growth, weight deficit should be quantified and expressed on a continuous scale, for example as a standard deviation score, instead of using a fixed cut-off value. The more severe the weight reduction the higher the risk of neonatal morbidity and mortality for SGA neonates, regardless of the cause of the growth deficit (25) and the higher the risk of low intellectual performance in adulthood (26). It is unclear if body proportionality—categorized as symmetric versus asymmetric growth retardation—is a relevant predictor of childhood growth in addition to weight deficit. Whereas term neonates with asymmetric IUGR were more likely to demonstrate catch-up growth than term neonates with symmetric IUGR, preterm SGA neonates had retarded childhood growth, regardless of having a symmetric or asymmetric growth retardation at birth (21). Reduced adipose tissue thickness is a more sensitive predictor for neonatal complications in SGA neonates than weight because symptomatic SGA neonates with hypoglycemia and/or polycythemia had a thinner subcutaneous fat layer than asymptomatic SGA neonates, whereas there was no difference in body weight or length between the two groups (27).

Extra- and Intracellular Fluid Volume

The total body water compartment can be subdivided into the extracellular volume (ECV) and the intracellular volume (ICV). Early in gestation the ECV is extremely large, accounting for 62% of body weight, and is more than twice the size of the ICV. This reflects early fetal growth, which occurs by cell division rather than by cell growth and produces tissues with small cells surrounded by a broad layer of extracellular fluid. During normal intrauterine growth in the second half of gestation, the intracellular space increases from 25% of body weight at mid-gestation to 32% at term, whereas the extracellular volume at the same time decreases from 62% of

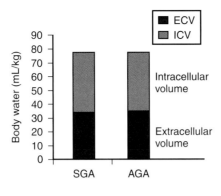

Figure 9-2 The distribution of total body water between extracellular (ECV) and intracellular volume (ICV) is similar in near-term and term small for gestational age (SGA) and appropriate for gestational age (AGA) neonates (After vd Wagen A, Okken A, Zweens J, Zijlstra WG: Body composition at birth of growth-retarded newborn infants demonstrating catch-up growth in the first year of life. Biol Neonate 49:121–125, 1986.)

body weight to 43%, reflecting the growth in cell size taking place in the second half of gestation (7).

Intrauterine growth restriction (IUGR), unless severe, seems to have little influence on the distribution of TBW between intra- and extracellular volume. ECV values, measured by sucrose dilution, and intracellular volume, calculated by TBW (D_2O dilution)−ECV, in near-term and term neonates were similar in SGA and AGA neonates and there were no differences in the ICV to ECV ratio (1.26 in SGA neonates versus 1.20 in AGA neonates) (18) (Fig. 9-2).

In a study in neonatal baboons (28) and two studies in human neonates (16,17), ECV (bromide space) and ICV (TBW (Antipyrine space)−ECV (bromide space)) were both increased by about 30–40 mL/kg in the SGA neonates, leaving the ICV to ECV ratio unchanged compared to AGA term neonates. A very pronounced and significant expansion of ECV of 73 mL/kg was found only in a subgroup of neonates with severe growth restriction, indicated by a reduced weight and length compared to neonates with a moderate growth retardation, indicated by reduced weight but normal length (29) (Table 9-1).

Plasma Volume and Red Cell Mass

Intrauterine growth restriction is not necessarily associated with an increased plasma volume or red cell mass. Plasma volume, measured by Evans Blue dilution in 14 term SGA neonates (37 ± 4 mL/kg), did not differ from AGA neonates (37 ± 6 mL/kg) and there was also no difference in red cell mass (SGA: 69 ± 17 mL/kg; AGA: 63 ± 12 mL/kg) or blood volume (SGA: 105 ± 18 mL/kg; AGA: 101 ± 16 mL/kg) calculated from plasma volume and hematocrit (30). Yet in the subgroup of SGA neonates who postnatally developed polycythemia, blood volume was increased. Blood volume in polycythemic SGA neonates calculated from hematocrit changes during exchange transfusion was 106 mL/kg compared to 86 mL/kg in AGA polycythemic neonates (31). The increased red cell mass can be the result of an adaptation to chronic intrauterine hypoxemia, as indicated by increased erythropoetin levels in SGA neonates (32) or of an acute placento-fetal transfusion. Total placento-fetal blood volume at term is about 120 mL/kg of which 70 mL/kg are in the fetus and 50 mL/kg in the placenta (33). The distribution of blood volume between neonate and placenta after delivery is influenced by a number of perinatal events. The most marked increase in neonatal blood volume can be achieved by delayed cord clamping while the neonate is held below the level of the placenta, resulting in a gravity-driven placento-fetal transfusion (34,35). SGA neonates are more frequently associated with perinatal events favoring placento–fetal transfusion, such as a decrease in umbilical blood flow, intrauterine asphyxia, or maternal hypertension (33).

Amniotic Fluid Volume

Strictly speaking, amniotic fluid volume (AFV) is not a fetal body fluid compartment. Yet AFV in the second half of gestation is largely dependent on fetal organ function, its volume is regulated within a narrow range and it is reduced during IUGR and increased with fetal macrosomia. Therefore it was included in this review.

During an uncomplicated pregnancy AFV shows a slow increase from 350 mL at 20 weeks' gestation to 700 mL at term (36). As gestation progresses, fetal organ function becomes more and more important for the regulation of AFV. The two primary sources of amniotic fluid after midgestation are the fetal urine production of approximately 300 mL/kg/day and the secretion of tracheal and pulmonary fluid of 60–100 mL/kg/day. Removal of amniotic fluid occurs by fetal swallowing of about 200–250 mL/kg per day and by intramembraneous absorption of amniotic fluid into the fetal blood, which perfuses the fetal surface of the placenta. Near term, the daily amniotic fluid turnover of 1000 mL is higher than the amniotic fluid volume of 700–800 mL. Therefore, AFV must be highly regulated to avoid oligo- or polyhydramnios. Changes (increasing or decreasing) in intra-membraneous absorption appear to be the main way of altering AFV, although the precise regulation mechanism remains elusive (37).

Intrauterine growth restriction is often associated with oligohydramnios. The rate of neonates with a birth weight < 10th percentile was 13% in low-risk singleton pregnancies at term with oligohydramnios compared to 5.5% in pregnancies without oligohydramnios (38). The causes of oligohydramnios during IUGR are not completely understood. Chronic fetal hypoxia without placental insufficiency does not cause oligohydramnios because AFV remained unchanged during prolonged hypoxia induced over 4 days in fetal sheep by lowering maternal inspired oxygen concentration. The marked fetal polyuria, with an excess urine volume of 4 L, induced by the fetal hypoxia, was compensated for by increased intramembraneous absorption (39). Yet, severe placental insufficiency induced in fetal sheep by embolisation of the umbilical artery reduced AFV by 62% without a reduction in fetal urine production. This suggests an increased absorption of amniotic fluid by the chorioamnion during placental insufficiency, but the mechanisms of this intra-membraneous absorption of amniotic fluid volume remain to be explained (40).

ADAPTATION OF BODY FLUID COMPARTMENTS IN SGA NEONATES IN THE IMMEDIATE POSTNATAL PERIOD

Transition from intrauterine to extrauterine life is an adaptation from aquatic to terrestrial life and encompasses marked changes in body water content and fluid homeostasis. During the first postnatal days a weight loss of about 10% of birth weight occurs in healthy term neonates caused by a reduction of the extracellular volume (16).

A postnatal weight loss of up to 15% of birth weight occurs in low birth weight infants (41) and in extremely low birth weight infants (42) with normal intrauterine growth (i.e., AGA infants). Measurements of body water compartments demonstrated that this weight loss is loss of total body water. In low birth weight neonates with RDS (mean birth weight 1558 g), mean postnatal weight loss was 181 g (=7.7% of birth weight). With weight loss there was a concurrent reduction in total body water by 183 mL and in extracellular volume by 204 mL (43). These findings were confirmed in a more recent study in preterm neonates after normal intrauterine growth (44). The postnatal weight loss of 7.8% of birth weight was caused by a reduction in the extracellular volume accompanied by a negative fluid and sodium balance. There was no evidence of tissue catabolism because body solids remained unchanged, the nitrogen retention and energy intake were sufficient to meet energy expenditure by day 2 (12).

Measurements of postnatal changes of body fluid compartments in SGA neonates are sparse because they are invasive and difficult to perform. There are no longitudinal measurements in term SGA infants and only two small studies of SGA preterm neonates.

Postnatal weight loss in 7 SGA preterm neonates (birth weight < 5th percentile) with a mean gestational age of 35 weeks was only 5% and was accompanied by a proportionate reduction in body water and body solids (45). This study included no information about fluid intake or diuresis and no AGA control group. In another study comparing 5 SGA preterm neonates (mean gestational age 35 weeks) with 14 weight matched AGA neonates (mean gestational age 31 weeks), the SGA neonates had a maximal postnatal weight loss of only 2% compared to a maximal postnatal weight loss of 8% in the AGA control infants. On days 4–6 of life the SGA neonates had already regained birth weight and there was no detectable change in total body water or body solids, whereas at the same postnatal age body weight and total body water in the AGA neonates were significantly lower than at birth (44). There were no differences in day-to-day fluid and energy intake during the first week of life in the SGA and AGA groups; however the AGA infants had a higher urine output during this time. A possible reason for the attenuated postnatal increase in urine output in SGA preterm neonates is their altered hemodynamic adaptation. SGA preterm neonates did not show the postnatal increase in cardiac output observed in the AGA neonates (46).

To summarize, the evidence thus far suggests that in AGA very low birth weight infants, the immediate postnatal weight loss is most likely a result of a reduction in total body water, primarily the extracellular compartment. In the SGA infant, the immediate postnatal weight loss appears to be of less magnitude than the AGA group and is likely a result of catabolism rather than body fluid contraction. It should be pointed out that the data on SGA infants is limited and the study is complicated by a lack of direct comparison with the AGA counterparts.

FLUID THERAPY IN SGA PRETERM NEONATES IN THE IMMEDIATE POSTNATAL PERIOD

Fluid therapy in the immediate neonatal period in AGA preterm neonates has the following objectives: (i) it allows for the physiologic postnatal contraction of the extracellular volume to occur, (ii) it aims at a postnatal weight loss of about 10% of body weight, (iii) it aims at a negative fluid and sodium balance on days 1–3 of life, and (iv) it minimizes transepidermal water loss (47). This can be achieved with a restricted water intake, which reduces the risk of PDA, NEC and death (48). There is also suggestive evidence that sodium restriction during the first week of life, to produce a negative sodium balance, can achieve the same goals as fluid restriction (49,50).

Unfortunately, there are no systematic clinical trials about fluid therapy for SGA neonates. From the body water measurements we know that despite their 'wrinkled' appearance, SGA neonates are not dehydrated at birth. Severely growth restricted neonates rather have an expanded extracellular volume. The only study providing data on fluid therapy in the immediate neonatal period reports an attenuated postnatal weight loss in SGA preterm infants receiving the same amount of fluid intake as weight-matched AGA preterm infants (44). This study suggests that SGA preterm neonates do not need extra fluid intake in the immediate neonatal period but rather a cautious approach to fluid prescription. The need to provide a continuous infusion of glucose to treat and prevent hypoglycemia is the only condition necessitating earlier or additional fluid intake in SGA neonates (51).

BODY FLUID COMPARTMENTS IN LGA NEONATES

Fetal overgrowth is defined either as fetal macrosomia (estimated fetal weight or birth weight > 4–4.5 kg) or large for gestational age (LGA) when birth weight exceeds the 90th or 95th percentile for a population-based intrauterine growth chart.

LGA neonates are associated with maternal diabetes, maternal adiposity, and fetal gene disorders or syndromes. Though maternal diabetes is the classical entity resulting in fetal overgrowth due to longstanding fetal insulin excess, 79% of LGA neonates are born to mothers who are not glucose intolerant. The incidence of LGA neonates is increasing due to the increase in maternal adiposity (52). Studies of body water compartments in LGA neonates are much more limited than in SGA neonates.

Total Body Water and Body Solids

Studies of TBW in LGA neonates are confined to small groups of neonates. TBW measured by D_2O dilution was reduced in 7 infants of diabetic mothers compared to controls (73% versus 80% of body weight). But this group was not confined to LGA neonates but included birth weights from 1430 g to 3495 g (53).

A decreased TBW indicates an increase in fat mass. Indeed, recently an increased fat mass was found using DEXA analysis in LGA neonates. Thirty LGA term infants, defined by a body weight > 90th percentile and including 9 infants of diabetic mothers, which were measured with DEXA, had a fat mass of 22.5% of body weight. Forty-seven term LGA neonates, defined by a body weight > 4000 g and including 11 infants of diabetic mothers, had, compared to 47 AGA neonates, a higher body fat content and a lower lean body mass. The changes were most marked in the LGA neonates of diabetic mothers (54) (Table 9-2). In support of these findings increases in fat mass have been demonstrated in fetuses of diabetic mothers using ultrasound measurements of both abdominal wall fat thickness as well as proximal extremity fat area (55).

Plasma volume and blood volume were not increased in LGA neonates (birth weight > 90th percentile) compared to AGA neonates as long as there was no polycythemia (30).

Amniotic Fluid Volume

Fetal macrosomia is associated with polyhydramnios. In singleton pregnancies with polyhydramnios the rate of neonatal macrosomia (birth weight > 4000 g) was three

Table 9-2	Body Composition of Large for Gestational Age (LGA) and Appropriate for Gestational Age (AGA) Human Neonates		
	LGA	**LGA**	**AGA**
	Normal	**Glucose tolerance impaired**	**Normal**
N	36	11	47
Body weight (g)	4244 ± 304	4475 ± 251	3224 ± 321
Total body fat (%)	20 ± 4	26 ± 3	16 ± 3
Lean body mass (%)	77 ± 5	71 ± 3	82 ± 3
Bone mineral content (%)	2 ± 0.2	2 ± 0.1	2 ± 0.2

After Hammami M, Walters JC, Hockman EM, Koo WWK: Disproportionate alterations in body composition of large for gestational age neonates. J Pediatr 38:817–821, 2001.

times higher than in uncomplicated pregnancies with normal AFV (19.2% versus 6.0%) (56). The physiologic process underlying the association between macrosomia and polyhydramnios is not clear.

SUMMARY

The effect of fetal growth aberrations on body fluid compartments (total body water, extracellular volume, intracellular volume, blood volume) is small and does not require specific postnatal fluid therapy. SGA neonates, despite their 'wrinkled' appearance, are not dehydrated. Rather their total body water, expressed as percentage of body weight, is increased. But this is not a true expansion of TBW due to fluid retention but the result of the reduced deposition of fat, protein and minerals following the intrauterine nutritional deficit. In mild to moderate SGA neonates the ratio of ECV/ICV is not altered; ECV is disproportionately expanded only after severe growth restriction. Blood volume is increased only when the growth restriction is associated with polycythemia requiring hemodilution. The only fluid compartment that is decreased by intrauterine growth restriction to a clinically relevant extent is amniotic fluid volume. The mechanism is incompletely understood. In experimental placental insufficiency in lambs the reduction in AFV was not due to reduced fetal urine output but due to increased absorption of AFV across the fetal membranes. Whether this mechanism applies to the human fetus is unknown. During postnatal adaptation SGA neonates have an attenuated weight loss. LGA neonates have a reduced TBW due to an increased fat deposition. AFV is increased.

The availability of non-invasive body composition measurements, such as DEXA, offers the opportunity to study larger groups of neonates with growth aberrations so that effects of body composition on outcome and effects of therapies aimed at normalization of body composition can be investigated.

REFERENCES

1. Das UG, Sysyn GD. Abnormal fetal growth: intrauterine growth retardation, small for gestational age, large for gestational age. Pediatr Clin North Am 51:639–654, 2004.
2. Bernstein I. Fetal body composition. Curr Opin Clin Nutr Metab Care 8:613–617, 2005.
3. Lafeber HN. Nutritional assessment and measurement of body composition in preterm infants. Clin Perinatol 26:997–1005, 1999.
4. Ellis KJ. Human body composition: in vivo methods. Physiol Reviews 80:649–680, 2000.
5. Brans YW, Andrew DS, Dutton EB, et al. Dilution kinetics of chemicals used for estimation of water content of body compartments in perinatal medicine. Pediatr Res 25:377–382, 1989.
6. Koo WWK. Body composition measurements during infancy. Ann NY Acad Sci 904:383–392, 2000.
7. Friis-Hansen B. Body water compartments in children: changes during growth and related changes in body composition. Pediatrics 28:169–181, 1961.
8. Catalano PM, Tyzbir ED, Allen SR, et al. Evaluation of fetal growth by estimation of neonatal body composition. Obestet Gynecol 79:46–50, 1992.
9. Butte NF, Hopkinson JM, Wong WW, et al. Body composition during the first two years of life: an updated reference. Pediatr Res 47:578–585, 2000.
10. Catalano PM, Drago NM, Amini SB. Factors affecting fetal growth and body composition. Am J Obstet Gynecol 172:1459–1463, 1995.
11. Ziegler EE, O'Donnell AM, Nelson SE, Fomon SJ. Body composition of the reference fetus. Growth 40:329–341, 1976.
12. Bauer K, Bovermann G, Roithmaier A, et al. Body composition, nutrition, and fluid balance during the first two weeks of life in preterm neonates weighing less than 1500 grams. J Pediatr 118:615–620, 1991.
13. Petersen S, Gotfredsen A, Knudsen FU. Lean body mass in small for gestational age and appropriate for gestational age infants. J Pediatr 113:886–889, 1988.
14. Hohenauer L, Oh W. Body composition in experimental intrauterine growth retardation in the rat. J Nutr 99:358–361, 1969.
15. Hartnoll G, Betremieux P, Modi N. Body water content of extremely preterm infants at birth. Arch Dis Child Fetal Neonatal Ed 83:F56–F59, 2000.
16. Cheek DB, Wishart J, MacLennan A, Haslam R. Cell hydration in the normally grown, the premature, and the low weight for gestational age infant. Early Hum Dev 10:75–84, 1984.

17. Cassady G, Milstead RR. Antipyrine space studies and cell water estimates in infants of low birth weight. Pediatr Res 5:673–682, 1971.
18. vdWagen A, Okken A, Zweens J, Zijlstra WG. Body composition at birth of growth-retarded newborn infants demonstrating catch-up growth in the first year of life. Biol Neonate 49:121–125, 1986.
19. Padoan A, Rigano S, Ferrazzi E, et al. Differences in fat and lean mass proportions in normal and growth restricted fetuses. Am J Obstet Gynecol 191:1459–1464, 2004.
20. Lal MK, Manktelow BN, Draper ES, Field DJ. Chronic lung disease of prematurity and intrauterine growth retardation: a population-based study. Pediatrics 111:483–487, 2003.
21. Strauss RS, Dietz WH. Growth and development of term children born with low birth weight: effects of genetic and environmental factors. J Pediatr 133:67–72, 1998.
22. Gardeil F, Greene R, Stuart B, Turner MJ. Subcutaneous fat in the fetal abdomen as a predictor of growth restriction. Obstet Gynecol 94:209–212, 1999.
23. Brans YW, Sumners JE, Dweck HS, Cassady G. A noninvasive approach to body composition in the neonate: dynamic skinfold measurement. Pediatr Res 8:215–222, 1974.
24. Lapillonne A, Braillon P, Claris O etal: Body composition in appropriate and in small for gestational age infants. Acta Paediatr 86:196–200, 1997.
25. Kramer MS, Olivier M, McLaen FH, et al. Impact of intrauterine growth retardation and body proportionality on fetal and neonatal outcome. Pediatrics 85:707–713, 1990.
26. Bergvall N, Iliadou A, Johannsson S, et al. Risks for low intellectual performance related to being born small for gestational age are modified by gestational age. Pediatrics 117:e460–e467, 2006.
27. Drossou V, Diamanti E, Noutsia H, et al. Accuracy of anthropometric measurements in predicting symptomatic SGA and LGA neonates. Acta Paediatr 84:1–5, 1995.
28. Brans YW, Kuehl TJ, Hayashi RH, Andrew DS. Body water estimates in intrauterine-growth-retarded versus normal grown baboons. Biol Neonate 50:231–236, 1986.
29. Cassady G. Body composition in intrauterine growth retardation. Pediatr Clin North Am 17:79–99, 1970.
30. Brans YW, Shannon DL, Ramamurthy RS. Neonatal polycythemia: II. Plasma, blood, and red cell volume estimates in relation to hematocrit levels and quality of intrauterine growth. Pediatrics 68:175–182, 1981.
31. Maertzdorf WJ, Aldenhuyzen-Dorland W, Slaaf DW, et al. Circulating blood volume in appropriate and small for gestational age full term and preterm polycythemic infants. Acta Paediatr Scand 80:620–627, 1991.
32. Snijders RJ, Abbas A, Melby O, et al. Fetal plasma erythropoietin concentrations in severe growth retardation. Am J Obstet Gynecol 168:615–619, 1993.
33. Linderkamp O. Placental transfusion: determinants and effects. Clin Perinatol 9:559–592, 1982.
34. Yao AC, Lind J. Placental transfusion. Am J Dis Child 127:128–141, 1974.
35. Alandangady N, McHugh S, Aitchison TC, et al. Infants' blood volume in a controlled trial of placental transfusion at preterm delivery. Pediatrics 117:93–98, 2006.
36. Magann EF, Bass JD, Chauhan SP, et al. Amniotic fluid volume in normal singleton pregnancies. Obstet Gynecol 90:524–528, 1997.
37. Brace RA. Physiology of amniotic fluid volume regulation. Clin Obstet Gynecol 2:280–289, 1997.
38. Locatelli A, Vergani P, Toso L, et al. Perinatal outcome associated with oligohydramnios in uncomplicated term pregnancies. Arch Gynecol Obstet 269:130–133, 2004.
39. Thurlow RW, Brace RA. Swallowing, urine flow, and amniotic fluid volume responses to prolonged hypoxia in the ovine fetus. Am J Obstet Gynecol 189:601–608, 2003.
40. Gagnon R, Harding R, Brace RA. Amniotic fluid and fetal urinary response to severe placental insufficiency in sheep. Am J Obstet Gynecol 186:1076–1084, 2002.
41. Shaffer SG, Quimiro CL, Anderson JV, Hall RT. Postnatal weight changes in low birth weight infants. Pediatrics 79:702–705, 1987.
42. Pauls J, Bauer K, Versmold H. Postnatal body weight curves for infants below 1000g birth weight receiving early enteral and parenteral nutrition. Eur J Pediatr 157:416–421, 1998.
43. Shaffer SG, Bradt SK, Hall RT. Postnatal changes in total body water and extracellular volume in the preterm infant with respiratory distress syndrome. J Pediatr 109:509–514, 1986.
44. Bauer K, Cowett RM, Howard GM, et al. Effect of intrauterine growth retardation on postnatal weight change in preterm infants. J Pediatr 123:301–306, 1993.
45. vdWagen A, Okken A, Zweens J, Zijlstra WG. Composition of postnatal weight loss and subsequent weight gain in small for dates newborn infants. Acta Paediatr Scand 74:57–61, 1985.
46. Leipäläja, Boldt T, Turpeinen U, et al. Cardiac hypertrophy and altered hemodynamic adaptation in growth-restricted preterm infants. Pediatr Res 53:989–993, 2003.
47. Modi N. Management of fluid balance in the very immature neonate. Arch Dis Child Fetal Neonatal Ed 89:F108–F111, 2004.
48. Bell EF, Acarregui MJ. Restricted versus liberal water intake for preventing morbidity and mortality in preterm infants. The Cochrane Database of Systematic Reviews 3: CD000503, 2001.
49. Hartnoll G, Betremieux P, Modi N. Randomized controlled trial of postnatal sodium supplementation on oxygen dependency and body weight in 25–30 week gestational age infants. Arch Dis Child 85:F29–F32, 2000.
50. Hartnoll G, Betremieux P, Modi N: Randomized controlled trial of postnatal sodium supplementation on body composition in 25–30 week gestational age infants. Arch Dis Child 82:F24–F28.
51. Cornblath M, Hawdon JM, Williams AF, et al. Controversies reagarding definition of neonatal hypoglycemia: suggested operational thresholds. Pediatrics 105:1141–1145, 2000.
52. Grassl AE, Guiliano MA. The neonate with macrosomia. Clin Obstet Gynecol 43:340–348, 2000.

53. Clapp WM, Butterfield LJ, O'Brien D. Body water compartments in the premature infant, with special reference to the effects of the respiratory distress syndrome and of maternal diabetes and toxemia. Pediatrics 29:883–889, 1962.

54. Hammami M, Walters JC, Hockman EM, Koo WWK. Disproportionate alterations in body composition of large for gestational age neonates. J Pediatr 38:817–821, 2001.

55. Larciprete G, Valensise H, Vasapollo B, et al. Fetal subcutaneous tissue thickness in healthy and gestational diabetic pregnancies. Ultrasound Obstet Gynecol 22:591–597, 2003.

56. Panting-Kemp A, Nguyen T, Chang E, et al. Idiopathic polyhydramnios and perinatal outcome. Am J Obstet Gynecol 181:1079–1082, 1999.

Chapter 10

Acute Problems of Prematurity: Balancing Fluid Volume and Electrolyte Replacements in Very Low Birth Weight (VLBW) and Extremely Low Birth Weight (ELBW) Neonates

Stephen Baumgart, MD

In this chapter we will discuss three problem areas for achieving fluid and electrolyte balance in the extremely low birth weight (ELBW) infant less than 1000 g at birth, and for his/her historical predecessor, the very low birth weight (VLBW) infant less than 1500 g at birth. The most recent clinical research on fluid and electrolyte therapy neatly addresses these groups as separate; however, the principles of achieving fluid balance in either group represent the same physiology, albeit at different phases of fetal development.

The first of these problems is poor epidermal barrier function. Especially in ELBW babies, thin, gelatinous skin promotes rapid transcutaneous evaporation, producing severe electrolyte disturbances in the first few days of life, as well as presenting a poor barrier to the invasion of infections, and is also subject to trauma from tape/adhesive injury and even more minor trauma from bedclothes and routine handling.

A second area of major concern is pulmonary edema formation. Increased lung water (pulmonary edema) has been suggested in the pathogenesis of several conditions (including patent ductus arteriosus (PDA), congestive heart failure, and broncopulmonary dysplasia, (BPD), leading to the controversy of fluid restriction versus fluid replenishment in preventing chronic lung disease in both VLBW and ELBW babies. Also controversial is the routine use of diuretics and steroids for the treatment of pulmonary edema with acute RDS, and with BPD and chronic lung disease.

Finally, a relatively new area of concern is the neurodevelopmental outcome of those infants manifesting severe electrolyte imbalances early in life, particularly in those who develop hyponatremia, or hypernatremia/hyperosmolality in the first few weeks.

IMMATURE EPIDERMAL BARRIER FUNCTION AND THE ELBW HABITUS

The tiny baby (ELBW, less than 1000 g at birth) experiences large transepidermal water loss immediately upon birth (1,2). The ELBW baby has little in the way of skin keratin content, and the skin appears translucent, gelatinous and shiny (Fig. 10-1). In addition, these infants have a proportionally larger extracellular pool with a nearly normal saline content in equilibrium with the plasma compartment (3) from which to evaporate body water leaving the sodium behind (Fig. 10-2) (4,5). During early fetal life, more than 85% of body mass may be comprised of water, two-thirds of which resides in the extracellular space; only one-third of this water resides in the intracellular space. In contrast, by term gestation, the infant is comprised of 75% water, with half of this water residing in the extracellular space and the other half in the intracellular space. By three months postnatal age, only 60% of body mass is water, with two-thirds residing in the intracellular compartment, and only one-third in the extracellular space. Finally, the ELBW neonate has a geometrically larger skin surface area exposed for evaporation from the extracellular compartment pool than in more mature infants and adults (Fig. 10-3) (6). Compared to adult physiology, the

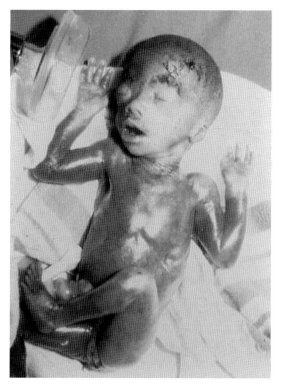

Figure 10-1 Photograph at birth of a 23–3/7 weeks' gestation 530 g birth weight extremely low birth weight (ELBW) infant born in 1980 showing that the extremely immature skin has little in the way of skin keratin content, and appears translucent, gelatinous and shiny as if moist with body water rapidly evaporating into the cool-dry delivery room air. Her eyelids are fused; she is pink, well perfused, and making breathing efforts. She is moving all extremities with apparently good postural tone and spontaneous activity. She went on to survive relatively intact.

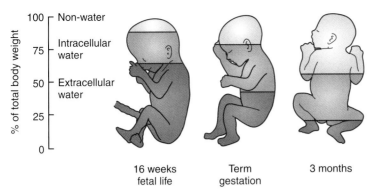

Figure 10-2 Changes in the composition of body fluids occurring during normal fetal and neonatal development. (From Costarino AT, Baumgart S: Modern fluid and electrolyte management of the critically ill premature infant. Ped Clin No Amer 33:153–178, 1986, with permission WB Saunders Co.) Derived from summary by Friis-Hansen B: Body water compartments in children. Pediatrics 28:169–81, 1961. Note the sizeable extracellular water compartment (an extension of the amniotic fluid space) during fetal life shown on the left.

ELBW baby proportionally has over six times the skin surface area exposed per kilogram of body weight, with at least three times the mass of water content vulnerable to evaporation (5,6). A 500 g infant has as much as 1400 cm^2 skin exposed per kilogram compared with about 750 cm^2/kg in a term infant, and 240 cm^2/kg in the adult. Remember, this exposed body mass is largely comprised of extracellular, sodium-rich water exposed for evaporation.

TRANSCUTANEOUS (INSENSIBLE) WATER LOSS

In 1981, we proposed a geometric model (Fig. 10-4) for estimating insensible water loss (IWL) in ELBW infants, using a metabolic balance (Potter Baby Scale, Hartford, CN) for the continuous measurement of body weight loss (insensible weight loss IL) over a 1–3 h period (1,7). Although not widely accepted at the time (IWL estimates in ELBW babies < 700 g were as high as 7.0 mL/kg/h, approaching 170 mL/kg/day), these findings were exactly reproduced by Hammerlund & Sedin in 1983 (2), using an entirely different method to measure water evaporation

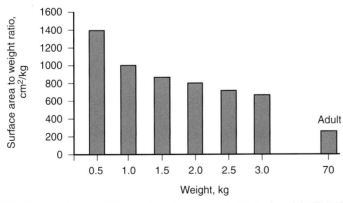

Figure 10-3 Compared with adult physiology, the extremely low birth weight (ELBW) baby proportionally has over 6 times the skin surface area exposed per kg of body weight, with at least 3 times the mass of water content vulnerable to evaporation. (After Baumgart S: Water and electrolyte balance in newborn infants. In Hay WW, Thureen PJ (eds): Neonatal Nutrition and Metabolism, 2nd edn, 2006 in press, with permission Cambridge University Press, Cambridge, UK.)

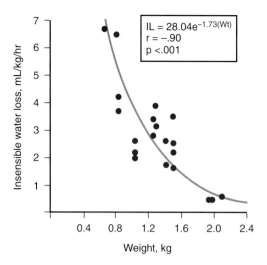

$$IL = 28.04e^{-1.73(Wt)}$$
$$r = -.90$$
$$p < .001$$

Figure 10-4 Concept of a geometric model for estimating insensible water loss in extremely low birth weight infants, using a metabolic balance for the continuous measurement of body weight loss over a 3-h period. (From Baumgart S, Langman CB, Sosulski R, Fox WW, Polin RA: Fluid, electrolyte and glucose maintenance in the very low birthweight infant. Clin Pediatr 21:199–206, 1982, with permission J.B. Lippincott Co.)

directly from the skin (transcutaneous water loss TEWL) by measuring vapor gradients (Transcutaneous Evaporimeter, Servomed, Stockholm) measured over the immature skin surface of ELBW and VLBW premature neonates during the first weeks of life. These investigators reported similar estimations of transcutaneous evaporation, yielding rates of 50–60 g/m²/h, or approximately 170–200 mL/kg/day in the first 1–3 days of life (Fig. 10-5) (2).

WATER LOSS AND PATHOGENESIS OF TRANSCUTANEOUS DEHYDRATION

Also in 1982, we reported a small series of ELBW infants who, despite fluid replenishment to as much as 250 mL/kg/day, nevertheless developed hypernatremic

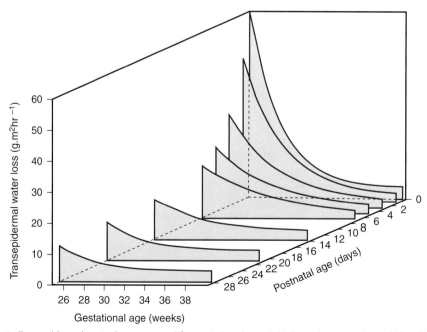

Figure 10-5 Transepidermal water loss measured for gestational age at birth, and postnatal age. (After Hammarlund K, Sedin G: Transepidermal water loss in newborn infants. VIII. Relation to gestational age and post-natal age in appropriate and small for gestational age infants. Acta Paediatr Scand 72:721, 1983, with permission Scandinavian University Press, Stockholm, Sweden.)

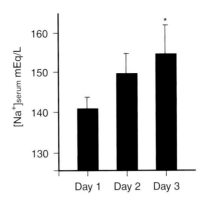

Figure 10-6 Extremely low birth weight (ELBW) babies are prone to developing hypernatremic serum sodium concentrations by day 3 of life, with values averaging 155 mEq/L, and peaking in the smallest babies at a serum sodium of nearly 180 mEq/L (2 standard deviations). (From Baumgart S, Langman CB, Sosulski R, Fox WW, Polin RA: Fluid, electrolyte and glucose maintenance in the very low birthweight infant. Clin Pediatr 21:199–206, 1982, with permission J.B. Lippincott Co.)

serum sodium concentrations by day 3 of life, with values averaging 155 mEq/L (Fig. 10-6), and peaking in the smallest babies at a serum sodium of nearly 180 mEq/L (1). These observations led to our first description of the pathogenesis of water depletion, with the development of hypernatremia, hyperglycemia, hyperosmolarity, and a hyperkalemic state peculiar to the ELBW baby, and developing in the first 72 h of life (Fig. 10-7) (8). In the figure, large free water loss through transcutaneous evaporation is balanced by clinicians increasing the rates of fluid replacement, usually adding sodium in the second day of life to match anticipated urinary sodium losses. These influxes contributed to an immense sodium load presented to an immature kidney glomerular apparatus. Added to this exogenous sodium load, the large salt reservoir in the extracellular space was subjected to rapid transcutaneous dehydration, and the low glomerular filtration rate (GFR) of the fetal kidney led to salt retention. Immature renal tubules with poor concentration ability tended to waste additional free water, and an osmolar diuresis may also have resulted from dextrose overload and hyperglycemia. The result was that by 48–72 h of life, a hyperosmolar, hypernatremic state evolved. This state contributed to the development of life-threatening hyperkalemia, as we shall see later.

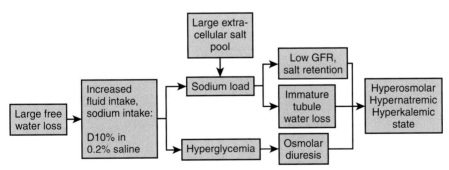

Figure 10-7 Large free water loss through transcutaneous evaporation is balanced by clinicians increasing the rates of fluid replacement, usually adding sodium in day 2 of life to match anticipated urinary sodium losses. These influxes contribute to an immense sodium load presented to an immature kidney glomerular apparatus. Added to this exogenous sodium load, the large salt reservoir in the extracellular space is subjected to rapid transcutaneous dehydration, and the low glomerular filtration rate (GFR) of the fetal kidney leads to salt retention. Immature renal tubules with poor concentration ability tended to waste additional free water, and an osmolar diuresis may also result from dextrose overload and hyperglycemia. The result is that by 48–72 h of life, a hyperosmolar, hypernatremic state evolves, and hyperkalemia is likely to occur as well. (After Baumgart S: Fluid and electrolyte therapy in the premature infant: Case management. In Burg F, Polin RA (eds): Workbook in Practical Neonatology (pp. 25–39). WB Saunders, Philadelphia, 1983, with permission W.B. Saunders Co.)

SALT RESTRICTION PROPHYLAXIS

To prevent this syndrome, Costarino et al conducted a randomized and blinded control trial of sodium restriction versus maintenance sodium administration during the first five days of life in infants born less than 1000 g and less than 28 weeks' gestation (9). Infants were randomly assigned to either a low sodium group who received no maintenance sodium additive with their parenteral nutrition, to a high sodium replenishment group who received 3–4 mEq/kg/day added to their daily maintenance fluids, and administered beginning on day 2 of life. A safety committee analyzed data at half-enrollment, and stopped the study. Two out of the nine infants in the sodium restricted group became hyponatremic with serum sodium concentrations < 130 mEq/L by day 5 of life, and were taken out of the study. Conversely, two of the eight infants in the sodium replenishment group became hypernatremic with a serum sodium > 150 mEq/L by day 4, and were also removed from the study. None of these occurrences were reversed. Daily assessments of serum sodium concentrations were significantly and consistently higher in the sodium supplemented infants after day 1 of life (Fig. 10-8) (9).

By study design, sodium intake (seen in the top graph, Fig. 10-9) ranged between 4–6 mEq/kg/day in the sodium supplemented maintenance group (shaded bars) (9). Infants in the restricted group inadvertently received between 1.0 and 1.75 mEq/kg/day of sodium as additives (shown as clear bars on the graph) with medications containing sodium (sodium heparin, sodium ampicillin, and sodium citrated transfusions, etc.). It was impossible to eliminate sodium intake entirely due to these often unrecognized sources of exogenously supplied salt. Sodium output in the urine (shown in the middle graph Fig. 10-9) remained the same for the first three days of the study, but began to increase after day 4 in infants in the sodium-supplemented group. As shown in the bottom graph (Fig. 10-9), calculated sodium balance was nearly zero in the sodium supplemented group (shaded bars) where intake matched urinary sodium excretion, but remained markedly negative in the sodium restricted group by as much as 6 mEq/kg/day net sodium loss (white bars).

Fluid intakes, prescribed independently of the study by the physicians (who did not know the group assignment), were similar in both groups of babies, ranging between 90–130 mL/kg/day throughout the first 3 days of life (Fig. 10-10, top graph). However, after 3 days, fluid volume exceeded 130 mL/kg/day in the sodium supplemented infants (indicated by black circles); and was significantly higher than the salt restricted babies who only received approximately 90 mL/kg/day (shown by open circles). These results suggest that infants in the sodium-supplemented group were prescribed increasing amounts of fluid to compensate for their rising serum sodium. Conversely, infants in the sodium-restricted group required relative fluid restrictions, probably in response to falling serum sodium concentrations. Failure to restrict fluid intake volume after 5 days may result in clinically significant hyponatremia.

Of interest (as seen in the bottom graph, Fig. 10-10), urine output was fixed throughout the study in both groups, at between 2–4 mL/kg/h (or about 50–100 mL/kg/day), and was not dependent on either the volume of fluid administered, or the amount sodium intake.

Survival was similar in both groups at about two-thirds, and the co-morbidities of intraventricular hemorrhage and patent ductus arteriosus were also similar. There was a trend, however, towards infants developing bronchopulmonary dysplasia in the high sodium/high fluid intake group: 7 of 7 infants versus 4 of 8 infants in the low sodium/low fluid intake group, p = 0.08. However, this safety analysis was underpowered to detect the impact of fluid volume administration on these co-morbidities.

Figure 10-8 Infants randomly assigned to either a low sodium group who received no maintenance sodium additive with their parenteral nutrition, or to a high sodium replenishment group who received 3–4 mEq/kg/day added to their daily maintenance fluids, and administered beginning on day 2 of life. Daily assessments of serum sodium concentrations were significantly and consistently higher in the sodium supplemented infants after day 1 of life (After Costarino AT, Gruskay JA, Corcoran L, Polin RA, Baumgart S: Sodium restriction vs. daily maintenance replacement in very low birthweight premature neonates, a randomized and blinded therapeutic trial. J Pediatr 120:99–106, 1992, with permission Elsevier, Inc.)

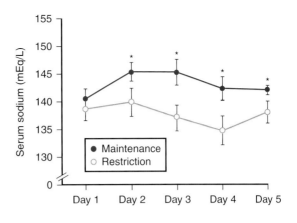

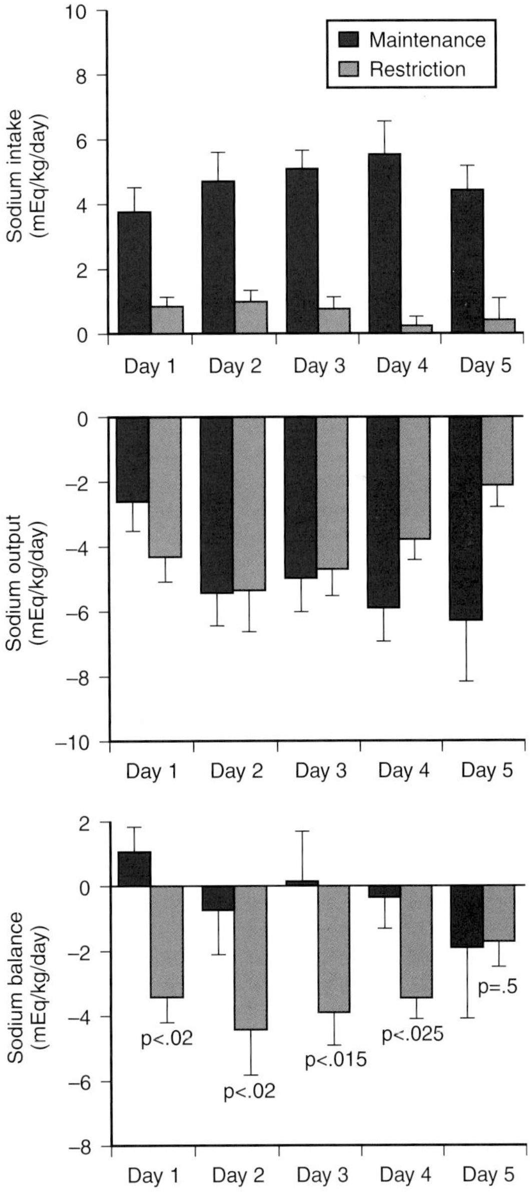

Figure 10-9 Sodium intake (top) ranged between 4–6 mEq/kg/day in the sodium supplemented maintenance group (2–4 mEq/kg/day shaded bars). Infants in the restricted group received between 1.0 and 1.75 mEq/kg/day of sodium as additives (shown as clear bars in the graph) with medications containing sodium (see text). It was impossible to eliminate sodium intake entirely due to these often unrecognized sources of exogenously applied salt. In the bottom graph, calculated sodium balance was nearly zero in the sodium supplemented group (shaded bars) where intake matched urinary sodium excretion, but remained markedly negative in the sodium restricted group by as much as 6 mEq/kg/day net sodium loss (2 standard deviations, white bars). (After Costarino AT, Gruskay JA, Corcoran L, Polin RA, Baumgart S: Sodium restriction vs. daily maintenance replacement in very low birthweight premature neonates, a randomized and blinded therapeutic trial. J Pediatr 120:99–106, 1992, with permission Elsevier, Inc.)

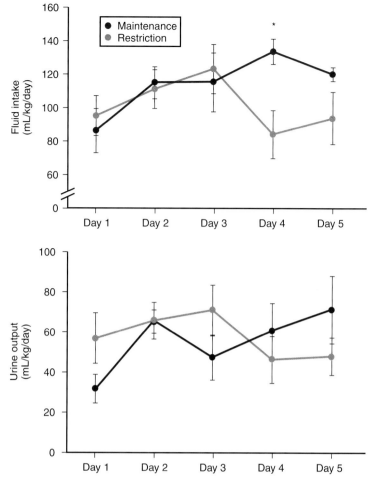

Figure 10-10 Fluid intakes prescribed by the physicians unaware of the sodium supplemental group assignment were similar in both groups of babies, ranging between 90–130 mL/kg/day throughout the first 3 days of life (top). However, after 3 days, fluid volume exceeded 130 mL/kg/day in the sodium supplemented infants (indicated by black circles); and was significantly higher than the salt restricted babies who only received approximately 90 mL/kg/day (shown by open circles). These results suggest that infants in the sodium-supplemented group were prescribed increasing amounts of fluid to compensate for their rising serum sodium. Conversely, infants in the sodium-restricted group required relative fluid volume restriction, probably in response to falling serum sodium concentrations. Failure to restrict fluid intake volume after 5 days, however, may result in clinically significant hyponatremia. Urine output (bottom) was fixed throughout the study in both groups, at between 2–4 mL/kg/h (or about 50–100 mL/kg/day), and was not dependent on either the volume of fluid administered, or the amount of sodium intake. (After Costarino AT, Gruskay JA, Corcoran L, Polin RA, Baumgart S: Sodium restriction vs. daily maintenance replacement in very low birthweight premature neonates, a randomized and blinded therapeutic trial. J Pediatr 120:99–106, 1992, with permission Elsevier, Inc.)

Hartnoll et al (10) observed that the timing of sodium supplementation after preterm birth does not affect the rate of fall in pulmonary arterial pressure. The increased risk of continuing oxygen requirement in ELBW infants is more likely, therefore, to be a direct consequence of persistent expansion of the extracellular compartment and increased pulmonary interstitial fluid, resulting from sodium intake. This adds further weight to the authors' view that the timing of routine sodium supplementation should be delayed until the onset of postnatal extracellular volume contraction, marked clinically by weight loss.

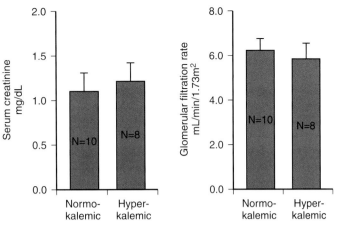

Figure 10-11 Eight hyperkalemic extremely low birth weight (ELBW) infants compared to 10 comparable ELBW infants who remained normokalemic. Renal functions for these two groups of babies demonstrated similar serum creatinine and glomerular filtration rates. (From Gruskay J, Costarino AT, Polin RA, Baumgart S: Non-oliguric hyperkalemia in the premature infant less than 1000 grams. J Pediatr 113:381–386, 1988, with permission Elsevier, Inc.)

NON-OLIGURIC HYPERKALEMIA IN ELBW BABIES

During these studies, we encountered an additional electrolyte disturbance that was further investigated by Gruskay et al, who first reported non-oliguric hyperkalemia in extremely low birth weight babies, in the absence of renal failure (11). These authors measured renal functions in a group of ELBW infants, some of whom developed serum potassium concentrations > 6.8 mEq/L, a level first identified by Usher that increases the risk for life-threatening cardiac arrhythmias in neonates (12). Gruskay et al (11) described 8 ELBW infants in a hyperkalemic group with slightly lower birth weights, and compared them to 10 comparable ELBW infants who remained normokalemic. Peak serum potassium levels averaged at $8.0 + 0.3$ mEq/L in the hyperkalemic babies, and all of these infants indeed developed electrocardiographic abnormalities requiring treatment.

Renal functions for these two groups of babies demonstrated similar serum creatinine and glomerular filtration rates (Fig. 10-11). In contrast, urine sodium excretion was markedly increased in hyperkalemic infants, with urine

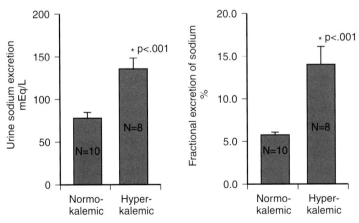

Figure 10-12 Urine sodium excretion was markedly increased in hyperkalemic infants, with urine concentrations of urine sodium sometimes exceeding 140 mEq/L (standard deviation), and mean fractional excretion of sodium was nearly 15% in the hyperkalemic group, compared to only 5% in the normokalemic infants. Both of these observations suggest a profoundly immature tubular conservation of filtered sodium. (From Gruskay J, Costarino AT, Polin RA, Baumgart S: Non-oliguric hyperkalemia in the premature infant less than 1000 grams. J Pediatr 113:381–386, 1988, with permission Elsevier, Inc.)

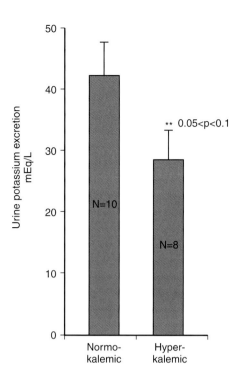

Figure 10-13 Potassium excess is normally secreted from the distal tubule. Hyperkalemic infants' urines had significantly less potassium excretion than normokalemic infants, suggesting an immaturity in renal tubular response to aldosterone, resulting in these electrolyte disturbances. (From Gruskay J, Costarino AT, Polin RA, Baumgart S: Non-oliguric hyperkalemia in the premature infant less than 1000 grams. J Pediatr 113:381–386, 1988, with permission Elsevier, Inc.)

concentrations of sodium exceeding 140 mEq/L (Fig. 10-12), and fractional excretion of sodium of nearly 15% in the hyperkalemic group, compared to only 5% in the normokalemic infants. Both of these observations suggest a profoundly immature tubular conservation of filtered sodium. Moreover, potassium excess is normally secreted from the distal tubule. Hyperkalemic infants' urines revealed significantly less potassium excretion than normal infants (Fig. 10-13). These authors suggested an immaturity in renal tubular response to aldosterone, resulting in these electrolyte disturbances.

However, Stefano et al (13) reported a similar investigation of 12 ELBW infants developing non-oliguric hyperkalemia and compared them to 27 babies of similar gestation who remained normokalemic. In addition to urine and renal function studies, these authors reported erythrocyte Na+/K+ ATP'ase activity that was significantly higher in normokalemic infants, suggesting that the cellular maturation of this enzyme was markedly more immature in the hyperkalemic babies, and contributed towards the exudation of potassium from the intracellular compartment. Potassium leakage can be exacerbated by high serum sodium levels, when sodium leaks into cells, and competitively exceeds the Na+/K+ ATP'ase pump's capacity to exclude sodium, further promoting intracellular potassium leakage into the extracellular compartment. These authors concluded that hyperkalemia was due to an intracellular-to-extracellular potassium shift with diminished Na+/K+ ATP'ase, and that glomerular-tubular imbalance in the kidney did not completely explain why hyperkalemia was developing in these babies. Subsequent observational studies by Lorenz & Kleinman (14) have confirmed their findings.

THE EPIDERMAL BARRIER: REDUCING TRANSCUTANEOUS EVAPORATION

Other than manipulating water and electrolyte administration to ELBW babies, an alternative strategy for preventing these disturbances is to reduce the large transepidermal water loss that creates electrolyte imbalances in the first place. Several techniques have been proposed to accomplish this, and include: incubator humidification, 'swamping' babies in mist either within incubators or within plastic body chambers under radiant warmers, application of petroleum based ointments used on the skin as an emollient, polyvinyl chloride plastic blankets or body bags, and non-occlusive semi-adherent polyurethane artificial skins. Native transepidermal water evaporation gradually lessens, as spontaneous keratinization of the epidermis develops over a 1–4 week period after birth in these babies, probably too late to prevent the acute dehydration syndrome described (15).

Environmental Humidification

Incubator humidification for premature babies is recommended by the American Academy of Pediatrics and the American College of Obstetricians guidelines (16). Levels suggested are between 40–50% relative humidity. Saturated environments for 'swamping' babies at 80–100% relative humidity may lead to 'rain-out' (a term used to describe 'swamp-like' condensation of water on the interior surfaces of incubators or other plastic covers for tiny babies, and raises our concern for water borne infections.

Harpin & Rutter (17) used 80–90% humidified incubators for 33 VLBW infants, and compared them to 29 historical controls nurtured in dry incubators. All infants were less than 30 weeks' gestation, and were studied for the first 2 weeks of life. Two infants developed pseudomonas sepsis in the humidified group and one died, and one developed pseudomonas in the dry group who died. These authors concluded that saturated humidification was effective, but may be associated with water borne nosocomial infection.

More recently, Gaylord (18) studied 70 infants in dry incubators, comparing them to 85 babies nursed in humidified incubators, again using historical controls. Despite similar fluid balance, dry incubator babies were significantly more likely to develop hypernatremia, hyperkalemia, azotemia, oliguria, and to receive more fluid volume replacements; whereas babies in humidified incubators did not have these problems; but had more gram negative isolates (62%) recovered from surface cultures.

Therefore, humidity should be employed cautiously, not exceeding 80% relative humidity during incubator care. Using the sophisticated humidification monitoring and control systems now incorporated into modern incubators is also suggested. 'Swamping' infants either within incubators or under radiant warmers is not recommended. Any visible water (even mist), is condensation, which promotes bacterial and fungal growth.

Skin Emollients

Research on petroleum based ointments to treat the skin of newborn babies began as early as 1981 when Rutter & Hull (19) first applied paraffin oil to premature infants every 4–6 h, reducing transepidermal water loss, but not significantly altering fluid balance over the first several days of life. In 1996, Nopper et al (20) conducted a small randomized trial in 16 infants, using Aquaphor®, a preservative-free petroleum ointment to reduce transepidermal water loss, bacterial colonization and sepsis. These authors claimed better skin integrity with this treatment, and many nurseries adopted this treatment as standard practice for ELBW babies. In 2000, however, Campbell & Baker (21) reported an increasing occurrence of candidiasis in their nurseries after the introduction of petroleum ointment use. And the multi-center Vermont Oxford trial (22) observed an increase in coagulase-negative staphylococcal sepsis occurring in babies who were treated with this petroleum preparation. Because of these concerns for infection, and the requirement for

Table 10-1	Transepidermal Evaporation (TEE, $g/m^2/h$) with and without a Flexible Polyurethane Plastic, Non-Occlusive Skin Barrier (OpSite®, Smith Nephew Inc., Columbia, SC, USA)				
	Day 1	**Day 2**	**Day 3**	**Day 4**	**Day 5, removal**
Naked	27.5	31.3	21.4	18.8	20.8
Dressed	8.9*	9.5*	9.0*	10.6*	18.8

(From Knauth A, Gordin M, McNelis W, Baumgart S. A semipermeable polyurethane membrane as an artificial skin in the premature neonate. Pediatrics 83:945–950, 1989. Copyright the American Academy of Pediatrics.)

*Indicates significant reduction in TEE.

more frequent handling (ELBW babies were required to be repeatedly re-applied with ointment to maintain an effective moisture barrier), we no longer use this technique in our nurseries.

Plastic Shields, Bags or Blankets

Alternatively, we have reported the use of a single layer of Saran® polyvinyl chloride to reduce insensible water loss during the first few days of life by more than half in low birth weight babies, and I have advocated the use of this technique, especially for tiny infants under radiant warmers during the first 24–48 h of life (23). To date, however, there have been no studies to evaluate the occurrence of infection or bacterial colonization with the use of these plastic 'blankets.' Knauth et al (24) alternatively suggested the use of a flexible polyurethane plastic, non-occlusive skin barrier (Tegaderm® or OpSite®). Some of these barriers are treated with anti-microbial suppressants, and are relatively infection neutral when used as TPN catheter site dressings. We evaluated transcutaneous evaporation using these materials, and produced a two-thirds reduction in transcutaneous water loss shown in Table 10-1 during the first 4 days of life in a series of premature babies. However, as seen on the right side of this table, after removal on the 5th day, evaporation again increased, either with re-exposure of the immature skin, or with the exfoliation of the developing keratin underneath this gently adhesive barrier.

Porat & Brodsky (25) recently published data on the use of polyurethane dressings covering low birth weight infants completely. They demonstrated significant reductions in hypernatremia, excessive fluid volume intake, weight loss, bronchopulmonary dysplasia, and mortality with the use of an artificial layer during the first few weeks of life.

Donahue et al (26), thereafter, conducted a randomized trial of this technique in 61 babies, but did not reveal changes in fluid volume requirements, although improved skin integrity was suggested by these authors. For any of these strategies, a consistent effect in reducing electrolyte disturbances has not been demonstrated. Humidification and emollient ointments may increase the risk of infection. Some randomized data exist, none of which supports their use. Alternatively, standard incubation at moderate humidity between 40–60%, with or without a plastic barrier, remains the most popular practice in our nurseries.

PULMONARY EDEMA FORMATION

After the initial first week of life, the risk for dehydration diminishes as the skin barrier matures. Thereafter, and usually during the second or third week of life in ELBW babies, many authors have now described water overload in the pathogenesis of pulmonary edema, probably resulting from continuing overzealous fluid replenishment therapy past the first week, when these babies were more subject to dehydration.

Suggested pathogenesis for water overload is depicted in Fig. 10-14 (8). Fluid replenishment volume, when administered too aggressively, may result in increased lung water, and contribute to the pathogenesis of bronchopulmonary dysplasia (27–29). Moreover, high fluid intakes, which have been associated with the development of clinically significant patent ductus arteriosus and congestive heart failure (30–32), also may contribute to the pathogenesis of BPD (33). Increased pulsatility and diastolic run-off with a clinically significant PDA may contribute to the development of necrotizing enterocolitis (34), and intraventricular hemorrhage (35).

Perhaps the root cause of this problem is the premature infant's markedly immature renal development. The fetal kidney at 25 weeks has a lobulated appearance, with a thin cortex predominated by small, less well developed juxta-medullary nephrons and lacking entirely the robust cortical nephron population. The result of diminutive anatomy is less glomerular surface available for filtration of any fluid volume or salt excess. We can only imagine even more immature nephrons, and the severe functional limitations present in the tiny kidneys of an extremely low birth weight infant between 500–1000 g in development.

Prevention of Iatrogenic Fluid Overload

In testing the prevention strategy of low versus high fluid volume administration for the development of fluid overload in premature infants, Bell & Acarregui recently reviewed a meta-analysis of four randomized controlled trials (Table 10-2) (30–34). Of the studies reported, fluid intakes ranged from as low as 50 mL/kg/day to as high as 200 mL/kg/day routinely, depending on the study designs used. All four were conducted primarily on VLBW (and not ELBW) populations; and only two of the studies demonstrated significant differences in the occurrences of PDA, congestive heart failure, BPD, NEC, or death in the high fluid groups. The meta-analysis of all randomized data, however, favored low fluid volume infusions, revealing that PDA with congestive heart failure and necrotizing enterocolitis were more frequently observed in the high fluid group; death was significantly higher as well. More recently, Kavvidia et al (36) reported the only randomized series including a number of extremely low birth weight infants, with gestational ages ranging between 23–33

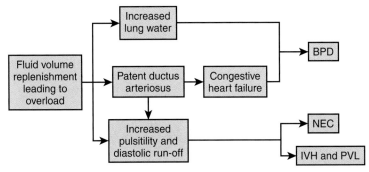

Figure 10-14 Fluid replenishment volume, when administered too aggressively, may result in increased lung water, and contribute to the pathogenesis of bronchopulmonary dysplasia (26–28). Moreover, high fluid intakes have been associated with the development of clinically significant patent ductus arteriosus and congestive heart failure (29–31), also contributing to the pathogenesis of broncopulmonary dysplasia (BPD) (32). Increased pulsatility and diastolic run-off, with a clinically significant PDA, may contribute to the development of necrotizing enterocolitis (33), and IVH or intraventricular hemorrhage (34). (After Baumgart S: Fluid and electrolyte therapy in the premature infant: Case management. In Burg F, Polin RA (eds): Workbook in Practical Neonatology (pp. 25–39). WB Saunders, Philadelphia, 1983, with permission W.B. Saunders Co.)

Table 10-2   Meta-analysis of Four Studies Evaluating High Versus Low Fluid Volume Intake Strategies for Maintenance Therapy in VLBW Infants. PDA, Congestive Heart Failure (CHF), and Necrotizing Enterocolitis (NEC) were Significantly More Common with High Fluid Volumes Administered

Study	Study design	Weights and gestations	High/low fluid volume limits	Outcomes
Bell et al (1980)	170 sequential matched pairs, 30 days	1.41 kg 31 weeks	122/169 mL/kg/day	PDA, CHF, NEC in high fluid group
Von Stackhauser et al (1980)	56 random pairs, 3 days	1.9/2.0 kg 34.6/34.2 weeks	60/150 mL/kg/day	No differences
Lorenz et al (1982)	88 random matched pairs, 5 days	1.20 kg 29 weeks	60–85 mL/kg/day 80–140 mL/kg/day	No differences
Tammela et al (1982)	100 random pairs, 28 days	1.30 kg 31 weeks	50–150 mL/kg/day 80–200 mL/kg/day	Death, BPD in high fluid group

After Bell EF, Acarregui MJ: Restricted versus Liberal Water Intake for Preventing Morbidity and Mortality in Preterm Infants. Cochrane Database of Systematic Reviews 3:CD000503, 2001.

Bell, EF, Warburton D, Stonestreet BS, Oh W: Effect of fluid administration on the development of symptomatic patent ductus arteriosus and congestive heart failure in premature infants. N Engl J Med 302:598–604, 1980.

von Stockhausen HB, Struve M: Die Auswirkungen einer stark unterschiedlichen parenteral en Flussigkeitszufuhr bei Fruh- und Neugeborenen in den ersten drei Lebenstagen. Klin Padiatr 192:539–46, 1980.

Lorenz JM, Kleinman LI, Kotagal UR, Reller MD: Water balance in very low-birth weight infants: relationship to water and sodium intake and effect on outcome. J Pediatr 101:423–32, 1982.

Tammella OKT, Koivisto ME: Fluid restriction for preventing bronchopulmonary dysplasia? Reduced fluid intake during the first weeks of life improves the outcome of low-birth-weight infants. Acta Paediatr 81:207–12, 1992.

weeks, and offered only modest differences in high versus low fluid volumes prescribed. No beneficial or adverse effects could be demonstrated.

Finally, Oh et al (29), for the Neonatal Research Network, summarized a cohort of 1382 ELBW babies born at between 401–1000 g who were followed prospectively at Network centers to characterize their prescribed daily fluid volume intakes (both parenteral and enteral, net intake mL/kg/day (Fig. 10-15)) and percent of birth weight loss daily over the first 10 days of life; and analyzed retrospectively for adverse outcomes of BPD and death. Multivariate logistic regression demonstrated that higher fluid intake volumes with weight retention over the first 10 days of life were significantly associated with higher risk of death or BPD. As in other studies, however, higher birth weight was associated with lower risk for death or BPD, suggesting that even slightly more developmentally mature infants are less likely to require excessive fluid replenishment to maintain electrolyte balance, described above in the sections on epidermal barrier and renal organogenesis in ELBW babies. Wide ranges of daily fluid volume prescriptions (41–389 mL/kg/day) were observed in this study, with average group differences of as little as 7–24 mL/kg/day.

It can be concluded from these published data that careful fluid volume restriction reduces death, PDA, and necrotizing enterocolitis in VLBW babies between 1000–1500 g, and may also be prudent for the ELBW population < 1000 g, and that there is also a trend towards less chronic lung disease in infants from both categories. However, we cannot readily extrapolate a fluid restriction strategy for the treatment of ELBW babies during the first 3–5 days of life because of the risk of dehydration with severe electrolyte disturbances, as described above. Randomized trials of either artificial epidermal barriers to circumvent hypernatremia/hyperkalemia, with or without free water restriction to avoid weight retention and to allow body water and sodium pool contraction over the first week after birth, are wanting and warranted.

Diuretic Therapy

Diuretic therapy to treat fluid overload and pulmonary edema after it occurs also remains controversial. In 2002, Brion et al (37) reported a meta-analysis of six randomized controlled trials for the combination of spironolactone and thiazide diuretics given for 3 weeks duration or longer, with some success in the treatment of chronic lung disease. A year later Brion & Sol (38) conducted a second meta-analysis, describing six randomized controlled trials for the use of furosemide in treating lung edema in acute RDS. Oxygenation was only transiently improved with furosemide. However, furosemide is also a vasodilator, and was associated with the development of symptomatic PDA in RDS babies. Moreover, in some cases, significant hypovolemia developed, requiring excess fluid administration to recover blood pressure. Brion and Sol concluded that furosemide should not be recommended for treating acute RDS. Of note, none of these studies was done in the era of prenatal prophylactic steroid therapy. Therefore, combinations of therapies effective for treating pulmonary edema and the development of BPD have not been adequately tested or reported in the present era.

Regarding lung edema, in a 1990 review Bland (39) summarized perinatal animal models, describing lung water physiology. Prenatally, the pulmonary epithelium actively secretes chloride ion with water; but postnatally the lung changes over to an active Na+/K+ exchange-mediated absorbing mechanism. This transitional change from a secretory organ to a dry organ may be disrupted by RDS, or a clinically significant PDA with congestive heart failure; becoming involved in the pathogenesis of pulmonary edema, and bronchopulmonary dysplasia.

Corticosteroid Therapy

Helve et al (40) reported the use of postnatal steroids on the epithelial sodium channel, and described mRNA expression as diminished in very low birth weight babies with RDS, comparing them to normal term control infants. All five RDS subjects' mothers had received prenatal β-methasone therapy. Subsequently, when given dexamethasone for the treatment of BPD occurring after 1 month of age in four of these subjects, increased sodium channel mRNA expression was again observed, suggesting a potential role for postnatal steroids in resorbing lung edema, and diminishing lung water.

In the only study of water and sodium homeostasis in ELBW babies exposed to prenatal steroids, Omar et al (41) reported prenatal corticosteroid effects on development in ELBW infants ranging from 565 g to 865 g. They noted higher urine output during the first two days of life in babies receiving prenatal steroids, when compared to controls. The authors speculated that natriuresis may be due to better mobilization of lung fluid through the augmentation of Na+/K+ ATP'ase in the pulmonary epithelium. These authors also commented on a lower calculated insensible water loss during the first 4 days of life in these infants, speculating that prenatal steroids may also have improved epidermal barrier function. It is the opinion of this author that results of studies on corticosteroids and fluid balance remain highly speculative at this time, and unfortunately, no recommendations for routine therapy should be made.

ELECTROLYTE IMBALANCES AND NEURODEVELOPMENT

Hyponatremia

In examining the effects of fluid and electrolyte imbalances on later neurodevelopment, Bhatty et al (42) has given us a preliminary description of hyponatremia occurring in a group of ELBW infants less than 1000 g. These authors defined a serum sodium concentration < 125 mEq/L as clinically significant hyponatremia. Thirty-five babies developing hyponatremia during the first few weeks of life were compared retrospectively to 43 non-hyponatremic birth weight-matched control infants using multivariate regression analysis. Although not statistically significant, hyponatremic babies, in general, seemed more critically ill—all subsequently developed BPD, had longer ventilator and oxygen courses, with longer hospital stays. Moreover, more severe IVH (grades 3 and 4) were observed in 23% of the hyponatremic subjects, and only 5% of the non-hyponatremic infants. Similarly, significant retinopathy (grades 3 and 4) was more prevalent in the hyponatremic subjects.

On follow-up through early infancy, Bhatty et al (42, 57) observed a higher occurrence of spastic cerebral palsy in infants who had developed hyponatremia, more hypotonia, and an increased occurrence of sensory-neural hearing loss, as well as behavioral problems reported by parents later in childhood. Using regression analysis, the authors suggested a specific association between recovery from hyponatremia and neurodevelopmental problems subsequently developing in the extremely low birth weight population.

When evaluating the degree of hyponatremia at onset, the degree of worst hyponatremia (lowest serum sodium concentration), and the duration of hyponatremia, they found no correlation to subsequent neurodevelopmental outcomes. In contrast, when looking at the speed of recovery from hyponatremia, the 11 infants with more rapid correction of serum sodium concentrations (by more than 10 mEq/L in 24 h), experienced the worst neurodevelopmental outcomes later on. The authors concluded that rapid correction of hyponatremia, particularly within the first 24 h of onset of serum sodium concentration < 125 mEq/L, may

Table 10-3 Published Studies Suggesting Hyponatremia is Associated with Adverse Neurodevelopmental Outcomes

Study	Study design	Population	Developmental deficits
Leslie et al (1995)	Case controls	ELBW	Sensory-neural hearing loss
Murphy et al (1997)	Case controls	VLBW	Cerebral palsy
Ertl & Sulyok (2001)	Multivariate analysis, case controls	VLBW	Sensory-neural hearing loss

Leslie GI, Kalaw MB, Bowen JR, Arnold JD: Risk factors for sensorineural hearing loss in extremely premature infants. J Paediatr Child Health 31:312–6, 1995.

Murphy DJ, Hope PL, Johnson A: Neonatal risk factors for cerebral palsy in very preterm babies: case-control study. BMJ 314:404–8, 1997.

Ertl T, Hadzsiev K, Vincze O, Pytel J, Szabo I, Sulyok E: Hyponatremia and sensorineural hearing loss in preterm infants. Biology of the Neonate 79:109–12, 2001.

be associated with adverse neurodevelopmental sequelae; and that the calculated sodium correction should provide a rate no more than 0.4 mEq/L/h, or at most 10 mEq/L/day. We presently do not recommend any more rapid correction, and in most situations we avoid entirely the use of 3% hypertonic saline acutely for correction of hyponatremia in ELBW or VLBW neonates.

Many other studies have suggested an association between hyponatremia and later neurodevelopmental problems (Table 10-3). Leslie et al (43) matched case controls revealing significant sensory-neural hearing deficits in ELBW babies under 28 weeks' gestation and 1000 g at birth. Hyponatremia in this study was also diagnosed at a sodium concentration < 125 mEq/L. Murphy et al (44) reported 134 case controls for 59 VLBW babies developing cerebral palsy, and associated

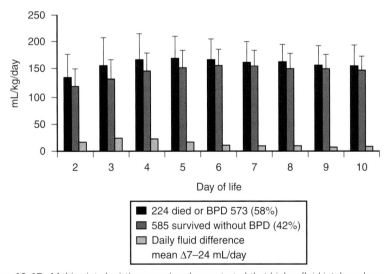

Figure 10-15 Multivariate logistic regression demonstrated that higher fluid intake volumes with weight retention over the first 10 days of life were significantly associated with higher risk of death or broncopulmonary dysplasia (BPD) in 1382 extremely low birth weight (ELBW) infants followed prospectively from day 1 of life. Wide ranges of daily fluid volume prescriptions (41–389 mL/kg/day) were observed in this study, with average group differences of as little as 7–24 mL/kg/day. (After Oh W, Poindexter BB, Perritt R, Lemons JA, Bauer CR, Ehrenkranz RA, Stoll BJ, Poole K, Wright LL, for the Neonatal Research Network: Association between fluid intake and weight loss during the first ten days of life and risk of bronchopulmonary dysplasia in extremely low birth weight infants. J Pediatr 147:786–90, 2005, with permission from Elsevier, Inc.)

cerebral palsy with hyponatremia. Ertl et al (45) matched 22 sensory-neural hearing loss babies to 25 case controls for multivariate analysis, and found an association between hearing impairment and hyponatremia specifically. None of these studies reported the course of development or treatment of hyponatremia, nor made recommendations for therapy.

And in a fascinating long-term follow-up study, Al-Dahan et al (46) reported that sodium supplemented VLBW babies < 32 weeks given 4–5 mEq/kg/day in their diets, and lasting from 4 to 14 days of life, had, at 10 years of age, better performance IQs, better motor and memory indices, and improved parental behavioral assessments. This report suggests that routine sodium restriction in premature babies, although expedient to prevent hypernatremia, may not be beneficial with respect to long term outcomes.

Hypernatremia

In contrast (and despite the frequent observation of hypernatremia in ELBW babies already described), the data associating hypernatremia with central nervous system disruptions have not been as closely examined. Simmons et al in (47) suggested restricting hypertonic sodium bicarbonate use, associating the resulting hypernatremia with significant intraventricular hemorrhages. However, Lupton et al (48) re-evaluated serum sodium concentrations during the first 4 days of life in VLBW prematures < 1500 g, who had developed IVH in that time period, and found no association with hypernatremia. Lupton et al's study, however, defined hypernatremia at serum sodium levels > 145 mEq/L, which may not comprise a critical threshold for evaluating neurological impairment. We certainly have seen more severe hypernatremia in the ELBW population, with serum sodium concentrations ranging from > 150 to as high as 180 mEq/L (1).

None of these reports on hypernatremia directly addresses the occurrences of developmental delays with electrolyte imbalance in the ELBW population, and further investigation is needed. Existing developmental follow-up data for this population should probably be examined for routinely recorded serum sodium concentrations.

AREAS FOR FURTHER INVESTIGATION

There are many areas for further investigation. For the ELBW baby, in whom virtually every therapy is experimental, protocols to standardize care should be developed in each provider's institution along with safety and outcome evaluations. Epidermal barrier augmentation seems to be a first, natural step in these investigations, to avoid the disruption of fluid and electrolyte balance in the first place. Materials for promoting a temporary artificial skin barrier that is neutral to infection are more elusive than we might have imagined.

Manipulations of both sodium and free water volume intake are also warranted. Comparing babies receiving high volume fluid intake vs low volume fluid restriction seems to me a naive approach to this problem. Rather, a more strict and precise definition of fluid balance is needed. Right now we depend on serial measurements of serum sodium concentration to evaluate whether ELBW babies need more or less water volume replenishment. The trouble with this approach is that serum sodium concentration must be abnormal before we can adjust fluid intake to offset changing losses. Further investigation of sodium channel development and the promotion of natural lung water resorption through endogenous means is a more complex area for basic science investigations. Clinical trials of diuretics and steroids should be performed before prescribing these therapies routinely. In the area of neurodevelopmental outcomes, hyponatremia, water restriction, and

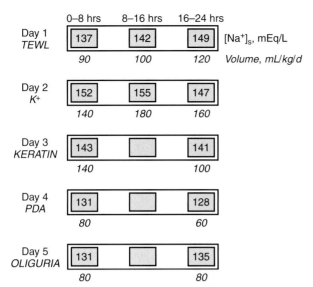

Figure 10-16 On day 1 of life, the primary problem is the tremendously high transepidermal water loss (TEWL). We recommend checking serum electrolytes every 8 h during day 1–2 of life, and adjusting an electrolyte-free solution upwards in 10–20 mL increments every 6–8 h, depending on the rate of rise in the measured serum sodium concentration. The key to this strategy is checking serum/urine electrolytes more frequently, because, once the serum sodium rises, the patient is already dehydrated. By day 2 the problem of hyperkalemia often emerges—volume replacement maximizes as serum sodium concentration peaks, and sodium leaks into the cells displacing potassium outwards from the intracellular compartment. Then on day 3 TEWL begins to diminish as keratin deposition occurs, or in response to incubator care with additional humidification. At this juncture, the serum sodium concentration may suddenly decrease. We should anticipate this change by diminishing water volume immediately when we first see the serum sodium concentrations fall, thus anticipating fluid overload and the risk for promoting a hemodynamically significant PDA by day 4 of life, imaging the ductus prospectively may be of consequential benefit. The occurrence of iatrogenic hyponatremia is most often observed at this time and may be associated with patent ductus physiology, (49) and is best addressed by aggressive water volume restriction to as little as 60 mL/kg/day, minimizing the rate of sodium correction and entirely avoiding the use of hypertonic salt infusions. Oliguria observed while treating for PDA and hyponatremia should not be addressed by liberalizing fluid volume administration, nor by the use of furosemide which may actually dilate the PDA. (36) Rather, maintenance fluid restriction should be continued while the PDA is addressed definitively, either with Indocin, or by surgical ligation. (After Sridhar S, Baumgart S: Water and electrolyte balance in newborn infants. In Hay WW, Thureen PJ (eds): Neonatal Nutrition and Metabolism, 2nd edn, 2006 in press, with permission Cambridge University Press, Cambridge, UK.)

sodium supplementation are hot topics for investigation, given the numerous associations with sensory-neural hearing loss and cerebral palsy reviewed previously. Randomized controlled trials for routine sodium replacement versus restriction therapy may now be warranted. Regarding life-threatening hypernatremia and hyperkalemia, no investigative reports to date have described late adverse neurodevelopmental outcomes, and such investigations should at least include multivariate analysis of presently existing databases in this regard.

BETWEEN A ROCK AND A HARD PLACE: SUGGESTIONS FOR VIGILENT FLUID BALANCE THERAPY IN ELBW BABIES

Maintenance fluid therapy is at best a moving target that should be addressed by adjusting required fluid volumes frequently, at least two or three times daily, depending on our periodic clinical assessment of hydration and balance (intake and output). We should try to anticipate and to avoid both extremes of under- and over-hydration in ELBW babies, by anticipating their physiological progress, as demonstrated in a hypothetical 600 g patient in Fig. 10-16 (49). On day 1 of life, the primary problem is the tremendously high transepidermal water loss (TEWL); We recommend checking serum electrolytes every 8 h during the first 1–2 days of life, and adjusting an electrolyte-free solution upwards in 10–20 mL increments every 6–8 h, depending on the rate of rise in the measured serum sodium concentration. The key to this strategy is checking serum/urine electrolytes more frequently, because once the serum sodium rises, you are already behind in water volume administration, as shown. By day 2 the problem of hyperkalemia often emerges—volume replacement maximizes as serum sodium concentration peaks, and sodium leaks into the cells displacing potassium outwards from the intracellular compartment. Then on day 3 TEWL begins to diminish as keratin deposition occurs, or in response to incubator care with additional humidification. At this juncture, the serum sodium concentration may suddenly decrease. We should anticipate this change by diminishing water volume immediately when we first see the serum sodium concentrations fall, thus anticipating fluid overload and the risk for promoting a hemodynamically significant PDA by day 4 of life, imaging the ductus prospectively may be of consequential benefit. The occurrence of iatrogenic hyponatremia is most often observed at this time and may be associated with ductal physiology (50), and is best addressed by aggressive water volume restriction to as little as 60 mL/kg/day, minimizing the rate of sodium correction and avoiding entirely the use of hypertonic salt infusions. Oliguria observed while treating for PDA and hyponatremia should not be treated by liberalizing fluid volume administration, nor by the use of furosemide, which may actually dilate the PDA (37). Rather, maintenance fluid restriction should be continued while the PDA is addressed definitively, either with Indocin, or by surgical ligation.

Monitoring changes in body weight is also an important means of assuring appropriate fluid balance. As a reflection of transitional physiologic contraction of extracellular fluid compartment, the VLBW infants experience a 2–3% per kg per day weight loss during the first 3 days (51). The body weight loss stabilizes during the 4th and 5th days of life, suggesting completion of the transitional ECF contraction. The weight gain at 2–3% per kg per day from day 6 and on is a reflection of the anabolic phase of infants' metabolic status. It is very useful to plot the daily weight changes on the postnatal weight grid in infants as published (52).

A Parting Shot at Aggressive PDA Management

Much of this discussion regarding fluids and electrolyte imbalances in ELBW premature infants revolves around the prevention of a clinically significant patent ductus arteriosus. In a recent and controversial opinion paper, Laughon et al (53) questioned the significance of a PDA and how it can and should be managed. These authors remind us of our assumption that a PDA is per se pathological. Indeed, the ductus before birth is essential to maintain systemic circulation in the fetus delivering oxygenated blood to vital organs while bypassing the lungs. After birth at term, the ductus usually closes within 3 days. In LBW premature infants > 30 weeks' gestation, the ductus usually closes within 5 days. In the ever troublesome VLBW premature newborn < 30 weeks' gestation, and certainly in the ELBW population < 1000 g birth weight, at least two thirds of infants have PDAs that do not close, and, incidentally, this is the group with serious pulmonary disease and high pulmonary vascular resistance to shunting left-to-right (that which results in lung congestion). The importance of diagnosis of a clinically significant PDA (i.e., pulmonary congestive) is raised by these authors. It seems echocardiography invariably demonstrates an anatomically patent ductus in these critically ill babies with refractory respiratory distress; however, identifying the significance of this finding when screening for a ductus with echocardiography routinely on day 4 of life, as suggested above, requires examining the patient, not just for the presence of a systolic heart murmur (difficult to auscultate while on an oscillatory ventilator), nor just for echogenic evidence of an otherwise normal structure, but for bounding pulses, a hyperactive precordium, and a widened pulse pressure (systolic value more than double the diastolic). Doppler evidence of a significant left-to-right ductal shunt is often vaguely represented as 'bi-directional' on an echocardiogram, and deleterious effects of diastolic run-off flow velocities seem exaggerated. Failure to improve oxygenation despite prenatal corticosteroid and postnatal surfactant therapies often leads to frustration when asking, 'what stone can be left unturned?' Therefore, treating the ductus aggressively seems prudent, even though a markedly premature lung morphology and fluid physiology (secretory versus dry organogenesis) may remain the true culprits of premature lung disease. Surgical ligation is the gold standard for premature ductal closure. Although 40% of murmurs observed remain asymptomatic, the majority of symptomatic murmurs become asymptomatic with fluid restriction alone (a strong recommendation for a 'dry' approach to parenteral fluid prescription during the first week of life in ELBW infants) (54). Surgery is not without risks for a hemodynamically unstable patient: bleeding, pneumothorax, vocal cord paralysis, grades 3–4 retinopathy and infection have all been associated with PDA surgical ligation.

Indomethacin medical therapy is used to avoid surgery in patients not responding to fluid restriction within 48 h. In the landmark multicenter collaborative trial, authored by Gersony et al (54), over 3500 infants with significant PDAs failing fluid restriction received indomethacin for one or two courses by 2 weeks' postnatal age (with 79% closure), before being offered surgery (35%). There were no differences in mortality or duration of mechanical ventilation or hospital stay; nor IVH or NEC in medical versus surgical treatment groups. At the end of the study, however, all ductuses were closed. Other landmark studies of indomethacin therapy have followed (e.g., prophylactic treatment for all vulnerable premature infants to prevent PDA and intraventricular hemorrhages, or only for those with asymptomatic PDAs having echocardiographic evidence of a ductus on screening), but amelioration of final adverse outcomes remains wanting (neurodevelopmental delays persist, as does chronic lung disease at > 36 weeks' post-conceptional age) (55,56).

Conclusion

If judicious fluid and electrolyte balance is achievable in ELBW babies, neither indomethacin nor surgery might be required.

REFERENCES

1. Baumgart S, Langman CB, Sosulski R, Fox WW, Polin RA. Fluid, electrolyte and glucose maintenance in the very low birthweight infant. Clin Pediatr 21:199–206, 1982.
2. Hammerlund K, Sedin G. Transepidermal water loss in newborn infants. VIII. Relation to gestational age and post-natal age in appropriate and small for gestational age infants. Acta Paediatr Scand 72:721, 1983.
3. Michel CC. Fluid movements through capillary walls. In Renkin EM, Michel CC, (eds.): Handbook of Physiology, Section II, Vol II. Bethesda, MD: American Physiologic Society 1984.
4. Costarino AT, Baumgart S. Modern fluid and electrolyte management of the critically ill premature infant. Ped Clin No Amer 33:153–178, 1986.
5. Friis-Hansen B. Body water compartments in children. Pediatrics 28:169–181, 1961.
6. Haycock GB, Schwartz GJ, Wisotsky DH. Geometric method for measuring body surface areas: A height-weight formula validated in infants, children and adults. J Pediatr 93:62–66, 1978.
7. Baumgart S, Engle WD, Fox WW, et al. Radiant warmer power and body size as determinants of insensible water loss in the critically ill neonate. Pediatr Res 15:1495–1499, 1981.

8. Baumgart S. Fluid and electrolyte therapy in the premature infant: Case management. In Burg F, Polin RA, (eds.): Workbook in Practical Neonatology (pp. 25-39). Philadelphia, PA: WB Saunders, 1983.

9. Costarino AT, Gruskay JA, Corcoran L, Polin RA, Baumgart S. Sodium restriction vs. daily maintenance replacement in very low birthweight premature neonates, a randomized and blinded therapeutic trial. J Pediatr 120:99–106, 1992.

10. Hartnoll G, Betremieux P, Modi N. Randomised controlled trial of postnatal sodium supplementation on body composition in 25 to 30 week gestational age infants. Arch Dis Child Fetal Neonatal Ed 82(1):F24–F28, 2000.

11. Gruskay J, Costarino AT, Polin RA, Baumgart S. Non-oliguric hyperkalemia in the premature infant less than 1000 grams. J Pediatr 113:381–386, 1988.

12. Usher RH. The respiratory distress syndrome of prematurity. I. Change in potassium in the serum and the electrocardiogram and effects of therapy. Pediatrics 24:562, 1959.

13. Stefano JL, Norman ME, Morales MC, et al. Decreased erythrocyte Na+, K+ ATPase activity associated with cellular potassium loss in extremely low birth weight infants with nonoliguric hyperkalemia. J Pediatr 122:276–284, 1993.

14. Lorenz JM, Kleinman LI. Nonoliguric hyperkalemia in preterm neonates (Letter). J Pediatr 114:507, 1989.

15. Kalia Yn, Nonato LB, Lund CH, Guy RH. Development of skin barrier function in premature infants. J Invest Derm 111:320–326, 1998.

16. Guidelines for Perinatal Care, 2nd edn. Elk Grove Village, IL: American Academy of Pediatrics and American College of Obstetricians and Gynecologists, 1988:278.

17. Harpin VA, Rutter N. Humidification of incubators. Arch Dis Child 60:219, 1985.

18. Gaylord MS, Wright K, Lorch K, Lorch V, Walker E. Improved fluid management utilizing humidified incubators in extremely low birth weight infants. J Perinatol 21:438–443, 2001.

19. Rutter N, Hull D. Reduction of skin water loss in the newborn. I. Effect of applying topical agents. Arch Dis Child 56:669, 1981.

20. Nopper AJ, Horii KA, Sookdeo-Drost S, Wang TH, Mancini AJ, Lane AT. Topical ointment therapy benefits premature infants. J Pediatr 128:660, 1996.

21. Campbell JR, Zaccaria E, Baker CJ. Systemic candidiasis in extremely low birth weight infants receiving topical petrolatum ointment for skin care: a case-control study. Pediatrics 105: 1041–1045, 2000.

22. Edwards WH, Conner JM, Soll RF/Vermont Oxford Network Neonatal Skin Care Study Group. The effect of prophylactic ointment therapy on nosocomial sepsis rates and skin integrity in infants with birth weights of 501–1000 g. Pediatrics 113:1195-1203, 2004.

23. Baumgart S. Reduction of oxygen consumption, insensible water loss and radiant heat demand with use of a plastic blanket for low birthweight infants under radiant warmers. Pediatrics 74:1022-1028, 1984.

24. Knauth A, Gordin M, McNelis W, Baumgart S. A semipermeable polyurethane membrane as an artificial skin in the premature neonate. Pediatrics 83:945–950, 1989.

25. Porat R, Brodsky N. Effect of Tegederm use on outcome of extremely low birth weight (ELBW) infants. Pediatr Res 33:231(A), 1993.

26. Donahue ML, Phelps DL, Richter SE, Davis JM. A semipermeable skin dressing for extremely low birth weight infants. Journal of Perinatology 16(1):20–26, 1996.

27. Palta M, Babbert D, Weinstein MR, Peters ME. Multivariate assessment of traditional risk factors for chronic lung disease in very low birth weight neonates. J Pediatr 119:285–292, 1991.

28. Van Marter LJ, Pagano M, Allred EN, Leviton A, Kuban KCK. Rate of bronchopulmonary dysplasia as a function of neonatal intensive care practices. J Pediatr 120:938–946, 1992.

29. Oh W, Poindexter BB, Perritt R, Lemons JA, Bauer CR, Ehrenkranz RA, Stoll BJ, Poole K, Wright LL, for the Neonatal Research Network. Association between fluid intake and weight loss during the first ten days of life and risk of bronchopulmonary dysplasia in extremely low birth weight infants. J Pediatr 147:786–790, 2005.

30. Bell EF, Warburton D, Stonestreet BS, Oh W. Effect of fluid administration on the development of symptomatic patent ductus arteriosus and congestive heart failure in premature infants. N Engl J Med 302:598–604, 1980.

31. von Stockhausen HB, Struve M. Die Auswirkungen einer stark unterschiedlichen parenteral en Flussigkeitszufuhr bei Fruh- und Neugeborenen in den ersten drei Lebenstagen. Klin Padiatr 192:539–546, 1980.

32. Lorenz JM, Kleinman LI, Kotagal UR, Reller MD. Water balance in very low-birth weight infants: relationship to water and sodium intake and effect on outcome. J Pediatr 101:423–432, 1982.

33. Tammella OKT, Koivisto ME. Fluid restriction for preventing bronchopulmonary dysplasia? Reduced fluid intake during the first weeks of life improves the outcome of low-birth-weight infants. Acta Paediatr 81:207–212, 1992.

34. Bell EF, Acarregui MJ. Restricted versus liberal water intake for preventing morbidity and mortality in preterm infants. Cochrane Database of Systematic Reviews 3: CD000503, 2001.

35. Perlman JM, McMenamin JB, Volpe JJ. Fluctuating cerebral blood flow velocity in respiratory distress syndrome: Relationship to the development of intraventricular hemorrhage. N Engl J Med 309:209–213, 1983.

36. Kavvidia V, Greenough A, Dimitriou G, Forsling ML. Randomized trial of two levels of fluid input in the perinatal period—effect on fluid balance, electrolyte and metabolic disturbances in ventilated VLBW infants. Acta Paediatr 89:237–241, 2000.

37. Brion LP, Primhak RA, Ambrosio-Perez I. Diuretics acting on the distal renal tubule for preterm infants with (or developing) chronic lung disease. Cochrane Database of Systematic Reviews 3: CD001817; PMID:10908511, 2000.

38. Brion LP, Sol RF. Diuretics for respiratory distress syndrome in preterm infants. Cochrane Database of Systematic Reviews 2:CD001454;PMID:10796265, 2000.

39. Bland RD. Lung epithelial ion transport and fluid movement during the perinatal period. Am J Physiol 259:L30–L37.

40. Helve O, Pitkanen OM, Andersson S, O'Brodovich H, Kirjavainen T, Otulakowski G. Low expression of human epithelial sodium channel in airway epithelium of preterm infants with respiratory distress. Pediatrics 113:1267–1272, 2004.

41. Omar SA, Decristofaro JD, Agarwal BI, La Gamma E, et al. Effects of prenatal steroids on water and sodium homeostasis in extremely low birth weight neonates. Pediatrics 104:482–488, 1999.

42. Bhatty SB, Tsirka A, Quinn PB, LaGamma EF, DeCristofaro JD: Rapid correction of hyponatremia in extremely low birth weight (ELBW) premature neonates is associated with long term developmental delay. Pediatr Res 41:140A–43, 1997.

43. Leslie GI, Kalaw MB, Bowen JR, Arnold JD. Risk factors for sensorineural hearing loss in extremely premature infants. J Paediatr Child Health 31:312–6, 1995.

44. Murphy DJ, Hope PL, Johnson A. Neonatal risk factors for cerebral palsy in very preterm babies: case-control study. BMJ 314:404–408, 1997.

45. Ertl T, Hadzsiev K, Vincze O, Pytel J, Szabo I, Sulyok E. Hyponatremia and sensorineural hearing loss in preterm infants. Biology of the Neonate 79:109–112, 2001.

46. Al-Dahan J, Jannoun L, Haycock G. Developmental risks and protective factors for influencing cognitive outcome at 5-1/2 years of age in very low birthweight children. Dev Med Child Neurol 44:508–516, 2002.

47. Simmons MA, Adcock EW 3rd, Bard H, Battaglia FC. Hypernatremia and intracranial hemorrhage in neonates. New Engl J Med 291:6–10, 1974.

48. Lupton BA, Roland EH, Whitfield MF, Hill A. Serum sodium concentration and intraventricular hemorrhage in premature infants. Am J Dis Child 144:1019–1021, 1990.

49. Baumgart S. Water and electrolyte balance in low birth weight infants. In Burg FD, Inglefinger JR, Polin RA, Gershon AA (eds): Current Pediatric Therapy, 18th edn (pp. 85–88). Philadelphia, PA: Elsevier Science, 2006.

50. Gupta J, Sridhar S, Baumgart S, DeCristofaro JD. Hyponatremia in extremely low birth weight (ELBW) infants may precede the development of a significant patent ductus arteriosus (PDA) in the first week of life. Pediatric Res 51:387A, 2002.

51. Stonestreet BS, Bell EF, Warburton D, Oh W. Renal response in low-birth-weight neonates. Results of prolonged intake of two different amounts of fluid and sodium. Am J Dis Child 137:215–219, 1983.

52. Tanis R, Fenton TR. A new growth chart for preterm babies: Babson and Benda's chart updated with recent data and a new format. BMC Pediatrics 3:13, 2003.

53. Laughon MM, Simmons MA, Bose CL. Patency of the ductus arteriosus in the premature infant: is it pathologic? Should it be treated? Curr Opin Pediatr 16:146–151, 2004.

54. Gersony WM, Peckham GJ, Ellison RC, Miettinen OS, Nadas AS. Effects of indomethacin in premature infants with patent ductus arteriosus: Results of a national collaborative study. J Pediatr 102:895–906, 1983.

55. Fowlie P, Davis PG: Prophylactic intravenous indomethacin for preventing mortality and morbidity in preterm infants. Cochrane Database of Systematic Reviews, 2002(3):CD000174.

56. Cooke L, Steer P, Woodgate P. Indomethacin for asymptomatic patent ductus arteriosus in preterm infants. Cochrane Database of Systematic Reviews, 2003(2):CD003745.

57. Bhatty SB, Tsirka A, Quinn PB, La Gamma EF, Baumgart S, DeCristofaro JD. Rapid correction of hyponatremia in extremely low birth weight premature neonates is associated with long term developmental delay. Pediatrics, 2007, in press.

Chapter 11

Lung Fluid Balance in Developing Lungs and its Role in Neonatal Transition

Lucky Jain, MD • Richard D. Bland, MD

Often signaled by a loud cry, the birth of a neonate marks a remarkable transition from its dependence for gas exchange on the placenta to an independent state of air breathing and gas exchange in the lungs. The fact that the lungs are filled with liquid during fetal life makes this transition particularly more challenging for the newborn. Scientists have known for a long time that fetal lungs are full of fluid, although it was presumed to be an extension of the amniotic fluid pool. However, studies have confirmed (1,2) that the fetal lung itself, rather than the amniotic sac, is the source of the liquid that fills the lung during development. Through an active process involving chloride secretion by the respiratory epithelium, this liquid forms a slowly expanding structural template that prevents collapse and promotes growth of the fetal lung (3,4). This active process can be inhibited by diuretics that block Na,K-2Cl co-transport (5,6). In vitro experiments using cultured explants of lung tissue and monolayers of epithelial cells harvested from human fetal lung have indicated that cation-dependent chloride transport, driven by epithelial cell Na,K-ATPase, is the mechanism responsible for liquid secretion into the lumen of the mammalian lung during fetal life (7–9).

For effective gas exchange to occur, rapid clearance of liquid from potential alveolar airspaces during and soon after birth is essential for establishing the timely switch from placental to pulmonary gas exchange. It is clear now that traditional explanations that relied on mechanical factors and Starling forces can only account for a small fraction of the fluid absorbed (10,11) and that the normal transition from liquid to air inflation is considerably more complex than the characteristic 'vaginal squeeze' theory might suggest. Physiologic events in the days before spontaneous delivery are accompanied by changes in the hormonal milieu of the fetus which pave the way for a smooth neonatal transition, including clearance of the large body of lung fluid. Respiratory morbidity resulting from failure to clear the lung fluid is not uncommon, and can be particularly problematic in some infants delivered prematurely, or when delivery occurs operatively before the onset of spontaneous labor. This review will consider some of the experimental work that provides the basis for our current understanding of lung liquid dynamics before, during and after birth, focusing on the various pathways and mechanisms by which this process occurs.

FETAL LUNG LIQUID AND ITS PHYSIOLOGICAL SIGNIFICANCE

As pointed out above, the lung is a secretory organ during development, displaying breathing-like movements but without any contribution to respiratory gas exchange. The small fraction of the combined ventricular output of blood from the heart that circulates through the pulmonary circulation (12) allows the delivery to the lung epithelium of the substrates needed to make surfactant and secretion of up to 5mL/kg/hour lung fluid at term gestation (13,14). Several studies have shown that the presence of an appropriate volume of secreted liquid within the fetal respiratory tract is essential for normal lung growth and development before birth (1,2,15). Conditions that interfere with normal production of lung liquid, such as pulmonary artery occlusion (16), diaphragmatic hernia with displacement of abdominal contents into the chest (17), and uterine compression of the fetal thorax from chronic leak of amniotic fluid (63), also inhibit lung growth. Conversely, excessive accumulation of lung fluid, such as that following tracheal occlusion, leads to excessive lung growth (1).

Fig. 11-1 is a schematic diagram showing the fluid compartments of the fetal lung. Potential air spaces are filled with liquid that is rich in chloride ($\sim$ 150 mEq/L) and almost free of protein (< 0.03 mg/mL) (18). The lung epithelium has tight intercellular junctions that provide an effective barrier to macromolecules, including albumin, whereas the vascular endothelium has wider openings that allow passage of large plasma proteins, including globulins and fibrinogen (19–21). Consequently, liquid in the interstitial space, which is sampled in fetal sheep by collecting lung lymph, has a protein concentration that is about 100 times greater than the protein concentration of liquid contained in the lung lumen (22). Despite the large trans-epithelial difference in protein osmotic pressure, which tends to inhibit fluid flow out of the interstitium into potential air spaces, active transport

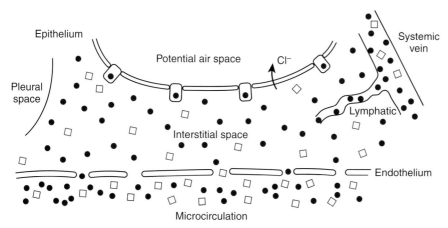

Figure 11-1 Schematic diagram of the fluid compartments in the fetal lung, showing the tight epithelial barrier to protein and the more permeable vascular endothelium, which restricts the passage of globulins (□) more than it restricts albumin (●). In the fetal mammalian lung, chloride secretion in the respiratory epithelium is responsible for liquid production within potential air spaces (After Bland RD: Adv Pediatr 34:175–222, 1989).

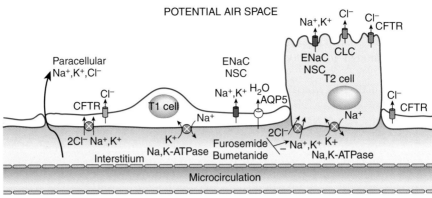

Figure 11-2 Schematic drawing of the fluid compartments of the fetal lung, highlighting the lung epithelium, consisting of type I cells that occupy most of the surface area of the lung lumen, and type II cells that manufacture and secrete surfactant. These cells also secrete Cl by a process that involves Na,K-2Cl co-transport and Na,K-ATPase (Na pump) activity. This energy-dependent process, which can be blocked by loop diuretics, furosemide and bumetanide, increases the concentration of Cl within the cell so that it exceeds its electrochemical equilibrium, with resultant extrusion of Cl through anion-selective channels on the apical membrane surface (cystic fibrosis transmembrane conductance regulator, CFTR or chloride channels, CLCs). Sodium (Na) and water follow the movement of Cl into the lung lumen.

of chloride (Cl) ions across the fetal lung epithelium generates an electrical potential difference that averages about -5 mV, luminal side negative (4). The osmotic force created by this secretory process drives liquid from the pulmonary microcirculation through the interstitium into potential air spaces.

Lung epithelial Cl transport, which in fetal sheep begins as early as mid-gestation (23), is inhibited by diuretics that block Na,K-2Cl co-transport (5,6). This finding supports the concept that the driving force for trans-epithelial Cl movement in the fetal lung is similar to the mechanism described for Cl transport across other epithelia. Accordingly, Cl enters the epithelial cell across its basal membrane linked to Na and to K (Fig. 11-2). Na enters the cell down its electrochemical gradient and is subsequently extruded in exchange for K (3 Na ions exchanged for 2 K ions) by the action of Na,K-ATPase located on the basolateral surface of the cell. This energy-dependent process increases the concentration of Cl within the cell so that it exceeds its electrochemical equilibrium. Cl then passively exits the epithelial cell through anion-selective channels that are located on the apical membrane surface. Na traverses the epithelium via paracellular pathways or via non-selective cation channels that have been identified in fetal distal airway epithelium, while water can flow either between epithelial cells or through water channels, one of which (aquaporin 5) is abundantly expressed in type I lung epithelial cells (24,25).

While the Cl concentration of liquid withdrawn from the lung lumen of fetal sheep is about 50% greater than that of plasma, the Na concentration is virtually identical to that of plasma (3,18). The concentration of bicarbonate in lung liquid of fetal sheep is <3 mEq/L, yielding a pH of ~ 6.3. This finding led to the notion that the lung epithelium of fetal sheep may actively transport bicarbonate out of the lung lumen. The demonstration that acetazolamide, a carbonic anhydrase inhibitor, blocks secretion of lung liquid in fetal sheep supports this view. Both physiologic and immunohistochemical studies have shown that H$^+$-ATPases are present on the respiratory epithelium of fetal sheep, where they likely provide an important mechanism for acidification of liquid within the lung lumen during development. In vitro electrophysiological studies using fetal rat lung epithelial cells provided evidence that exposure to an acid pH might activate Cl channels and thereby contribute to the production of fetal lung liquid (26). In fetal dogs and monkeys, however, the bicarbonate concentration of lung luminal liquid is not significantly different

Table 11-1	Factors that Can Delay Clearance of Fetal Lung Fluid
Failure of antenatal decrease in fetal lung fluid	• Delivery without labor
	• Prematurity
Excessive production of fluid	• Elevated transvascular pressure (e.g., cardiogenic edema)
	• Increased vascular permeability
Decreased epithelial transport of sodium and water	• Decreased number/function of type I and II cells
	• Decreased sodium-channel expression and activity
	• Loss of function mutations of ENaC
	• Decreased Na^+-K^+-ATPase function

from that of fetal plasma (27). Thus, the importance of lung liquid pH and acidification mechanisms during mammalian lung development in utero remains unclear.

The volume of liquid within the lung lumen of fetal sheep increases from 4 mL/kg to 6 mL/kg at mid-gestation (23) to more than 20 mL/kg near term (21,22). The hourly flow rate of lung liquid increases from ~ 2 mL/kg body weight at mid-gestation (23) to ~ 5 mL/kg body weight at term (13,14,28). Increased production of luminal liquid during development reflects a rapidly expanding pulmonary microvascular and epithelial surface area that occurs with proliferation and growth of lung capillaries and respiratory units (23,29). The observation that unilateral pulmonary artery occlusion decreases lung liquid production in fetal sheep by at least 50% (30) shows that the pulmonary circulation, rather than the bronchial circulation, is the major source of fetal lung liquid. Intravenous infusion of isotonic saline at a rate sufficient to increase lung microvascular pressure and lung lymph flow in fetal lambs had no effect on liquid flow across the pulmonary epithelium (31). Thus, transepithelial Cl secretion appears to be the major driving force responsible for the production of liquid in the fetal lung lumen. In vitro studies of epithelial ion transport across the fetal airways indicate that the epithelium of the upper respiratory tract also secretes Cl, thereby contributing to lung liquid production (32–34). However, most of this liquid forms in the distal portions of the fetal lung, where total surface area is many times greater than it is in the conducting airways.

Several studies have demonstrated that both the rate of lung liquid production and the volume of liquid within the lumen of the fetal lung normally decrease before birth, most notably during labor (22,28,35–37). Thus, lung water content is $\sim 25\%$ greater after premature delivery than it is at term, and newborn animals that are delivered by cesarean section without prior labor have considerably more liquid in their lungs than do animals that are delivered either vaginally or operatively after the onset of labor (Table 11-1) (38,39). In studies with fetal sheep, extravascular lung water was 45% less in mature fetuses that were in the midst of labor than in fetuses that did not experience labor, and there was a further 38% decrease in extravascular lung water measured in term lambs that were studied 6 h after a normal vaginal birth (22).

HOW IS THE FETAL LUNG FLUID CLEARED?

Studies performed over the last two decades to understand the mechanism(s) responsible for fetal lung fluid clearance at birth have shown that active Na^+ transport across the pulmonary epithelium drives liquid from lung lumen to the interstitium, with subsequent absorption into the vasculature (40–43). In the lung, Na^+ reabsorption is a two-step process (Fig. 11-3) (44). The first step is passive movement of Na^+ from the lumen across the apical membrane into the cell through Na^+ permeable ion channels. The second step is active extrusion of Na^+ from the cell

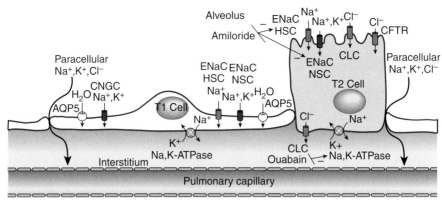

Figure 11-3 Epithelial sodium absorption in the fetal lung near birth. Na enters the cell through the apical surface of both ATI and ATII cells via amiloride-sensitive epithelial Na channels (ENaC), both highly selective channels (HSCs) and non-selective channels (NSCs), and via cyclic nucleotide gated channels (seen only in ATI cells). Electroneutrality is conserved with chloride movement through the cystic fibrosis transmembrane conductance regulator (CFTR) or through chloride channels (CLCs) in ATI and ATII cells, and/or paracellularly through tight junctions. The increase in cell Na stimulates Na,K-ATPase activity on the basolateral aspect of the cell membrane, which drives out 3 Na ions in exchange for 2 K ions, a process that can be blocked by the cardiac glycoside ouabain. If the net ion movement is from the apical surface to the interstitium, an osmotic gradient would be created, which would in turn direct water transport in the same direction, either through aquaporins or by diffusion.

across the basolateral membrane into the serosal space. Several investigators have demonstrated that the initial entry step involves apical Na^+ channels (ENaC) that are sensitive to amiloride, a diuretic. This is consistent with studies by O'Brodovich et al (45) who have shown that intraluminal instillation of amiloride in fetal guinea pigs delays lung fluid clearance.

More recent studies using the patch-clamp technique have confirmed the role of ENaC channels in ATI and ATII cells in the vectorial transport of Na^+ from the apical surface (46–48). Indeed, cDNAs which encode amiloride-sensitive Na^+ channels in other Na^+ transporting epithelia have also been cloned from airway epithelial cells (48–50). The lung epithelium is believed to switch from a predominantly Cl^- secreting membrane at birth to a predominantly Na^+ absorbing membrane after birth. These changes have also been correlated with an increased production of the mRNA for amiloride-sensitive epithelial Na^+ channels (ENaC) in the developing lung (51). Much of this information has come from studies using AT-II cells. Recent studies have shown that ATI cells also express functional Na^+ channels and other transporters capable of salt and fluid transport (52–54). In addition to ENaC channels, which account for the amiloride-sensitive portion of the alveolar fluid clearance, cyclic nucleotide gated channels (CNG) are also present in alveolar cells and contribute to the amiloride-insensitive sodium and fluid uptake.

SODIUM CHANNEL PATHOLOGY IN THE LUNG

Hummler et al (55) have shown that inactivating the alpha-ENaC (a-subunit of the epithelial Na^+ channel) leads to defective lung liquid clearance and premature death in mice. Inactivating β and γ ENaC subunits also leads to early death in newborn mice, albeit due to fluid and electrolyte imbalances, showing that α-ENaC expression is critical for fetal lung fluid absorption. This is the first direct evidence that in vivo ENaC constitutes the limiting step for Na^+ absorption in epithelial cells of the lung, and in the adaptation of newborn lung to air breathing. It also supports the hypothesis that in many newborns that have difficulty in the transition to air breathing, Na^+ channel activity may be diminished, albeit transiently.

Table 11-2   Pathologic States Associated with Abnormal Lung Ion Transport

Decreased sodium and water transport	• Respiratory distress syndrome • Transient tachypnea of the newborn • Pulmonary edema
Excessive sodium and water transport	• Cystic fibrosis

Studies in human neonates have also shown that immaturity of Na^+ transport mechanisms contributes to the development of transient tachypnea of the newborn (TTN) and respiratory distress syndrome (Table 11-2) (RDS) (56,57). Gowen et al (57) were the first to show that human neonates with TTN had an immaturity of the lung epithelial transport, measured as an amiloride induced drop in potential difference between the nasal epithelium and subcutaneous space. The potential difference was reduced in infants with TTN (suggesting a defect in Na^+ transport) and recovery from TTN in 1–3 days was associated with an increase in potential difference to normal level.

Similar studies have now been conducted in premature newborns with RDS and the results are consistent with impaired Na^+ transport in these infants (56). Barker et al (56) measured nasal transepithelial potential difference in premature infants < 30 weeks' gestation. Nasal potential difference is a good measure of the net electrogenic transport of Na^+ and Cl^- (dominant ion) across the epithelial layer (PD = Resistance × Current), and has been shown to mirror image ion transport occurring in the lower respiratory tract. It is recorded as the potential difference between the mucosal surface of a specific region of the nasal epithelium and the subcutaneous space. Authors found that maximal nasal epithelial potential difference increased with birth weight and was lower in infants with RDS. Premature infants without RDS had a nasal potential difference similar to normal full term infants. Further, the ability of amiloride to affect the potential difference was lower in preterm infants with RDS on day 1 of life, reflecting lower amiloride-sensitive Na transport. This study provides important evidence for the role of decreased Na channel activity in the pathogenesis of RDS and the accompanying pulmonary edema.

There is additional evidence that the ability of various agents to increase lung fluid absorption in fetal lambs is gestational age dependent (35,58–63) The mechanism for poor response of immature lungs to agents that stimulate Na^+ transport is not known. Deficiencies could exist in one or more of several steps including β-receptor, GTP-binding proteins, adenyl cyclase, protein kinase-A, or the Na^+ channel and its regulatory proteins. Studies have shown that the expression of a-subunit of ENaC is developmentally regulated in rats (51) and in humans (61). However, several questions remain to be answered. For example, pseudo-hypoaldosteronism type I (a renal salt-wasting disease), has been reported to be associated with mutations involving the α-subunit of ENaC (64). One would have expected these patients to have trouble clearing fluid from their spaces considering that the α-subunit is so critical for ENaC function. However, the incidence of RDS or TTN is not increased in infants who have this syndrome.

A complex and yet incompletely defined relationship exists between Na^+ and Cl^- channels. Cystic fibrosis (CF) is a genetic disease caused by mutations of the cystic fibrosis transmembrane conductance regulator (CFTR), which has been identified as a cAMP-dependent Cl channel (65). In the lungs of CF patients, amiloride-sensitive Na^+ absorption is increased, and aerosolized amiloride has been employed to reverse this imbalance (55,66,67). However, despite the absence of functional CFTR activity in fetuses that will go on to develop cystic fibrosis, fetal lung fluid production during gestation is unaffected and lungs are normally developed at birth. These findings are in contrast to recent studies that link the presence of CFTR to lung growth in congenital diaphragmatic hernia. Therefore, examining the molecular mechanisms and the cellular regulation of Na^+ reabsorption are important in understanding both normal lung development and physiology, but also abnormalities in lung Na and water balance in both fetal and adult lungs.

WHAT CAUSES THE NEONATAL LUNG EPITHELIUM TO SWITCH TO AN ABSORPTIVE MODE?

Developmental changes in transepithelial ion and fluid movement in the lung can be viewed as occurring in three distinct stages (68). In the first (fetal) stage, the lung epithelium remains in a secretory mode, relying on active Cl secretion via Cl channels and relatively low reabsorption activity of Na^+ channels. The second (transitional) stage involves a reversal in the direction of ion and water movement. A multitude of factors may be involved in this transition, including exposure of epithelial cells to an air interface and to high concentrations of steroids and cyclic nucleotides. This stage involves not only increased expression of Na^+ channels in the lung epithelia, but possibly a switch from nonselective cation channels to highly selective Na channels. The net increase in Na movement into the cell can also cause a change in resting membrane potential, leading to a slowing, and eventually a reversal of the direction of Cl movement through Cl channels. The third and final (adult) stage represents lung epithelia with predominantly Na reabsorption through Na channels and possibly Cl reabsorption through Cl channels, with a fine balance between the activity of ion channels and tight junctions. Such an arrangement can help ensure adequate humidification of alveolar surface while preventing excessive buildup of fluid. There is also recent evidence to show that fetal lung fluid clearance is facilitated by ciliary function (69) and that term neonates with genetic defects of cilia structure and/or function (Primary Cliary Dyskinesia, PCD) have a high prevalence of neonatal respiratory disease (69).

A considerable amount of research effort in this area has focused on physiologic changes that trigger the change in lung epithelia from a Cl secretory to a Na reabsorption mode (5,42,46,68,70–72). While several endogenous mediators (Table 11-3), including catecholamines, vasopressin, and prolactin, have been proposed to increase lung fluid absorption, none explains this switch convincingly (62,73,74). Mechanical factors, such as stretch and exposure of the epithelial cells to air interface, are other probable candidates that have not been well studied. Jain et al (46) have shown that alveolar expression of highly selective Na channels in the lung epithelia is regulated by the lung microenvironment, especially the presence of glucocorticoids, air interface, and oxygen concentration (75). Further, regulation

---

Table 11-3   Endogenous Factors that Can Enhance Lung Fluid Clearance

β-adrenergics/catecholamines
Dopamine
Arginine vasopressin
PGE_2
Prolactin
Surfactant
Oxygen
TNFα
Epidermal growth factor
Steroids
Alveolar expansion (stretch)

of Na channels is mediated through these factors in a tissue specific manner (76,77). For example, aldosterone is a major factor in the kidney and colon, but probably not in the lung (78). In the kidneys, it works by activating transcription of genes for ENaC subunits (78). Of the several factors that have been proposed to have a lung specific effect on Na reabsorption, some have been investigated, including glucocorticoids, oxygen, β-adrenergics, and surfactant (71,73,79).

High doses of glucocorticoids have been shown to stimulate transcription of ENaC in several Na transporting epithelia as well as in the lung (61). In the alveolar epithelia, glucocorticoids were found to induce lung Na reabsorption in the late gestation fetal lung (62). In addition to increasing transcription of Na channel subunits, steroids increase the number of available channels by decreasing the rate at which membrane associated channels are degraded, and increase the activity of existing channels. Glucocorticoids have also been shown to enhance the responsiveness of lungs to β-adrenergic agents and thyroid hormones (80). The enhanced Na reabsorption induced by glucocorticoids can be blocked by amiloride, suggesting a role for ENaC. This effect was not observed with triiodothyronine (T_3) or with cAMP. Glucocorticoid induction was found to be receptor mediated and primarily transcriptional. This observation is important because it provides an alternate explanation for the beneficial effect of antenatal steroids on the lung.

In the rat fetal lung, O'Brodovich et al (45,51) have previously shown that the expression of α-ENaC is markedly increased at ~20 days' gestation (corresponding to the saccular stage of lung development) and can be accelerated by exposure to dexamethasone and increased levels of thyroid hormone. Such an effect would translate into accelerated fetal lung fluid reabsorption at birth. Jain et al (46) have shown that steroids are highly effective in enhancing the expression of highly selective Na channels in lung epithelial cells. Under conditions of steroid deprivation, alveolar cells express predominantly a non-selective cation channel that is unlikely to transport the large load of Na and alveolar fluid clearance imposed at birth. However, when these steroid deprived (both fetal and adult) cells are exposed to dexamethasone, there is a rapid transition to highly selective Na channels, which are readily seen in other Na and fluid transporting systems such as the kidney and colon (46). In addition, steroids have been shown to have beneficial effects on the surfactant system as well as pulmonary mechanics (80–85).

There is considerable evidence to show that high levels of endogenous catecholamines at birth may be important for accelerating alveolar fluid clearance (86–88). We (73) have shown that β-agonists increase the activity of Na channels in the lung though a cAMP-PKA mediated mechanism. It would be logical to conclude, that in the absence of an endogenous surge in fetal catecholamines, exogenous catecholamines would be effective in initiating fetal lung fluid clearance. However, recent studies (surprisingly) show that exogenous addition of epinephrine in guinea pigs failed to stimulate fluid clearance in the newborn lungs (88). There are several possible explanations for this finding. First, catecholamines work on the fetal Na channel (mostly non-selective) by increasing its activity, not by increasing the gene transcription or translation of the proteins required to assemble the channel (68,73). Thus, if the developmentally regulated ENaC channels are not available in adequate numbers at birth, no amount of extra catecholamines are going to make a difference. Steroids, on the other hand, increase the transcription of the ENaC genes and, through another mechanism involving proteosomal degradation, increase the total number of ENaC channels available at birth; however, a longer duration (4–24 h) of exposure is required for such an effect. Indeed, if these in vitro findings were to hold true in vivo, then neonates exposed to antenatal steroids would be more responsive to other exogenous agents that enhance Na channel activity (i.e. catecholamines). Helms et al (52,89) have recently shown that dopamine can greatly enhance Na^+ channel activity working via a non cAMP dependent post-translational mechanism. However, since a significant ($\sim$40%) reduction in fetal lung fluid occurs prior to spontaneous delivery, and rapid clearance of the remaining fluid has to occur within hours after birth, it is doubtful if postnatal steroid treatment initiated after the infant has become symptomatic will be a successful alternate strategy.

SUMMARY

The transition from placental gas exchange to air breathing is a complex process that requires adequate removal of fetal lung fluid and a concomitant increase in perfusion of the newly ventilated alveoli. In neonates who are unable to make this transition, varying degrees of respiratory distress and impairment of gas exchange are not uncommon. Therapeutic approaches that can facilitate fetal lung fluid clearance are likely to reduce pulmonary morbidity in the neonatal period and help in designing therapies to combat lung edema formation in postnatal life.

REFERENCES

1. Alcorn D, Adamson TM, Lambert TF, Maloney JE, Ritchie BC, Robinson PM. Morphological effects of chronic tracheal ligation and drainage in the fetal lamb lung. J Anat 123:649–660, 1977.
2. Moessinger AC, Singh M, Donnelly DF, Haddad GG, Collins MH, James LS. The effect of prolonged oligohydramnios on fetal lung development, maturation and ventilatory patterns in the newborn guinea pig. J Dev Physiol 9:419–427, 1987.
3. Adams FH, Fujiwara T, Rowshan G. The nature and origin of the fluid in the fetal lamb lung. J Pediatr 63:881–888, 1963.
4. Olver RE, Strang LB. Ion fluxes across the pulmonary epithelium and the secretion of lung liquid in the foetal lamb. J Physiol 241:327–357, 1974.
5. Carlton DP, Cummings JJ, Chapman DL, Poulain FR, Bland RD. Ion transport regulation of lung liquid secretion in foetal lambs. J Dev Physiol 17:99–107, 1992.
6. Cassin S, Gause G, Perks AM. The effects of bumetanide and furosemide on lung liquid secretion in fetal sheep. Proc Soc Exp Biol Med 181:427–431, 1986.
7. Barker PM, Boucher RC, Yankaskas JR. Bioelectric properties of cultured monolayers from epithelium of distal human fetal lung. Am J Physiol 268:L270–L277, 1995.
8. McCray PB, Jr, Bettencourt JD, Bastacky J. Developing bronchopulmonary epithelium of the human fetus secretes fluid. Am J Physiol 262:L270–L279, 1992.
9. McCray PB, Jr, Bettencourt JD, Bastacky J. Secretion of lung fluid by the developing fetal rat alveolar epithelium in organ culture. Am J Respir Cell Mol Biol 6:609–616, 1992.
10. Karlberg P, Adams FH, Geubelle F, Wallgren G. Alteration of the infant's thorax during vaginal delivery. Acta Obstet Gynecol Scand 41:223–229, 1962.
11. Olver RE, Walters DV, Wilson, SM. Developmental regulation of lung liquid transport. Annu Rev Physiol 66:77–101, 2004.
12. Rudolph AM, Heymann MA. Circulatory changes during growth in the fetal lamb. Circ Res 26:289–299, 1970.
13. Adamson TM, Brodecky V, Lambert TF, Maloney JE, Ritchie BC, Walker AM. Lung liquid production and composition in the 'in utero' foetal lamb. Aust J Exp Biol Med Sci 53:65–75, 1975.
14. Mescher EJ, Platzker AC, Ballard PL, Kitterman JA, Clements JA, Tooley WH. Ontogeny of tracheal fluid, pulmonary surfactant, and plasma corticoids in the fetal lamb. J Appl Physiol 39:1017–1021, 1975.
15. Harding R, Hooper SB. Regulation of lung expansion and lung growth before birth. J Appl Physiol 81:209–224, 1996.
16. Wallen LD, Kulisz E, Maloney JE. Main pulmonary artery ligation reduces lung fluid production in fetal sheep. J Dev Physiol 16:173–179, 1991.
17. Harrison MR, Bressack MA, Churg AM, de Lorimier AA. Correction of congenital diaphragmatic hernia in utero. II. Simulated correction permits fetal lung growth with survival at birth. Surgery 88:260–268, 1980.
18. Adamson TM, Boyd RD, Platt HS, Strang LB. Composition of alveolar liquid in the foetal lamb. J Physiol 204:159–168, 1969.
19. Body RD, Hill JR, Humphreys PW, Normand IC, Reynolds EO, Strang LB. Permeability of lung capillaries to macromolecules in foetal and new-born lambs and sheep. J Physiol 201:567–588, 1969.
20. Normand IC, Olver RE, Reynolds EO, Strang LB. Permeability of lung capillaries and alveoli to non-electrolytes in the foetal lamb. J Physiol 219:303–330, 1971.
21. Normand IC, Reynolds EO, Strang LB. Passage of macromolecules between alveolar and interstitial spaces in foetal and newly ventilated lungs of the lamb. J Physiol 210:151–164, 1970.
22. Bland RD, Hansen TN, Haberkern CM, Bressack MA, Hazinski TA, Raj JU, Goldberg RB. Lung fluid balance in lambs before and after birth. J Appl Physiol 53:992–1004, 1982.

23. Olver RE, Schneeberger EE, Walters DV. Epithelial solute permeability, ion transport and tight junction morphology in the developing lung of the fetal lamb. J Physiol 315:395–412, 1981.
24. Borok Z, Lubman RL, Danto SI, Zhang XL, Zabski SM, King LS, Lee DM, Agre P, Crandall ED. Keratinocyte growth factor modulates alveolar epithelial cell phenotype in vitro: expression of aquaporin 5. Am J Respir Cell Mol Biol 18:554–561, 1998.
25. Dobbs LG, Gonzalez R, Matthay MA, Carter EP, Allen L, Verkman AS. Highly water-permeable type I alveolar epithelial cells confer high water permeability between the airspace and vasculature in rat lung. Proc Natl Acad Sci USA 95:2991–2996, 1998.
26. Blaisdell CJ, Edmonds RD, Wang XT, Guggino S, Zeitlin PL. pH-regulated chloride secretion in fetal lung epithelia. Am J Physiol Lung Cell Mol Physiol 278:L1248–L1255, 2000.
27. O'Brodovich H, Merritt TA. Bicarbonate concentration in rhesus monkey and guinea pig fetal lung liquid. Am Rev Respir Dis 146:1613–1614, 1992.
28. Kitterman JA, Ballard PL, Clements JA, Mescher EJ, Tooley WH. Tracheal fluid in fetal lambs: spontaneous decrease prior to birth. J Appl Physiol 47:985–989, 1979.
29. Schneeberger EE. Plasmalemmal vesicles in pulmonary capillary endothelium of developing fetal lamb lungs. Microvasc Res 25:40–55, 1983.
30. Shermeta DW, Oesch I. Characteristics of fetal lung fluid production. J Pediatr Surg 16:943–946, 1981.
31. Carlton DP, Cummings JJ, Poulain FR, Bland RD. Increased pulmonary vascular filtration pressure does not alter lung liquid secretion in fetal sheep. J Appl Physiol 72:650–655, 1992.
32. Cotton CU, Lawson EE, Boucher RC, Gatzy JT. Bioelectric properties and ion transport of airways excised from adult and fetal sheep. J Appl Physiol 55:1542–1549, 1983.
33. Krochmal EM, Ballard ST, Yankaskas JR, Boucher RC, Gatzy JT. Volume and ion transport by fetal rat alveolar and tracheal epithelia in submersion culture. Am J Physiol 256:F397–F407, 1989.
34. Zeitlin PL, Loughlin GM, Guggino WB. Ion transport in cultured fetal and adult rabbit tracheal epithelia. Am J Physiol 254:C691–C698, 1988.
35. Brown MJ, Olver RE, Ramsden CA, Strang LB, Walters DV. Effects of adrenaline and of spontaneous labour on the secretion and absorption of lung liquid in the fetal lamb. J Physiol 344:137–152, 1983.
36. Chapman DL, Carlton DP, Nielson DW, Cummings JJ, Poulain FR, Bland RD. Changes in lung lipid during spontaneous labor in fetal sheep. J Appl Physiol 76:523–530, 1994.
37. Dickson KA, Maloney JE, Berger PJ. Decline in lung liquid volume before labor in fetal lambs. J Appl Physiol 61:2266–2272, 1986.
38. Bland RD. Dynamics of pulmonary water before and after birth. Acta Paediatr Scand Suppl 305:12–20, 1983.
39. Bland RD, Bressack MA, McMillan DD. Labor decreases the lung water content of newborn rabbits. Am J Obstet Gynecol 135:364–367, 1979.
40. Bland RD. Loss of liquid from the lung lumen in labor: more than a simple 'squeeze'. Am J Physiol Lung Cell Mol Physiol 280:L602–L605, 2001.
41. Guidot DM, Folkesson HG, Jain L, Sznajder JI, Pittet JF, Matthay MA. Integrating acute lung injury and regulation of alveolar fluid clearance. Am J Physiol Lung Cell Mol Physiol 291:L301–6, 2006.
42. Jain L, Eaton DC. Alveolar fluid transport: a changing paradigm. Am J Physiol Lung Cell Mol Physiol 290:L646–L648, 2006.
43. Uchiyama M, Konno N. Hormonal regulation of ion and water transport in anuran amphibians. Gen Comp Endocrinol 147:54–61, 2006.
44. Matthay MA, Folkesson HG, Verkman AS. Salt and water transport across alveolar and distal airway epithelia in the adult lung. Am J Physiol 270:L487–L503, 1996.
45. O'Brodovich H, Hannam V, Seear M, Mullen JB. Amiloride impairs lung water clearance in newborn guinea pigs. J Appl Physiol 68:1758–1762, 1990.
46. Jain L, Chen XJ, Ramosevac S, Brown LA, Eaton DC. Expression of highly selective sodium channels in alveolar type II cells is determined by culture conditions. Am J Physiol Lung Cell Mol Physiol 280:L646–L658, 2001.
47. O'Brodovich H. Epithelial ion transport in the fetal and perinatal lung. Am J Physiol 261:C555–C564, 1991.
48. Voilley N, Lingueglia E, Champigny G, Mattei MG, Waldmann R, Lazdunski M, Barbry P. The lung amiloride-sensitive Na^+ channel: biophysical properties, pharmacology, ontogenesis, and molecular cloning. Proc Natl Acad Sci USA 91:247–251, 1994.
49. Canessa CM, Horisberger JD, Rossier BC. Epithelial sodium channel related to proteins involved in neurodegeneration [see comments]. Nature 361:467–470, 1993.
50. Canessa CM, Schild L, Buell G, Thorens B, Gautschi I, Horisberger JD, Rossier BC. Amiloride-sensitive epithelial Na^+ channel is made of three homologous subunits. Nature 367:463–467, 1994.
51. O'Brodovich H, Canessa C, Ueda J, Rafii B, Rossier BC, Edelson J. Expression of the epithelial Na^+ channel in the developing rat lung. Am J Physiol 265:C491–C496, 1993.
52. Helms MN, Self J, Bao HF, Job LC, Jain L, Eaton DC. Dopamine activates amiloride-sensitive sodium channels in alveolar type 1 cells in a lung slice preparation. Am J Physiol Lung Cell Mol Physiol 291:L610–18, 2006.
53. Johnson MD, Bao HF, Helms MN, Chen XJ, Tigue Z, Jain L, Dobbs LG, Eaton DC. Functional ion channels in pulmonary alveolar type I cells support a role for type I cells in lung ion transport. Proc Natl Acad Sci USA 103:4964–4969, 2006.
54. Johnson MD, Widdicombe JH, Allen L, Barbry P, Dobbs LG. Alveolar epithelial type I cells contain transport proteins and transport sodium, supporting an active role for type I cells in regulation of lung liquid homeostasis. Proc Natl Acad Sci USA 99:1966–1971, 2002.

55. Hummler E, Barker P, Gatzy J, Beermann F, Verdumo C, Schmidt A, Boucher R, Rossier BC. Early death due to defective neonatal lung liquid clearance in alpha-ENaC-deficient mice. Nat Genet 12:325–328, 1996.

56. Barker PM, Gowen CW, Lawson EE, Knowles MR. Decreased sodium ion absorption across nasal epithelium of very premature infants with respiratory distress syndrome [see comments]. J Pediatr 130:373–377, 1997.

57. Gowen CW, Jr, Lawson EE, Gingras J, Boucher RC, Gatzy JT, Knowles MR. Electrical potential difference and ion transport across nasal epithelium of term neonates: correlation with mode of delivery, transient tachypnea of the newborn, and respiratory rate. J Pediatr 113:121–127, 1988.

58. Barker PM, Brown MJ, Ramsden CA, Strang LB, Walters DV. The effect of thyroidectomy in the fetal sheep on lung liquid reabsorption induced by adrenaline or cyclic AMP. J Physiol 407:373–383, 1988.

59. Barker PM, Gowen CW, Lawson EE, Knowles MR. Decreased sodium ion absorption across nasal epithelium of very premature infants with respiratory distress syndrome. J Pediatr 130:373–377, 1997.

60. Perks AM, Cassin S. The effects of arginine vasopressin and epinephrine on lung liquid production in fetal goats. Can J Physiol Pharmacol 67:491–498, 1989.

61. Venkatesh VC, Katzberg HD. Glucocorticoid regulation of epithelial sodium channel genes in human fetal lung. Am J Physiol 273:L227–L233, 1997.

62. Wallace MJ, Hooper SB, Harding R. Regulation of lung liquid secretion by arginine vasopressin in fetal sheep. Am J Physiol 258:R104–R111, 1990.

63. Walters DV, Ramsden CA, Olver RE. Dibutyryl cAMP induces a gestation-dependent absorption of fetal lung liquid. J Appl Physiol 68:2054–2059, 1990.

64. Chang SS, Grunder S, Hanukoglu A, Rosler A, Mathew PM, Hanukoglu I, Schild L, Lu Y, Shimkets RA, Nelson-Williams C, Rossier BC, Lifton RP. Mutations in subunits of the epithelial sodium channel cause salt wasting with hyperkalaemic acidosis, pseudohypoaldosteronism type 1. Nat Genet 12:248–253, 1996.

65. Liedtke CM. Electrolyte transport in the epithelium of pulmonary segments of normal and cystic fibrosis lung. Faseb J 6:3076–3084, 1992.

66. Knowles MR, Olivier K, Noone P, Boucher RC. Pharmacologic modulation of salt and water in the airway epithelium in cystic fibrosis. Am J Respir Crit Care Med 151:S65–S69, 1995.

67. Mall M, Grubb BR, Harkema JR, O'Neal WK, Boucher RC. Increased airway epithelial Na^+ absorption produces cystic fibrosis-like lung disease in mice. Nat Med 10:487–493, 2004.

68. Jain L, Eaton DC. Physiology of fetal lung fluid clearance and the effect of labor. Semin Perinatol 30:34–43, 2006.

69. Noone PG, Leigh MW, Sannuti A, Minnix SL, Carson JL, Hazucha M, Zariwala MA, Knowles MR. Primary ciliary dyskinesia: diagnostic and phenotypic features. Am J Respir Crit Care Med 169:459–467, 2004.

70. Jain L. Alveolar fluid clearance in developing lungs and its role in neonatal transition. Clin Perinatol 26:585–599, 1999.

71. Jain L, Chen XJ, Brown LA, Eaton DC. Nitric oxide inhibits lung sodium transport through a cGMP-mediated inhibition of epithelial cation channels. Am J Physiol 274:L475–L484, 1998.

72. Jain L, Chen XJ, Malik B, Al-Khalili O, Eaton DC. Antisense oligonucleotides against the alpha-subunit of ENaC decrease lung epithelial cation-channel activity. Am J Physiol 276:L1046–L1051, 1999.

73. Chen XJ, Eaton DC, Jain L. Beta-adrenergic regulation of amiloride-sensitive lung sodium channels. Am J Physiol Lung Cell Mol Physiol 282:L609–L620, 2002.

74. Cummings JJ, Carlton DP, Poulain FR, Fike CD, Keil LC, Bland RD. Vasopressin effects on lung liquid volume in fetal sheep. Pediatr Res 38:30–35, 1995.

75. Bouvry D, Planes C, Malbert-Colas L, Escabasse V, Clerici C. Hypoxia-induced cytoskeleton disruption in alveolar epithelial cells. Am J Respir Cell Mol Biol 35:519–27, 2006.

76. Anantharam A, Tian Y, Palmer LG: Open probability of the epithelial sodium channel is regulated by intracellular sodium. J Physiol 574:333–47, 2006.

77. Renard S, Voilley N, Bassilana F, Lazdunski M, Barbry P. Localization and regulation by steroids of the alpha, beta and gamma subunits of the amiloride-sensitive Na^+ channel in colon, lung and kidney. Pflugers Arch 430:299–307, 1995.

78. Eaton D, Ohara A, Ling BN. Cellular regulation of amiloride blockable Na^+ channels. Biomed Res 12:31–35, 1991.

79. Guidot DM, Modelska K, Lois M, Jain L, Moss IM, Pittet JF, Brown LA. Ethanol ingestion via glutathione depletion impairs alveolar epithelial barrier function in rats. Am J Physiol Lung Cell Mol Physiol 279:L127–L135, 2000.

80. Jobe AH, Ikegami M, Padbury J, Polk DH, Korirnilli A, Gonzales LW, Ballard PL. Combined effects of fetal beta agonist stimulation and glucocorticoids on lung function of preterm lambs. Biol Neonate 72:305–313, 1997.

81. Ervin MG, Berry LM, Ikegami M, Jobe AH, Padbury JF, Polk DH. Single dose fetal betamethasone administration stabilizes postnatal glomerular filtration rate and alters endocrine function in premature lambs. Pediatr Res 40:645–651, 1996.

82. Pillow JJ, Hall GL, Willet KE, Jobe AH, Hantos Z, Sly PD. Effects of gestation and antenatal steroid on airway and tissue mechanics in newborn lambs. Am J Respir Crit Care Med 163:1158–1163, 2001.

83. Smith LM, Ervin MG, Wada N, Ikegami M, Polk DH, Jobe AH. Antenatal glucocorticoids alter postnatal preterm lamb renal and cardiovascular responses to intravascular volume expansion. Pediatr Res 47:622–627, 2000.

84. Willet KE, Jobe AH, Ikegami M, Kovar J, Sly PD. Lung morphometry after repetitive antenatal glucocorticoid treatment in preterm sheep. Am J Respir Crit Care Med 163:1437–1443, 2001.
85. Willet KE, Jobe AH, Ikegami M, Newnham J, Brennan S, Sly PD. Antenatal endotoxin and glucocorticoid effects on lung morphometry in preterm lambs. Pediatr Res 48:782–788, 2000.
86. Baines DL, Folkesson HG, Norlin A, Bingle CD, Yuan HT, Olver RE. The influence of mode of delivery, hormonal status and postnatal O_2 environment on epithelial sodium channel (ENaC) expression in perinatal guinea-pig lung. J Physiol 522 Pt 1:147–157, 2000.
87. Berthiaume Y, Staub NC, Matthay MA. Beta-adrenergic agonists increase lung liquid clearance in anesthetized sheep. J Clin Invest 79:335–343, 1987.
88. Finley N, Norlin A, Baines DL, Folkesson HG. Alveolar epithelial fluid clearance is mediated by endogenous catecholamines at birth in guinea pigs. J Clin Invest 101:972–981, 1998.
89. Helms MN, Chen XJ, Ramosevac S, Eaton DC, Jain L. Dopamine regulation of amiloride-sensitive sodium channels in lung cells. Am J Physiol Lung Cell Mol Physiol 290:L710–L722, 2006.

Chapter 12

Edema

Caroline D. Boyd, MD • Andrew T. Costarino, MD

Physiology of Water Control
Pathophysiology of Edema
Relevance to Critically Ill Infants

Edema is abnormal accumulation of body water. In health, total body water (TBW) volume comprises over 60% of body mass in the adult, and close to 80% in newborns (1,2). Semi-permeable plasma membranes establish two large divisions of the TBW: (i) intracellular water (ICW) contained within the cells; and (ii) the surrounding extra-cellular water (ECW), which is further subdivided by the capillary endothelium into plasma water and non-plasma water (the interstitial, intercellular or 'third' water space) (1). The ECW shields the internal cellular compartment from direct interface with the external environment, providing a buffer from sudden changes in environmental stresses, therefore protecting the cell from acute fluxes in water (and solute) concentrations. This arrangement requires the organism to have systems that monitor the volume and composition of the ECW, and mechanisms that correct for the water losses or gains that result from contact with the environment and metabolism (3–5).

In illness, these systems may become stressed or dysfunctional and the TBW balance is disrupted. While edema is any abnormal accumulation of tissue water, most clinicians are referring to ECW interstitial water (third space) accumulation when using the term edema.

PHYSIOLOGY OF WATER CONTROL

Regulation of Body Water Distribution

Water moves spontaneously from a region of high concentration to one of low concentration. Osmosis is the movement of water down its concentration gradient through the cell's semi-permeable membrane. Osmolality is the number of solute particles per kg of water solvent, with one osmole constituting one g-molecular-weight of a substance. A solution of 'pure' water contains 55.5 osmoles of water per kg, but when sodium chloride or another solute is added to the solution, the water concentration will be reduced. Since water is the solvent in all body fluids, water concentration is expressed conversely; that is, body fluid osmolality refers to the concentration of the solutes. Body water solute osmolality is usually 280–295 milliosms per kg.

The water movements across semi permeable plasma membranes are important in regulating cell volume. The force driving water through a semi permeable membrane is the osmotic pressure and its magnitude is proportional to the difference in the concentration of water on either side of the membrane. The Van't Hoff equation expresses this force in terms of millimeters of mercury (6).

$$P = cRT \tag{1}$$

where: P = osmotic pressure (mmHg), c = solute concentration (Osmoles/L), R = the universal gas constant (62.3 mmHg*L/Osm+°K), T = the absolute temperature (°K).

Solving equation 1 at body temperature demonstrates that one milliosmole per L of solution will exert 19.3 mmHg of osmotic pressure (6). The osmolality of both the ECW and the ICW is normally between 270–300 mOsm, so on average, the osmotic pressure in each compartment is 5500 mmHg. Since each compartment has the same or similar osmolality, there is no net movement of water. However, if a cell was suddenly placed into pure water, a force equal to 5500 mmHg would drive water into the cell. This is why hypotonic extra-cellular states may disrupt normal cell function, as when intravenous infusion of sterile water causes hemolysis.

The intracellular water compartment is regulated by passive movement of water (solvent), and by active transport of solutes across plasma membranes. The driving force for water movement is osmotic pressure generated by the many differences in solute concentrations (6,7) across the cell membrane. Intracellular, non-permeable macromolecules (mostly proteins) produce osmotic and electrochemical forces that result in unequal distribution of small molecular weight permeable ions (Na^+, Cl^- and K^+) inside the cell. A return to equilibrium might cause cells to swell with water if not for active transport of Na^+ (with Cl^-) out of the cell by the cell membrane Na^+/K^+ ATPase pump. The Na^+/K^+ ATPase pump is the most important regulator of the ICW (8,9), and makes the cell effectively impermeable to sodium. In the setting of cellular energy failure the Na^+/K^+ ATPase pump becomes dysfunctional and cellular edema (swelling) will occur.

While cell volume and ICW concentration are actively regulated by ion transport at the cell membrane, this system is not, by itself, suitable for sustained or severe challenges to cell volume because the large shifts in the concentration of intracellular potassium would have troublesome consequences on cell function. The ECW serves to shield the ICW from direct interface with the external environment and dramatically reduces the range of osmotic gradients that confront most tissue. In some tissues, where greater and more sudden changes in solute concentrations occur (e.g., the renal medulla) or where the consequence of cellular volume changes is more harmful (the brain) additional mechanisms exist to adjust intracellular solute concentration (8,9). These tissues can produce and metabolize organic osmolytes, small organic molecules found in high concentrations in the cytoplasm that reduce the cross membrane gradient for water movement (9). The concentration of these compounds can change dramatically without harmful effects on cell constituents or enzymatic processes. The organic osmolytes are of three classes: the polyols (sorbitol and myo-inostol), amino acids (taurine, alanine and proline) and the methylamines (betaine and glycerylphosphorylcholine) (8,9). An osmotic challenge that tends to reduce cell volume results in an accumulation of the organic osmolytes through uptake from the extracellular space or a change in cell production or their degradation. This is a process that occurs over hours. In the opposite occurrence of cellular swelling a decrease in organic osmolytes occurs in two steps: first the osmolytes are lost through cell membrane channels activated by the swelling, then a reduction in the uptake or production of the compounds follows.

Extracellular Water Regulation

The ECW serves to buffer the stress that confronts the ICW, but interaction with the environment and energy production are reflected in changes in size of the ECW, therefore the whole organism must have a regulatory system to respond to these changes. The ECW regulatory response is designed to: (i) assure the integrity of the circulation (vascular pressure); and (ii) keep the osmolality of the ECW compartment within 3% of the osmolar set point (280–290 mOsm). A broad overview of the ECW feedback control is as follows: an increase in ECW is reflected in an increase in the plasma volume, which in turn increases blood flow and vascular pressure. The increased vascular pressure leads to an increase in renal glomerular filtrate and urinary flow, which then returns the ECW volume to baseline. If the increased ECW volumes lowered plasma osmolality, modulation by hormonal controls will result in a dilute diuresis. Decreased ECW volume results will decrease vascular pressure and glomerular filtration, leading to decreased urinary flow that lasts until intake replenishes the lost volume. Hypertonicity, which accompanies many low-volume states, stimulates thirst and hormonal renal resorption of water.

The description above provides the general overview of ECW control but each component is equipped with negative and positive feedback mechanisms which 'fine tune' the physiologic response. Thus, cardiac output, perfusion distribution, urine flow and the hormonal responses, including renin-angiotensin-aldosterone system, arginine vasopressin and atrial natriuretic peptide, all interact to maintain homeostasis. As a result, in health, little variation in organ perfusion and vital signs are observable despite wide variation in the external stress to the ECW. Alternatively, in the critically ill infant, disease and treatment alter the normal response of the vasomotor, renal and hormonal components of the ECW control system maintaining homeostasis. Additionally, gastrointestinal intake is usually completely controlled by others, therefore thirst mechanisms controlling voluntary intake are nonfunctional. As a result of these consequences of disease and treatment it is very common for the critically ill patient to have abnormal ECW water balance and third space water accumulation—edema.

Distribution of Water within the ECW

The ECW compartment is subdivided into plasma water and interstitial water. The distribution of water, electrolytes and proteins between these subcompartments of the ECW is a function of the interaction among hydrostatic pressure generated by cardiovascular function, oncotic pressure, endothelial membrane functions and the lymphatics.

Starling Forces

Water movement across an idealized capillary wall was described qualitatively by Starling in 1896 (10), then quantitatively refined by Pappenheimer & Soto-Rivera (11), Landis & Pappanheimer (12) and Landis (13).

$$JV = K_F[P_{capillary} - P_{interstitium}] - \delta[\pi_{plasma} - \pi_{tissue}] \tag{2}$$

Where JV is the net flow across the capillary, K_F is the hydrostatic filtration coefficient across the capillary endothelium, $P_{capillary}$ is the capillary hydrostatic pressure, $P_{interstitium}$ is the hydrostatic pressure in the interstitial space, δ is the Stavermann reflection coefficient, π_{plasma} is the plasma oncotic pressure, and π_{tissue} is the interstitial oncotic pressure.

This relationship demonstrates that the movement of fluid out of the blood vessel is dependent on the product of the water permeability intrinsic to the capillaries (K_F), and the net driving pressure out of or into the capillary. That net driving pressure, $[(P_{capillary} - P_{interstitium}) - \delta (\Pi_{plasma} - \Pi_{tissue})]$, is a balance between the hydrostatic forces on either side of the capillary membrane ($P_{capillary} - P_{interstitium}$), and the oncotic pressure on either side ($\Pi_{plasma} - \Pi_{tissue}$) (7,10–13).

Normally, the balance among forces results in a small amount of water leaving the plasma at the arterial end (higher pressure) of the capillary bed, with most re-entering the plasma as the hydrostatic pressure falls at the venous end (7). The small amount of fluid remaining in the interstitium is removed by lymphatic drainage. In disease, these balanced forces within the capillary bed may be disrupted favoring accumulation of fluid in the interstitium of some, or all, organs. Imbalance may be due to: (i) conditions of high plasma hydrostatic pressure; (ii) decreased interstitial hydrostatic pressure; (iii) increased vascular permeability for water (4) increased vascular permeability to proteins; (iv) low plasma oncotic pressure; (v) high interstitial oncotic pressure; (vi) lymphatic drainage abnormalities.

PATHOPHYSIOLOGY OF EDEMA

The balance among the Starling forces is maintained in the infant but the normal values for the constituents of equation 2 can vary in the older child and adult. Additionally, the common diseases that lead to intensive care can alter the balance, quickly leading to edema.

Plasma Hydrostatic Pressure (P$_{capillary}$)

The average capillary hydrostatic pressure is determined by arterial and venous pressures (Pa and Pv), and by the ratio of the capillary resistances from post to pre-capillary (Rv/Ra). Increasing either arterial or venous pressure will increase capillary pressure. However, a given change in Pv is about one-fifth more effective in changing Pc than the same change in Pa. Venous resistance is relatively low, therefore changes in Pv are readily transmitted back to the capillary. Because arterial resistance is relatively high, changes in Pa are poorly transmitted downstream to the capillary.

Fetal central venous pressure, as estimated by the umbilical venous pressure, is approximately 5.0–6.5 cmH$_2$O (range 2–9 cmH$_2$O). This is generally higher than in the spontaneously breathing healthy newborn (14). At birth, central venous pressure falls then normal resting central venous pressure increases over the first week of life (15), which may be related to adaptation to the loss of supra-atmospheric pressure and the buoyancy provided by the amniotic fluid.

Vascular hypertension may be present on the arterial or the venous side of the capillary bed. Clinically encountered arterial hypertension is generally regulated by the pre-capillary sphincters, and is not usually a source of tissue edema. In malignant arterial hypertension the pressure exceeds the tissue auto regulation and organ edema may occur.

More common is capillary bed hypertension associated with increased venous pressures. This can be due to increased blood volume (e.g. excessive fluid administration or transfusion) or some impediment to venous drainage (e.g. pulmonary edema due to left ventricular dysfunction, postural edema of the lower extremities). In congestive heart failure, the chronically increased venous volume and pressure leads to a viscous cycle of accumulation of venous blood volume, decreased arterial volume and a triggering of compensatory mechanisms that promote renal water and solute retention with significant corporeal and pulmonary edema.

Mechanical ventilation causes positive intra-thoracic pressure, relative to extra-thoracic venous pressures causing corporeal venous hypertension to varying degrees.

This pathologic respiratory–cardiac interaction has the added feature of reducing venous return to the heart, necessitating extra fluid administration to maintain cardiac output. As a result, critically ill patients have clinically notable edema. Depending on the disease that requires treatment with mechanical ventilation, these patients usually have abnormalities in the other components of the Starling relationship, which result in systemic or pulmonary edema.

Interstitial Hydrostatic Pressure ($P_{interstitium}$)

The interstitium is the space located between the capillary walls and the cells, and can be termed the extracellular matrix (ECM). It is a complex, dynamic structural entity surrounding and supporting cells and is a hydrated gel composed of three different classes of biomolecules; (i) structural proteins (collagen, elastin), (ii) specialized proteins (fibrillin, fibronectin), and (iii) proteoglycans (16). Proteoglycans are composed of a protein core to which long chains of repeating disaccharide units termed glycosaminoglycans (GAGS) are attached. Glycosaminoglycans are located primarily on the surfaces of cells or in the ECM, and are highly negatively charged molecules (16). Fig. 12-1 illustrates the composition of the ECM and the forces involved in controlling net capillary filtration discussed above (17).

There are various forms of GAGS that differ from tissue to tissue, including hyaluronic acid (present in most tissues), heparin (liver, mast cells), heparin sulfate (basement membranes), keratin sulfate (bone), chondroitin sulfate (cartilage, bone), and dermatan sulfate (skin, blood vessels) (16). These substances are produced by tissue fibroblasts and their function remains a matter of speculation. However, they do contribute to the shape of the various organs and appear to be involved in cell signaling. In relation to the transfer of water between the plasma and the non-plasma water, the interstitial gel is important because it determines the pressure–volume relationship (compliance) of the interstitial space. The interstitial pressure–volume relationship is demonstrated in Fig. 12-2 (17).

Animal studies in newborn lambs suggest that the hydrostatic pressure in the pleural interstitial tissue of the lung increases from just above atmospheric pressure at birth up to $6 + 0.7$ cmH$_2$O at 2 h postnatal. Over the next 6 h the pulmonary interstitial pressure decreases, becoming sub-atmospheric ($-6.0 + 1.6$ cmH$_2$O). In contrast, extra-pleural interstitial pressure did not change, remaining just under atmospheric at -1.5 to -2.0 cmH$_2$O. These authors speculate that the increased

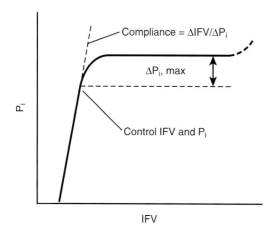

Figure 12-1 Overview of the control of interstitial fluid volume illustrating the composition of the ECM as well as the Starling forces acting to maintain fluid balance (From Aukland K, Reed RK: Interstitial-lymphatic mechanisms in the control of extracellular fluid volume. Physiological Reviews 73:1–78, 1993).

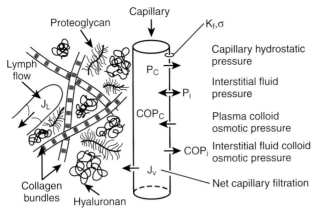

Figure 12-2 Interstitial compliance is defined as the ratio between the change in interstitial fluid volume and the resultant change in interstitial fluid pressure. The interstitium is usually in a state of mild dehydration and compliance is low. In this situation, a change in interstitial fluid volume is readily reflected by a change in interstitial fluid pressure. At some point during overhydration, compliance increases and the pressure–volume relationship becomes linear. At this point, large changes in interstitial fluid volume have little impact on interstitial fluid pressure (From Aukland K, Reed RK: Interstitial-lymphatic mechanisms in the control of extracellular fluid volume. Physiological Reviews 73:1–78, 1993).

pulmonary interstitial pressure helps promote fluid clearance from the lung interstitium into the pulmonary capillaries in the first hours after birth (18).

Increased Vascular Permeability for Water K$_F$ (Filtration Coefficient)

The filtration coefficient is proportional to two physical characteristics of the capillary bed (i) permeability for water, or water conductance for the capillaries of a given tissue, and (ii) the available capillary surface area (7,19). The first characteristic, the capillary permeability, is in turn determined by the number of pores (gaps) per cm^2 between endothelial cells that provide a channel for the water molecule (paracellular water transport) and the function of membrane proteins. Three dimensional integral membrane proteins, called aquaporins, seem to function to help control bidirectional water movement (20). These recently discovered compounds have multiple isoforms that vary depending on the tissue, facilitate movement down its concentration (osmolar) gradient created by energy-dependent cation transport via Na$^+$, K$^+$-ATPase. Additionally, water movement is aided by co-transporters such as Na$^+$-glutamate or Na$^+$-glucose co-transporter. Paracellular water transport can vary greatly depending on tissue type and disease state. The co-transporters are less efficient than the aquaporins but, in some tissues, for example the intestinal mucosa, they serve as the main mechanism for water uptake. Alternatively, water transport via aquaporins is much faster than diffusion of water via the lipid bilayer of the plasma membrane and allows a more specific regulation of water distribution than water movement via other pathways.

During development aquaporin expression and function is in part regulated by hormones. In the lung, aquaporins are abundantly expressed. There appear to be at least four isoforms, including AQP1, AQP3, AQP4 and AQP5, but the differing function of each is unclear (21). The AQP1 seems to be the primary form expressed in capillary endothelium, whereas the others are localized in the airway epithelial cells. In a rodent model, AQP1 deletion greatly reduced transcapillary osmotic water permeability and human studies in AQP1-null individuals suggest that AQP1 is the major determinant of vascular water permeability in the lung (22,23).

During the perinatal period, aquaporin expression in the lung endothelium changes dramatically. These changes are associated with the transition from water secretion to water absorption by the lung epithelium. The level of AQP1 in the lung endothelium increases perinatally and is upregulated by maternal corticosteroid treatment (22). Expression of AQP4 peaks immediately after birth (24,25), and AQP4 mRNA can be induced by glucocorticoids and β-adrenergic agonists. Alveolar AQP5 protein level also gradually increases after birth (25) and β-adrenergic agonist exposure increases AQP5 expression and membrane localization. Alveolar AQP3 function (26) is pH-regulated (27,28). Extracellular acidification significantly decreases the water permeability of AQP3 expressed in human bronchial epithelial cells. Thus, in conditions of acidemia, for example asphyxiated or acidotic infants, AQP3-mediated water permeability will be inhibited. These observations suggest a role for these compounds in abnormal lung water clearance in the lung of infants with hyaline membrane disease, perinatal asphyxia and bronchopulmonary dysplasia, as well as the mechanism by which antenatal steroids reduce lung water in critically ill infants (20).

The second determinant of capillary permeability, the available capillary surface area, varies greatly among tissue beds and changes during development. Thus, experimental data places values for KF anywhere from 0.01 to 0.3 ml/min/mmHg/100 g tissue depending on the model (5). Additionally, disease states, drugs and inflammatory mediators will alter K_F by affecting both the water conductance and the available surface area of the capillary bed (29–31).

Increased Vascular Permeability to Proteins δ (Stavermann Reflection Coefficient)

The reflection coefficient is the property of the capillary membrane that describes its permeability to plasma proteins. If the membrane is completely impermeable to protein, the value for δ will be 1.0 (5,19). Similar to the filtration coefficient (K_F), the value for δ differs greatly among capillary beds of different tissues and is influenced by medications and mediators of inflammation (29–31). In the fetus and newborn, protein permeability has been most closely examined in the lung. The permeability of lung epithelium decreases with increasing gestational age (32). Acute changes in lung epithelial permeability may also occur with the onset of breathing. In the newborn lamb model, following delivery of mature animals, the calculated protein pore size radius of approximately 6 angstroms increases transiently to 35–56 angstroms (33). Subsequently, the pore size decreases to 7–14 angstroms in the spontaneously breathing lamb. Immediately after birth albumin and water are absorbed at the same rate over the first 20 min of breathing. Subsequently, the protein flux from the airways of the term and premature animals with surfactant stopped, whereas those with less surfactant continued to leak (33,34).

Plasma Oncotic Pressure

Osmolality of body fluids is affected by the presence of large molecular weight plasma proteins (colloids) that do not pass freely through semi permeable membranes. The primary plasma colloid is albumen. Albumen, and most other plasma proteins are ionized at physiologic pH, so they have an associated electromotive force that causes an unequal distribution of the smaller diffusible ions (crystalloids) between body compartments (the Gibbs–Donnan Equilibrium) (7). The difference in osmotic pressure associated with colloid proteins is the oncotic pressure. Approximately two thirds is directly related to the nondiffusible proteins and one third is a result of the Gibbs–Donnan difference in diffusible particles. The osmotic gradient between plasma and interstitial water is a result of the differences in oncotic pressure. Plasma oncotic pressure is 25–28 mmHg in adults, 15–17 mmHg in term neonates (35,36). It is likely lower in premature infants because plasma proteins, including albumen, increase with increasing gestational age (35–37). Infants with acute and chronic lung disease have lower plasma protein levels (37).

In disease, extracorporeal losses (e.g., bleeding, proteinuria), sequestration (e.g., ascites) and decreased production will reduce serum proteins, plasma oncotic pressure and increase the tendency for edema (35,36)

Interstitial Oncotic Pressure

The oncotic pressure of the interstitial fluid depends on the interstitial protein concentration and the reflection coefficient of the capillary wall—the more permeable the barrier the higher the interstitial oncotic pressure. Fluid filtration into the interstitium also factors into determining the interstitial oncotic pressure. Increased capillary filtration decreases interstitial protein concentration, thus reducing the oncotic pressure. Increased capillary filtration decreases interstitial protein concentration, thus reducing the oncotic pressure. The lowered interstitial oncotic pressure will act to decrease the net capillary filtration pressure and thus return the net capillary filtration toward normal, thereby limiting changes in interstitial fluid volume. Typically, tissue oncotic pressure is about 50% of plasma oncotic pressure (38–40).

Lymphatic Drainage

Under conditions where the other components of Starling's relationship allow interstitial water accumulation the lymphatic drainage must increase or tissue edema will occur (7). Since the ability to increase lymphatic drainage varies among the different tissue beds, the propensity to become edematous varies among organs. Other factors affecting lymphatic drainage include: (i) body movement, where lymphatic flow depends in part on tissue movement; (ii) lymphatic obstruction due to tissue injury; (iii) mechanical factors.

RELEVANCE TO CRITICALLY ILL INFANTS

The example patient scenario below illustrates the physiologic principles discussed above and contributes to understanding common problems confronting the clinician caring for critically ill infants.

Case

A two-week-old infant boy who was born at 34 weeks' gestational age presents with increasing respiratory distress and diffuse radiodensity on chest radiograph. This patient was noted to be tachypneic immediately after birth and a chest X-ray at that time showed diffuse but mild radiodensity, small lung volumes and prominent vascular markings. The rest of the patient's physical examination was remarkable only for mild oxygen desaturation while breathing air. At that time, these findings were thought to be due to transient tachypnea of the newborn (TTN).

This patient's respiratory distress, after initial improvement, worsened in the second week of life. The chest X-ray appearance changed with increased lung radiodensity and the heart size remained normal to small. An echocardiogram was obtained that demonstrated total anomalous pulmonary venous connection to the inferior vena cava below the diaphragm.

Discussion 1

The initial presentation and the diagnosis of TTN suggest that poor clearance of pulmonary water may have contributed to the early respiratory signs. In utero, at the end of gestation, human fetal lung secretes approximately 0.5 L of fluid a day. At birth, most of the fluid in the lung is expelled mechanically. The fluid that remains is absorbed during the first postnatal days as aeration of the lung is established, surfactant reduces alveolar surface tension, and the initiation of regular spontaneous respiration promotes lymphatic drainage of alveolar and pulmonary interstitial water. Additionally, the lung epithelium switches from a secretory to absorptive epithelium and this switch involves increased expression of the epithelial sodium channel, the sodium pump, and lung aquaporins (20), as evidenced by postnatal increases in mRNA for these membrane constituents in the newborn rat model. The most specific perinatal induction pattern is the sharp and transient increase of AQP4 mRNA specific to lung tissue, occurring just after birth and coinciding with the time course for clearance of lung liquid and stimulated by β-agonists.

In some children this transition is delayed (with higher incidence in children born by elective caesarean section). The lung water and microatelectesis affect respiratory mechanics and respiratory gas exchange with resultant tachypnea and V/Q mismatch causing mild hypoxemia. One of the most prominent features of RDS and BPD is the lung edema believed to be caused by inadequate lung water clearance (41).

It is more likely that the anomalous venous connection to vascular structures below the diaphragm was associated with obstructed venous flow and venous hypertension. The venous hypertension results in changes in the Starling relationship that promote fluid movement into the intestitium and ultimately the alveoli. The pulmonary edema will dilute alveolar surfactant worsening microatelectesis, which in turn will reduce interstitial hydrostatic pressure and impede lymphatic drainage (33,34). The result is a vicious cycle of increasing lung water and abnormalities of lung mechanics and respiratory gas exchange. This pathophysiology accounts for the clinical presentation of respiratory distress, abnormal chest X-ray and absence of evidence of cardiomegaly.

Case Continuation

On day 16 of life this infant was taken to surgery for repair of the anomalous venous connection under general anesthesia and cardiopulmonary bypass. The infant returned to the neonatal intensive care unit (NICU) following surgery sedated on mechanical ventilation and with residual neuromuscular blockade. During the first postoperative hours, hypotension and oliguria required intravenous fluid boluses and blood product administration. The following morning's chest X-ray showed increased lung volumes and less radiodensity; however, the patient had dramatic edema of the face abdomen and extremities.

The edema so commonly present in this post surgical setting is the result of the many unavoidable clinical stresses on the components of the Starling relationship. For example, many anesthetic agents are venodilating and the increased venous capacitance requires that additional intravenous fluids be administered intraoperatively to maintain cardiac preload. Positive pressure ventilation has the combined effect of impeding venous return to the heart, necessitating intravenous fluid administration and increasing the hydrostatic pressure in the veins outside the pleura. Capillary hydrostatic pressure is increased by the fluid administration necessary to compensate for the decreased preload associated with anesthetic agents and the positive pressure ventilation, as well as the direct effect of the positive pressure ventilation. The increased capillary hydrostatic pressure promotes edema formation.

During surgery this patient was placed on cardiopulmonary bypass (CPB). The physical trauma to the blood and the need for administration of stored blood products associated with CPB variably triggers the release of inflammatory mediators. These compounds, including TNF-α, Il-6 and others, and the associated activation of white blood cells and other components of the immune system affect the permeability of the endothelium to water and protein (42–44). The diffusely increased permeability of the capillary beds leads to edema.

Low plasma oncotic pressure is likely to be present in this patient. Plasma proteins are often low in the critically ill infant (45), due to compromised nutrition, increased metabolism, protein consumption in inflammation and tissue injury, and blood coagulation. Plasma proteins are also lost and not replaced during surgical bleeding and are lost from serous surfaces through drainage catheters. The low oncotic pressure promotes water movement out of the vascular space into the interstitium.

Discussion 2

The oncotic pressure of the interstitium may be increased in critically ill infants similar to our patient example. Depending on the type and magnitude of the injury, diffusely increased permeability of the capillary beds to water may extend to permeability to proteins. Loss of plasma protein into the interstitium will promote edema formation.

Any process in critically ill neonates, resulting in a systemic inflammatory response, will likely result in edema (42–45) These processes include sepsis, anaphylaxis, and CPB, to name a few (42–44,46,47) The edema observed in this clinical setting is multifactorial, but the role of fluid administration, high venous hydrostatic pressure and increased capillary permeability are the key contributors. However, more recently, it is increasingly clear that other processes also contribute to the degree of edema, and the speed at which the edema develops (39,40). An in vitro phenomenon known as collagen gel contraction, which is the ability of fibroblasts to compact a collagen gel matrix to a fraction of its 'normal' size over a period of time (39,40). β1-integrins are receptors that mediate the interaction between fibroblasts and components of the ECM involved in this process. The contractile ability of the ECM, noted in in vitro studies, opposes the tendency for the ECM to swell. Inflammation may alter the function of β1-integrin receptors, leading to tissue expansion by decreasing the number or integrity of connections between components of the ECM. Tissue expansion will result in decreased interstitial fluid pressure, drawing fluid into the ECM and worsening edema (39,40).

Tissue injury and the resulting inflammatory cascade may disrupt the usual breakdown and remodeling processes of the ECM, leading to, or allowing for, further edema formation. Matrix metalloproteinases (MMPs) are enzymes that hydrolyze components of the ECM, and likely play a role in numerous biological processes, including degradation and remodeling of the ECM (48–50). The activity of MMPs are balanced by tissue inhibitors of metalloproteinases (TIMPs). This balance is important in many biological processes, including embryogenesis, normal tissue remodeling, angiogenesis and wound healing. The homeostasis that exists between MMPs and TIMPs can become deranged in certain disease processes. This has been demonstrated in hearts subjected to chronic volume overload, in which ventricular chambers remodel and dilate over time (48). Matrix metalloproteinases are upregulated and overwhelm the balance provided by TIMPs. It is possible that tissue injury leading to edema will disrupt this balance between MMPs and TIMPs and perhaps promote excessive degradation and remodeling of tissue. For instance, increased quantities of lung-specific MMPs have been demonstrated in experimental models of pulmonary edema (50,51).

Lymphatic drainage is also likely to be reduced in dependant and extremity areas, of this and similar patients, particularly when neuromuscular blockade is needed for extended periods. Although unlikely in this example patient, in others congenital anomalies of lymphatic drainage may be present. More commonly, the surgical procedure itself, vascular catheters or other interventions may injure or obstruct the central lymphatics. Under these circumstances variable amounts of edema may occur generally or in the tissues near the compromised lymphatics. Chylus pleural effusions may be present in infants following cardiothoracic surgery secondary to injury to the thoracic duct.

Our patient example illustrates how a number of common disease states and interventions may promote edema development in the neonatal population. Edema may be generalized, or may be localized to a specific organ. The most common site of localized edema is in the lungs; pulmonary edema. Our patient had a number of reasons to develop both pulmonary and generalized edema, and all of these inciting factors are ones seen on a regular basis in neonatal critical care. The Starling equation is a useful starting point in understanding fluid balance, and thus edema. However, it is clear that there are complex molecular and biochemical processes in the development of edema that are incompletely understood and require further investigation.

REFERENCES

1. Edelman IS, Liebman J. Anatomy of body electrolytes. Am J Med 27:256–277, 1959.
2. Friis-Hansen B. Body water compartments in children. Pediatrics 28:169–181, 1961.
3. Dahlstrom H. Basal metabolism and extracellular fluid. Acta Physio Scand 21(suppl 71):5–80, 1950.
4. Wedgewood RJ, Bass DE, Klincis JA, Kleeman CR, Quinn M. Relationship of body composition to basal metabolic rate in normal man. J Appl Physiol 6:317–334, 1953.
5. Speakman JR. The history and theory of the doubly labled water technique. Am J Clin Nutr 68(suppl):932S–938S, 1998.
6. Michel CC: Fluid movements through capillary walls. In Renkin EM, Michel CC (eds), Handbook of Physiology, Section II, Vol II. Bethesda, MD: American Physiologic Society, 1984.
7. Michel CC, Curry FE. Microvascular permiability. Physiol Review 79:703–761, 1999.
8. Trachtman H, Barbour R, Sturman JA, Finburg L. Taurine and osmoregulation: taurine is a cerebral osmoprotective molecule in chronic hypernatremic dehydration. Pediatr Res 23:35–39, 1988.
9. McManus MI, Churchwell KB, Strange K. Regulation of cell volume in health and disease. N Engl J Med 333:1260–1266, 1995.
10. Starling EH. On the absorption of fluid from the connective tissue spaces. J Physiol (London) 19:312–326, 1896.
11. Pappenheimer JR, Soto-Rivera. Effective osmotic pressure of the plasma proteins and other quantities associated with capillary circulation in the hind limb of cats and dogs. Am J Physiol 152:471–491, 1948.
12. Landis EM, Pappenheimer JR. Exchange of substances through capillary walls. In Handbook of Physiology. Circulation Section 2, Vol. 2 (pp. 961–1034). Washington, DC: American Physiologic Society, 1963.
13. Landis EM. Capillary pressure and capillary permeability. Physiol Rev 14:404–481, 1934.
14. Ville Y, Sideris I, Hecher K, Snijders RJ, et al. Umbilical venous pressure in normal, growth-retarded, and anemic fetuses. Am J Obstet Gyn 170:487–494, 1994.
15. Buckner PS, Quail AW, David BF, Cottee DBF, et al. Venous hydrostatic indifference point as a marker of postnatal adaptation to orthostasis in swine. J Appl Physiol 87:882–888, 1999.
16. Comper WD, Laurent TC. Physiologic function of connective tissue polysaccharides. Physiol Rev 58:255–315, 1978.
17. Aukland K, Reed RK. Interstitial-lymphatic mechanisms in the control of extracellular fluid volume. Physiological Reviews 73:1–78, 1993.
18. Miserocchi G, Poskurica BH, del Fabbro M. Pulmonary interstitial pressure in anesthetized paralysed neborn rabbits. J Appl Physiol 77:2260–2268, 1994.
19. Taylor AE. Capillary fluid filtration. Circ Res 49:557–575, 1981.
20. Zelenina M, Zelenin S, Aperia A. Water channels (aquaporins) and their role for postnatal adaptation. Ped Research 57:47R–53R, 2005.
21. Verkman AS. Aquaporin water channels and endothelial cell function. J Anatomy 200:617–627, 2002.

22. King LS, Nielsen S, Agre P, et al. Aquaporin-1 water channel protein in lung: ontogeny, steroid-induced expression, and distribution in rat. J Clin Invest 97:2183–2191, 1996.

23. Borok Z, Verkman AS. Lung edema clearance: 20 years of progress: invited review: role of aquaporin water channels in fluid transport in lung and airways. J Appl Physiol 93:2199–2206, 2002.

24. Yasui M, Serlachius E, Lofgren M, Belusa R, Nielsen S, Aperia A. Perinatal changes in expression of aquaporin-4 and other water and ion transporters in rat lung. J Physiol 505:3–11, 1997.

25. King LS, Nielsen S, Agre P. Aquaporins in complex tissues. I. Developmental patterns in respiratory and glandular tissues of rat. Am J Physiol Cell Physiol 273:C1541–C1548, 1997.

26. Kreda SM, Gynn MC, Fenstermacher DA, et al. Expression and localization of epithelial aquaporins in the adult human lung. Am J Respir Cell Mol Biol 24:224–234, 2001.

27. Zeuthen T, Klaerke DA. Transport of water and glycerol in aquaporin 3 is gated by H(+). J Biol Chem 274:21631–21636, 1999.

28. Zelenina M, Bondar AA, Zelenin S, Aperia A. Nickel and extracellular acidification inhibit the water permeability of human aquaporin-3 in lung epithelial cells. J Biol Chem 278:30037–30043, 2003.

29. Brigham KL, Bowers RE, Owen PS. Effects of antihistamines on lung vascular response to histamine in unanesthetized sheep. J Clin Invest 58:391–398, 1976.

30. Seghaye M-C, Grabitz RG, Duchateau J, et al. Inflammatory reaction and capillary leak syndrome related to cardiopulmonary bypass in neonates undergoing cardiac operations. J Thorac Cardiovasc Surg 112:687–697, 1996.

31. Neuhof C, Walter O, Dapper F, et al. Bradykinin and histamine generation with generalized enhancement of microvascular permeability in neonates, infants and children undergoing cardio-pulmonary bypass surgery. Ped Crit Care Med 4:299–304, 2003.

32. Goodman BE, Wangensteen D. Alveolar epithelium permeability to small solutes: developmental changes. J App Physiol 52:3–8, 1982.

33. Egan EA, Dillon WP, Zorn S. Fetal lung liquid absorption and alveolar epithelial solute permeability in surfactant deficient, breathing fetal lambs. Pediatr Res 18:566–570, 1984.

34. Jobe A, Jacobs H, Ikegami M, et al. Lung protein leaks in ventilated lambs: effect of gestational age. J Appl Physiol 1246–1251, 1985.

35. Bhat R, Javed S, Malalis L, et al. Colloid osmotic pressure in healthy and sick neonates. Crit Care Med 9:563–567, 1981.

36. Sola SA, Gregory GA. Colloid osmotic pressure of normal newborns and premature infants. Crit Care Med 9:568–572, 1981.

37. Moison RMW, Haasnoot AA, Zoeren-Grobben D, et al. Plasma proteins in acute and chronic lung disease of the newborn. Free Rad Biol Med 25:321–328, 1988.

38. Reed RK, Berg A, Gjerde EA, Rubin K. Control of interstitial fluid pressure: role of beta1-integrins. Seminars in Nephrology 21:222–230, 2001.

39. Reed RK, Rubin K, Wiig H, et al. Blockade of [beta]1-integrins in skin causes edema through lowering of interstitial fluid pressure. Circ Res 71:978–983, 1992.

40. Reed RK, Woie K, Rubin K. Integrins and control of interstitial fluid pressure. News Physiol Sci 12:42–48, 1997.

41. Modi N. Clinical implications of postnatal alterations in body water distribution. Semin Neonatol 8:301–306, 2003.

42. Seghaye M-C, Grabitz RG, Duchateau J, et al. Inflammatory reaction and capillary leak syndrome related to cardiopulmonary bypass in neonates undergoing cardiac operations. J Thorac Cardiovasc Surg 112:687–697, 1996.

43. Neuhof C, Walter O, Dapper F, et al. Bradykinin and histamine generation with generalized enhancement of microvascular permeability in neonates, infants and children undergoing cardio-pulmonary bypass surgery. Ped Crit Care Med 4:299–304, 2003.

44. Zhang P, Wang S, Li Q, et al. Capillary leak syndrome in children with C4A-deficiency undergoing cardiac surgery with cardiopulmonary bypass: a double-blind, randomized controlled study. The Lancet 366:556–562, 2005.

45. Durward A, Mayer A, Skellett S, et al. Hypoalbuminaemia in critically ill children: incidence, prognosis, and influence on the anion gap. Arch Dis Child 88:419–422, 2003.

46. Siflinger-Birnboim A, Johnson A. Protein kinase C modulates pulmonary endothelial permeability: a paradigm for acute lung injury. Am J Physiol Lung Cell Mol Physiol 284:L435–L451, 2003.

47. Davis AE. The pathophysiology of hereditary angioedema. Clinical Immunology 114:3–9, 2005.

48. Libby P, Lee RT. Matrix matters. Circulation 102:1874–1876, 2000.

49. Visse R, Hideaki N. Matrix metalloproteinases and tissue inhibitors of metalloproteinases. Circulation Research 92:827–839, 2003.

50. Passi A, et al. Involvement of lung interstitial proteoglycans in development of hydraulic- and elastase-induced edema. Am J Physiol Lung Cell Mol Physiol 275:L631–L635, 1998.

51. Miserocchi G, et al. Development of lung edema: interstitial fluid dynamics and molecular structure. News Physiol Sci 16:66–71, 2001.

Chapter 13

Renal Failure in the Neonate

Sharon P. Andreoli, MD

Definition
Epidemiology and Incidence of Renal Failure in the Newborn
Etiology of Renal Failure in the Newborn
Medical Management of Acute Renal Failure in the Newborn
Acute and Chronic Renal Replacement Therapy
Prognosis

Acute and chronic renal failure in the neonate is a very common problem and there are many different causes of renal failure in the newborn (Fig. 13-1). While many cases of acute renal failure can resolve with return of renal function to normal, some causes of acute renal failure result in permanent renal injury that is apparent immediately while others may result in renal disease years after the initial insult. It is well known that renal diseases such as renal dysplasia, obstructive uropathy, and cortical necrosis can lead to chronic kidney disease. In contrast, it has been thought in the past that acute kidney injury caused by hypoxic ischemic and nephrotoxic insults was reversible with return of renal function to normal. However, recent studies have demonstrated that hypoxic and ischemic insults can result in physiologic and morphologic alterations in the kidney that can lead to kidney disease at a later time (1,2). Thus, as will be discussed in more detail later, acute renal failure from any cause is a risk factor for later development of kidney disease.

Acute renal failure is classified as prerenal, intrinsic renal disease including vascular insults, and obstructive uropathy. In the newborn, renal failure may have a prenatal onset in congenital diseases such as renal dysplasia with or without obstructive uropathy and in genetic diseases such as autosomal recessive polycystic kidney disease. Newborns with congenital and genetic renal diseases that have a prenatal onset may have stigmata of Potter's syndrome due to in utero oliguria with resultant oligohydramnios. Newborns with Potter's syndrome may have life threatening pulmonary insufficiency, flattened nasal bridge, low-set ears, joint contractures and other orthopedic anomalies due to fetal constraint as a result of the oligohydramnios.

Acute and chronic renal disease can also result from the in utero exposure of the developing kidneys to agents that may interfere with nephrogenesis such as angiotensin converting enzyme inhibitors, angiotensin II receptor blockers and perhaps cylcooxygenase inhibitors (3–7). Exposure of the developing fetus to angiotensin converting enzyme inhibitors and angiotensin receptor blockers have each been associated with renal dysfunction that is acute and chronic, fetal death and under mineralization of the calvarial bones (3–5). Exposure to angiotensin converting enzyme inhibitors or angiotensin receptor blockers is most detrimental for

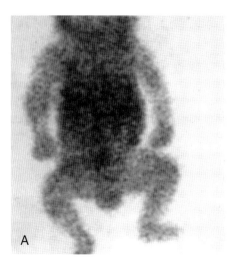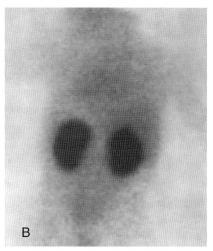

Figure 13-1 Mag-3 renal scan in a newborn with cortical necrosis (A) and ATN (B). Each scan is at 4 h after injection of isotope. A demonstrates no renal parenchymal uptake of isotope in a neonate with cortical necrosis while B shows delayed uptake of isotope with parenchymal accumulation of isotope with little to no excretion of isotope into the collecting system.

renal development when the fetus is exposed in the second and third trimesters but it has recently been shown that exposure during the first trimester is also associated with congenital defects (6).

Renal failure in the newborn is also commonly acquired in the postnatal period due to hypoxic ischemic injury and toxic insults. As in older children, hospital acquired acute renal failure in newborns is frequently multifactorial in origin (8–14). Since nephrogenesis proceeds through approximately 34 weeks' gestation, ischemic/hypoxic and toxic insults to the developing kidney in a premature newborn can result not only in acute renal failure but long term complications associated with potential interrupted nephrogenesis. Whether renal failure is congenital or acquired, it is important to appropriately manage the fluid and electrolyte imbalances and other side effects of renal failure in the newborn.

DEFINITION

Acute and chronic renal failure is characterized by an increase in the blood concentration of creatinine and nitrogenous waste products, a decrease in the glomerular filtration rate and by the inability of the kidney to appropriately regulate fluid and electrolyte homeostasis. Following birth, the serum creatinine in the newborn is a reflection of maternal renal function and cannot be used as a measure of renal function in the newborn shortly after birth (15,16). In full term healthy newborns, the glomerular filtration rate rapidly increases and the serum creatinine declines to about 0.4–0.6 mg/dL at about two weeks of age while the serum creatinine declines at a slower rate in premature infants (14–16). Thus, use of the serum creatinine as a determinate of renal insufficiency requires that the gestational age at time of birth and the postnatal age as well as maternal factors need to be taken into account. It is clear that a change in the serum creatinine is a rough measure of changes in renal function and current studies are under way to define early biomarkers of acute renal injury so that acute renal injury can be defined before changes in the serum creatinine are detected (17). A decrease in urine output is a common clinical manifestation of acute renal failure but many forms of acute renal failure are associated with normal urine output (4). Newborns with prerenal failure, or acute renal failure due to hypoxic/ischemic insults, or cortical necrosis are more likely to have oligo/anuria (urine output less than 1.0 cc/kg/h), while newborns with nephrotoxic renal insults, including aminoglycoside nephrotoxicity and contrast nephropathy, are more likely to have acute renal failure with normal urine output. The morbidity and mortality of nonoliguric acute renal failure is substantially less than oliguric renal failure (9–14). This chapter will review the epidemiology of renal failure in the newborn, the common causes of acute and chronic renal failure in the newborn, with a focus on hypoxic ischemic and nephrotoxic insults, management of acute and chronic renal failure in the newborn, and long term follow up of the neonate who has had acute renal failure.

EPIDEMIOLOGY AND INCIDENCE OF RENAL FAILURE IN THE NEWBORN

The precise incidence and prevalence of renal failure in the newborn is unknown, but several studies have demonstrated that renal failure is common in the neonatal intensive care unit (NICU) (9–19). The incidence of renal failure ranged from 6% to 24% of newborns in NICUs, and in at least one study acute renal failure was particularly common in neonates who had undergone cardiac surgery (9,11,14–16,18). Neonates with severe asphyxia had a high incidence of acute renal failure while acute renal failure is less common in neonates with moderate asphyxia and the acute renal failure was non-oliguric, oliguric, and anuric in 60%, 25%, and 15%, respectively (12). Other studies have demonstrated that very low birth weight (less than 1500 g), a low Apgar Score, a patent ductus arteriosis and maternal administration of antibiotics and nonsteroidal antiinflammatory drugs, was associated with the development of acute renal failure (19). Other studies have also shown that low Apgar score and maternal ingestion of nonsteroidal antiinflammatory drugs is associated with decreased renal function in preterm infants (20,21). The incidence of acute renal failure in newborns in a developing country was 3.9/1000 live births and 34.5/1000 newborns admitted to the neonatal unit (22).

Several very interesting studies have demonstrated that some newborns may have genetic risk factors for acute renal failure. Polymorphism of the angiotensin converting enzyme (ACE) gene or the angiotensin receptor gene with resultant alterations in activity of the renin angiotensin system might play a role in the development of acute renal failure (23). In studies on newborns, polymorphisms of tumor necrosis factor alpha, interleukin 1b, interleukin 6 and interleukin 10 genes were investigated in newborns to determine if polymorphisms of these genes would lead to a more intense inflammatory response and predispose newborns to acute renal failure (24). The allelic frequency of the individual genes did not differ between newborns with acute renal failure and those without acute renal failure, but the TNFa/IL-6 AG/GC haplotypes were present in 26% of newborns who developed acute renal failure compared to 6% of newborns who did not develop acute renal failure. The investigators suggested that the combination of these polymorphisms might lead to a greater inflammatory response and the development of acute renal failure in neonates with infection (24). In other studies, the incidence of ACE I/D allele genotypes or the variants of the angiotensin I receptor gene did not differ in neonates with acute renal failure compared to neonates without acute renal failure, but they may be associated with patent ductus arteriosis and heart failure and indirectly contribute to renal failure (23,25).

Acute renal failure occurred more commonly in very low birth weight neonates carrying the heat shock protein 72 (1267) GG genetic variation, which is associated with low inductability of heat shock protein 72 (26). Given the important role of heat shock proteins in ischemic renal injury, these findings suggest that some neonates are more susceptible to ischemic injury (27). Future studies of the genetic background of the neonate at risk for acute renal failure due to medication exposure, toxin exposure, ischemic hypoxic insults or other insults will likely impact the management of the child at risk for acute renal failure and the management of acute renal failure.

ETIOLOGY OF RENAL FAILURE IN THE NEWBORN

There are many different etiologies of acute renal failure in the neonate (Table 13-1) and the most common are related to prerenal mechanisms, including hypotension, hypovolemia, hypoxemia, perinatal and postnatal asphyxia, and sepsis (28,29). This chapter will highlight the more common causes of renal failure in neonates, including prerenal failure, vasomotor nephropathy/acute tubular necrosis, nephrotoxic insults, and vascular insults.

Prerenal Failure

In prerenal failure, renal function is decreased due to decreased renal perfusion and the kidney is intrinsically normal. Restoration of normal renal perfusion results in a return of renal function to normal while acute tubular necrosis implies that the kidney has suffered intrinsic damage. However, the evolution of prerenal failure to intrinsic renal failure is not sudden and a number of compensatory mechanisms work together to maintain renal perfusion when renal perfusion is compromised (30,31). When renal perfusion is decreased, the afferent arteriole relaxes its vascular tone to decrease renal vascular resistance and maintain renal blood flow. Decreased renal perfusion results in increased catecholamine secretion, activation of the renin angiotensin system and the generation of prostaglandins. During renal hypoperfusion, the intrarenal generation of vasodilatory prostaglandins, including prostacyclin, mediates vasodilatation of the renal microvasculature to maintain renal perfusion (30,31). Administration of aspirin or nonsteroidal antiinflammatory drugs can inhibit this compensatory mechanism and precipitate acute renal insufficiency during renal hypoperfusion. As discussed below, administration of indomethacin for closure of the patent ductus arteriosus in premature newborns is associated with a substantial risk of renal insufficiency (32–36). It was originally thought that selective COX-2 inhibitors would be renal sparing but it has been recognized that the selective COX -2 inhibitors can adversely affect renal hemodymanics similar to the effects of non selective COX inhibitors (37). In addition, clinical use of selective COX-2 inhibitors has been associated with acute renal failure in adult patients (38). Similarly, when renal perfusion pressure is low as in renal artery stenosis, the intraglomerular pressure necessary to drive filtration is in part mediated by increased intrarenal generation of angiotensin II to increase efferent arteriolar resistance (30,39,40). Administration of angiotensin converting enzyme inhibitors in these conditions can eliminate the pressure gradient needed to drive filtration and precipitate acute renal failure (30,39–42). Thus, administration of medications that can interfere with compensatory mechanisms to maintain renal perfusion can precipitate acute renal failure in certain clinical circumstances.

Prerenal failure results from renal hypoperfusion due to true volume contraction or from a decreased effective blood volume (30). Volume contraction results from hemorrhage, dehydration due to gastrointestinal losses, salt wasting renal or adrenal diseases, central or nephrogenic diabetes insipidus, increased insensible losses, and in disease states associated with third space losses such as sepsis, traumatized tissue and capillary leak syndrome, while decreased effective blood volume occurs when the true blood volume is normal or increased but renal perfusion is

Table 13-1   Etiology of Acute Renal Failure in the Neonate

Prerenal failure
Decreased true intravascular volume
  Dehydration
  Gastrointestinal losses
  Salt wasting renal or adrenal disease
  Central or nephrogenic diabetes insipidus
  Third space losses (sepsis, traumatized tissue)
Decreased effective intravascular volume blood volume
  Congestive heart failure
  Pericarditis, cardiac tamponade

Intrinsic renal disease
Acute tubular necrosis
  Ischemic/hypoxic insults
  Drug induced
    Aminoglycosides
    Intravascular contrast
    Non-steroidal anti-inflammatory drugs
  Toxin mediated
    Endogenous toxins
      Rhabdomyolysis, hemoglobinuria
Interstitial nephritis
  Drug induced—antibiotics, anticonvulsants
  Idiopathic
Vascular lesions
  Cortical necrosis
  Renal artery thrombosis
  Renal venous thrombosis
Infectious causes
  Sepsis
  Pyelonephritis

Obstructive uropathy
Obstruction in a solitary kidney
Bilateral ureteral obstruction
Urethral obstruction

Congenital renal diseases
Dysplasia/hypoplasia
Cystic renal diseases
  Autosomal recessive polycystic kidney disease
  Autosomal dominant polycystic kidney disease
  Cystic dysplasia
In utero exposure to ACEI or ARBs

decreased due to diseases such as congestive heart failure and cardiac tamponade (30). Whether prerenal failure is caused by true volume depletion or decreased effective blood volume, correction of the underlying disturbance will return renal function to normal.

The urine osmolality, urine sodium concentration, the fractional excretion of sodium, and the renal failure index have all been proposed to be used to help differentiate prerenal failure from vasomotor nephropathy/acute tubular necrosis (ATN). This differentiation is based on the premise that the tubules are working appropriately in prerenal failure and are therefore able to conserve salt and water appropriately, whilst in vasomotor nephropathy tubules have progressed to irreversible injury and are unable to appropriately conserve sodium (30,48,49).

During prerenal failure, the tubules are able to respond to decreased renal perfusion by appropriately conserving sodium and water such that the urine osmolality is greater than 400–500 mOsm/L, the urine sodium is less than 10–20 meq/L, and the fractional excretion of sodium is less than 1% in children. Since the renal tubules in newborns and premature infants are relatively immature compared to older infants and children, the corresponding values suggestive of renal hypoperfusion are urine osmolality greater than 350 mOsm/L, urine sodium less than 20–30 meq/L, and a fractional excretion of sodium of less than 2.5% (48,49). When the renal tubules have sustained injury, as occurs in acute tubular necrosis, they cannot appropriately conserve sodium and water such that the urine osmolality is <350 mOsm/L, the urine sodium is >30–40 meq/L and the fractional excretion of sodium is > 2.0%. However, the use of these numbers to differentiate prerenal failure from acute tubular necrosis requires that the patient has normal tubular function initially. While this may be the case in some pediatric patients, newborns (particularly premature newborns whose tubules are immature) may have prerenal failure with urinary indices suggestive of ATN. Therefore, it is important to consider the state of the function of the tubules prior to the potential onset that might precipitate vasomotor nephropathy/ATN.

Acute Ischemic Renal Failure and Nephrotoxic Renal Failure

Ischemic acute renal failure (also known as acute tubular necrosis and/or vasomotor nephropathy) can evolve from prerenal failure if the insult is severe and sufficient enough to result in vasoconstriction and acute tubular necrosis. The pathophysiology of ischemic/hypoxic ATN is thought to be related to early vasoconstriction followed by patchy tubular necrosis. The urinalysis may be unremarkable or demonstrate low grade proteinuria and granular casts while urine indices of tubular function demonstrate an inability to conserve sodium and water as described above. The creatinine typically increases by about 0.5–1.0 mg/dL per day. Radiographic studies demonstrate kidneys of normal size with loss of corticomedullary differentiation, while a radionucleotide renal scan with technetium–99-MAG3 or technetium–99-DTPA will demonstrate normal or slightly decreased renal blood flow with poor function and delayed accumulation of the radioisotope in the renal parenchyma without excretion of the isotope in the collecting system (Fig. 13-1B).

In the past it has been thought that the prognosis of ischemic acute renal failure is good except in cases when the insult is of sufficient severity to lead to vasculature injury and microthrombi formation with the subsequent development of cortical necrosis. However, recent studies demonstrate that chronic changes can occur and that such patients are at risk for later complications (1,2). As discussed later, acute renal failure before nephrogenesis is complete may also result in disrupted nephrogenesis and reduced nephron number (43–47).

The recovery of the neonate and the recovery of the renal function depend upon the underlying events that precipitated the ischemic/hypoxic insults. The mortality and morbidity of newborns with acute renal failure are much worse in neonates with multiorgan failure (9,10,12,18,48–52). In neonates who recover from ATN, the renal function returns to normal but the length of time before recovery is quite variable. Some neonates will begin to recover renal function within days of the onset of renal failure while recovery may not occur for several weeks in other newborns. Return of renal function may be accompanied by a diuretic phase with excessive urine output at a time when the tubules have begun to recover from the insult but have not recovered sufficiently to appropriately reabsorb solute and water. When the diuretic phase occurs during recovery, close attention to fluid and electrolyte balance is very important to ensure adequate fluid management to promote recovery from acute tubular necrosis and to prevent additional renal injury. As described below, long term follow up of newborns with acute renal failure is warranted to evaluate for late complications.

Many different drugs and agents may result in nephrotoxic acute renal failure. Nephrotoxic acute renal failure may result from the administration of a number of different medications as well as from indigenous compounds such as hemoglobinuria or myoglobinuria. Nephrotoxic acute renal failure in newborns is commonly associated with aminoglycoside antibiotics, nonsteroidal antiinflammatory medications, intravascular contrast media, amphotericin B while other medications have been implicated less commonly. Aminoglycoside nephrotoxicity usually presents with nonoliguric acute renal failure with a urinalysis showing minimal urinary abnormalities. The incidence of aminoglycoside antibiotic nephrotoxicity is related to the dose and duration of the antibiotic therapy as well as the level of renal function prior to the initiation of aminoglycoside therapy. The etiology of aminoglycoside nephrotoxicity is thought to be related to the lysosomal dysfunction of proximal tubules and is reversible once the aminoglycoside antibiotics have been discontinued (53). However, after the aminoglycoside is discontinued, the serum creatinine may continue to increase for several days due to ongoing tubular injury from continued high parenchymal levels of the aminoglycoside. Acute renal failure may also occur after administration of angiotensin converting enzyme inhibitors, probably by alteration in intrarenal hemodymanics (41).

Nonsteroidal antiinflammatory drugs may also precipitate acute renal failure by their effect on intrarenal hemodynamics (30–38). Indomethacin therapy, to promote closure of the patent ductus arteriosus in premature neonates, is associated with renal dysfunction including a 56% reduction in urinary flow rate, a 27% reduction in glomerular filtration rate and a 66% reduction in free water clearance (32,33). Other physiologic alterations following administration of indomethacin and ibuprofen include a decrease in urinary endothelin-1 (ET-1) and arginine vasopressin (AVP), along with a reduction in urinary sodium excretion and fractional excretion of sodium (34). Alterations in renal function occur in approximately 40% of premature newborns who have received indomethacin and such alterations are usually reversible (35). In a large study of more than 2500 premature newborns treated with indomethacin to promote closure of the patent ductus arteriosus, infants with pre-existing renal and electrolyte abnormalities and infants whose mothers had received indomethacin tocolysis, or who had chorioamnionitis, were at significantly increased risk for the development of renal impairment (36).

Hemolysis and rhabdomyolysis from any cause can result in sufficient hemoglobinuria or myoglobinuria to induce tubular injury and precipitate acute renal failure (54,55). Risk factors for acute renal failure during an episode of rhabdomyolysis in children include dehydration, the serum concentration of myoglobin, the presence of other organ failure, and the presence of the systemic inflammatory response syndrome (55). The mechanisms of injury are complex but may be related to vasoconstriction, precipitation of the pigments in the tubular lumen and/or heme-protein induced oxidant stress (55,56).

Vascular Injury

Renal artery thrombosis and renal vein thrombosis will result in renal failure if bilateral or if either occurs in a solitary kidney. Renal artery thrombosis is strongly associated with an umbilical artery line and a patent ductus arteriosus (57,58). In addition to acute renal failure, children may demonstrate hypertension, gross or microscopic hematuria, thrombocytopenia and oliguria. In renal artery thrombosis, the initial ultrasound may appear normal or demonstrate minor abnormalities, while a renal scan will demonstrate little to no blood flow. In renal vein thrombosis, the ultrasound demonstrates an enlarged, swollen kidney, while the renal scan typically demonstrates decreased blood flow and function. Therapy should be aimed at limiting extension of the clot by removal of the umbilical arterial catheter and anticoagulate or fibrinolytic therapy can be considered particularly if the clot is large (57–60).

Cortical necrosis is associated with hypoxic/ischemic insults due to perinatal anoxia, placenta abruption and twin–twin or twin–maternal transfusions with resultant activation of the coagulation cascade (61,62). Interestingly, intrauterine laser treatment in 18 sets of twins with twin–twin transfusion resulted in no long term renal impairment despite severe alterations of renal function, including anuria and polyuria before the laser treatment (63). Newborns with cortical necrosis usually have gross or microscopic hematuria, oliguria and may have hypertension as well (64). In addition to laboratory features of an elevated blood urea nitrogen (BUN) and creatinine, thrombocytopenia may also be present due to the microvascular injury. Radiographic features include a normal renal ultrasound in the early phase while ultrasound in the later phases may show that the kidney has undergone atrophy and has substantially decreased in size. A radionucleotide renal scan will show decreased to no perfusion with delayed or no function (Fig. 13-1A) in contrast to delayed uptake of the radioisotope, which is observed in ATN (Fig. 13-1B). The prognosis of cortical necrosis is worse than that of acute tubular necrosis. Children with cortical necrosis may have partial recovery or no recovery at all. Typically, children with cortical necrosis will need short or long-term dialysis therapy but children who do recover sufficient renal function are at risk for the late development of chronic renal failure.

MEDICAL MANAGEMENT OF ACUTE RENAL FAILURE IN THE NEWBORN

Once intrinsic renal failure has become established, management of the metabolic complications of acute renal failure involves appropriate management of fluid balance, electrolyte status, acid-base balance, nutrition and the initiation of renal replacement therapy when appropriate. Diuretic therapy to stimulate urine output eases management of acute renal failure but the conversion of oliguric to nonoliguric acute renal failure has not been shown to alter the course of acute renal failure (65). Diuretic therapy has potential theoretical mechanisms to prevent, limit or improve renal function. Mannitol (0.5–1.0 g/kg over several minutes) may increase intratubular urine flow to limit tubular obstruction, may limit cell damage by prevention of swelling or by acting as a scavenger of free radicals or reactive oxygen molecules. Lasix (1–5 mg/kg/dose) will also increase urine flow rate to decrease intratubular obstruction and will inhibit $Na^+K^+ATPase$, which will limit oxygen consumption in already damaged tubules with a low oxygen supply. When using mannitol in neonates with acute renal failure, a lack of response to therapy can precipitate congestive heart failure, particularly if the newborn's intravascular volume is expanded before mannitol infusion. In addition, lack of excretion of mannitol may also result in substantial hyperosmolality. Similarly, administration of high doses of lasix in renal failure has been associated with ototoxicity (65). When using diuretic therapy in newborns with acute renal failure, potential risks and benefits need to be considered. When the neonate is unresponsive to therapy, continued high doses of diuretics are not justified and unlikely to be beneficial to the neonate. In neonates who do respond to therapy, continuous infusions may be more effective and may be associated with less toxicity than bolus administration.

The use of 'renal' dose dopamine (0.5 to 3–5 µg/kg/min) to improve renal perfusion following an ischemic insult has become very common in intensive care units. While dopamine increases renal blood flow by promoting vasodilatation and may improve urine output by promoting natriuresis, there are no definitive studies to demonstrate that low dose dopamine is effective in decreasing the need for dialysis or improving survival in patients with acute renal failure (66,67). In fact, a placebo controlled randomized study of low dose dopamine in adult patients demonstrated that low dose dopamine was not beneficial and did not confer clinically significant protection from renal dysfunction (68). Other studies have demonstrated that renal dose dopamine is not effective in the therapy of acute renal failure and one study demonstrated that low dose dopamine worsened renal perfusion and renal function (69–71).

Intravenous infusion of theophylline in severely asphyxiated neonates given within the first hour after birth was associated with improved fluid balance, creatinine clearance, and reduced serum creatinine levels with no effects on neurological and respiratory complications (72). Other studies in asphyxiated neonates also demonstrated improved renal function and decreased excretion of β-2 microglobulin in the neonates given theophylline within 1 h of birth (73,74). However, the clinical significance of the improved renal function was not clear and the incidence of persistent pulmonary hypertension was higher in the neonates who had received theophylline (75). Additional studies are needed to determine the significance of these findings and the potential side effects of theophylline.

Mild hyponatremia is very common in acute renal failure and may be due to hyponatremia dehydration but fluid overload with dilutional hyponatremia is much more common. If the serum sodium is >120 meq/L, fluid restriction or water removal by dialytic therapy will correct the serum sodium. However, if the serum sodium is <120 meq/L, the child is at higher risk for seizures due to hyponatremia, and correction to a sodium level of approximately 125 meq/L with hypertonic saline should be considered. Since the kidney tightly regulates potassium balance and excretes approximately 90% of dietary potassium intake, hyperkalemia is a common and potentially life threatening electrolyte abnormality in acute renal failure (76). The serum potassium level may be falsely elevated if the technique of the blood drawing is traumatic and/or if the specimen is hemolyzed. Hyperkalemia results in disturbances of cardiac rhythm by its depolarizing effect on the cardiac conduction pathways. The concentration of serum potassium that results in arrhythmia is dependent upon the acid base balance and the other serum electrolytes. Hypocalcemia, which is common in renal failure, exacerbates the adverse effects of the serum potassium on cardiac conduction pathways. Tall peaked T-waves are the first manifestation of cardiotoxicity while prolongation of the PR interval, flattening of P waves and widening of QRS complexes are later abnormalities. Severe hyperkalemia will eventually lead to ventricular tachycardia and fibrillation and requires prompt therapy with sodium bicarbonate, intravenous glucose and insulin, intravenous calcium gluconate and albuterol (77,78). Albuterol infusions of 400 µg, given every 2h as needed, have been shown to rapidly lower serum potassium levels (78). Each of these therapies are temporizing measures and do not remove potassium from the body. Kayexalate given orally, per nasogastric tube or per rectum, will exchange sodium for potassium in the gastrointestinal tract and result in potassium removal (76,79). Complications of kayexalate therapy include possible hypernatremia, sodium retention and constipation. In addition, kayexalate therapy has been associated with intestinal necrosis (80). Depending upon the degree of hyperkalemia and the need for correction of other metabolic derangements in acute renal failure, hyperkalemia frequently requires the initiation of dialysis or hemofiltration. Since the kidney excretes net acids generated by diet and intermediary metabolism, acidosis is very common in acute renal failure. Severe acidosis can be treated with intravenous or oral sodium bicarbonate, oral sodium citrate solutions, and/or with dialysis therapy. When considering treatment of acidosis, it is important to consider the serum ionized calcium level. Under

Table 13-2   Comparison of Renal Replacement Therapies

	PD	HD	CVVH(D)
Solute removal	+++	++++	+(+++)
Fluid removal	++	+++	+++(+++)
Toxin removal	+	++++	− (+)
Removal of potassium	++	++++	+(++)
Removal of ammonia	+	++++	+(+++)
Need for hemodynamic stability	−	+++	−(−)
Need for anticoagulation	−	++	−/+(−/+)
Ease of access	+++	−	−
Continuous	+++	−	+++(+++)
Respiratory compromise	++	−	−(−)
Peritonitis	++++	−	−
Hypotension	+	+++	+++(+++)
Disequilibrium	−	+++	−(−)
Reverse osmosis water	−	++++	−(−)

PD, peritoneal dialysis; HD, hemodialysis; CVVH(D), continuous venovenous hemofiltration (diafiltration).

normal circumstances, approximately half the total calcium is protein bound while half is free and in the ionized form, which is what determines the transmembrane potential and electrochemical gradient. Hypocalcemia is common in acute renal failure and acidosis will increase the fraction of total calcium to the ionized form. Treatment of acidosis can then shift the ionized calcium to the more normal ratio, decreasing the amount of ionized calcium and precipitating tetany and/or seizures.

Since the kidney excretes the large amount of ingested phosphorus, hyperphosphatemia is a very common electrolyte abnormality noted during acute renal failure. Hyperphosphatemia should be treated with dietary phosphorus restriction and with oral calcium carbonate or other calcium compounds to bind phosphorus and prevent gastrointestinal absorption of phosphorus (81). Since most patients with acute renal failure have hypocalcemia, the use of calcium containing phosphate binders provides a source of calcium as well as phosphate binding capacity.

In many instances acute renal failure is associated with marked catabolism and malnutrition can develop rapidly, leading to delayed recovery from acute renal failure. Prompt and proper nutrition is essential in the management of the newborn with acute and chronic renal failure. If the gastrointestinal tract is intact and functional, enteral feedings with formula (PM 60/40) should be instituted as soon as possible. If the newborn is oligo/anuric and sufficient calories cannot be achieved while maintaining appropriate fluid balance, the earlier initiation of dialysis should be instituted.

ACUTE AND CHRONIC RENAL REPLACEMENT THERAPY

Renal replacement therapy is provided to remove endogenous and exogenous toxins, and to maintain fluid, electrolyte and acid base balance until renal function returns or to maintain the neonate until renal transplantation is possible. Renal replacement therapy may be provided by peritoneal dialysis, intermittent hemodialysis, and hemofiltration with or without a dialysis circuit. Peritoneal dialysis and hemodialysis are options for long term dialysis in infants whose renal function does not improve, while hemofiltration is used for acute renal failure. Each mode of renal replacement therapy has specific advantages and disadvantages (Table 13-2). For acute renal failure the preferential use of hemofiltration by pediatric nephrologists is increasing and the use of peritoneal dialysis is decreasing except for neonates and small infants (82).

There are no studies in newborns comparing the outcome of acute or chronic renal failure when different renal replacement therapies are used in the treatment of acute or chronic renal failure. A recent study of the choice of renal replacement therapy by pediatric nephrologists demonstrated that the use of peritoneal dialysis, hemodialysis, and hemofiltration in children with acute renal failure was approximately 30%, 20%, and 40%, respectively (82). Many factors, including the age and size of the child, the cause of renal failure, the degree of metabolic derangements, blood pressure and nutritional needs were considered in deciding when to initiate renal replacement therapy and the modality of therapy (82).

The indications to initiate renal replacement therapy are not absolute and take into consideration a number of factors, including the cause of renal failure, the rapidity of the onset of renal failure, the severity of fluid and electrolyte abnormalities and the nutritional needs of the neonate. Since neonates and infants have less muscle mass compared to older children, they require initiation of renal replacement therapy at lower serum levels of serum creatinine and BUN compared to older children. The presence of fluid overload unresponsive to diuretic therapy and the need for enteral feedings or hyperalimentation to support nutritional needs is an important factor in considering the initiation of renal replacement therapy.

Peritoneal Dialysis

Peritoneal dialysis has been a major modality of therapy for acute and chronic renal failure in the neonate since vascular access is difficult to maintain in newborns (9,10,82–85). Advantages of peritoneal dialysis is that it is relatively easy to perform, does not require heparinization, and the newborn does not need to be hemodynamically stable to undergo peritoneal dialysis. The disadvantages include a slower correction of metabolic parameters and the potential for peritonitis. To increase the efficiency of peritoneal dialysis, frequent exchanges as often as every hour and use of dialysate with higher glucose concentrations will remove more solute and water, respectively. Relative contraindications include recent abdominal surgery and massive organomegaly or intra–abdominal masses as well as ostomies, which may increase the risk of peritonitis.

Access to the peritoneal cavity is usually through a Tenckhoff catheter. Commercially available 1.5%, 2.5% and 4.25% glucose solutions are available for use in peritoneal dialysis. In older children, peritoneal dialysis is usually initiated with volumes of 15–20 cc/kg body weight, while neonates usually initiate peritoneal dialysis with slightly lower volumes of 5–10 cc/kg body weight. Low volume peritoneal dialysis will have a milder effect on the hemodynamic status of the neonate and has been shown to effectively control uremia and promote ultrafiltration in neonates and older children (85,86). The dialysate volume can be increased depending upon the need for additional solute and fluid removal and the cardiovascular and respiratory status. If the neonate has lactate acidosis, dialysis with the standard solutions will increase the lactate load and aggravate the acidosis. Peritoneal dialysis with a bicarbonate buffered dialysate solution should be used in the neonate with lactate acidosis (86).

Substantial fluid and electrolyte imbalances can occur during peritoneal dialysis, especially when using frequent exchanges, while prolonged use of hypertonic glucose solutions can result in hyperglycemia, hypernatremia and hypovolemia. Peritonitis (dialysate WBC > 100/mm^3) is another complication of acute peritoneal dialysis and can be treated with intraperitoneal antibiotics. If the neonate develops hypokalemia or hypophosphatemia during the course of dialysis, then 3–5 meq/L of KCL or 2–3 meq/L KPO_4 can be added to the dialysate. To avoid hypothermia in the neonates, the dialysate should be warmed to body temperature prior to infusion into the peritoneal cavity.

Although technically challenging, long term peritoneal dialysis has been carried out in very low birth weight infants with a weight as low as 930 g (84) while short term peritoneal dialysis has been used in smaller premature newborns (83). Peritoneal dialysis has been shown to provide adequate clearance in neonates with acute renal failure following cardiopulmonary bypass (87). The majority of infants who have undergone long term peritoneal dialysis were found to have normal developmental milestones or attended school regularly and had good growth and development (88). Neonates and infants with oliguria and with extra-renal abnormalities had a higher mortality rate compared to infants with isolated renal disease and nonoliguric renal failure (89).

Hemodialysis

Hemodialysis has also been used for several years in the treatment of acute and chronic renal failure during childhood (82,90,91). Hemodialysis has the advantage that metabolic abnormalities can be corrected rather quickly and hypervolemia can be corrected by rapid ultrafiltration as well (90,91). The disadvantages of hemodialysis include the requirement for heparinization, the need for maximally purified water by a reverse osmosis system and the need for skilled nursing personnel. Hemodialysis is commonly used for the treatment of metabolic disorders associated with hyperammonemia from urea cycle defects (92). Relative contraindications include hemodynamic instability or severe hemorrhage. When hemodialysis is needed in the child who has active hemorrhage or who is at high risk of hemorrhage, regional heparinization, citrate anticoagulation, and/or heparin free dialysis can be used to minimize the risk of hemorrhage (93).

During hemodialysis, rapid ultrafiltration may also result in hypotension, which has also been shown to result in additional renal ischemia and potentially prolongs the episode of acute renal failure (94). Rapid removal of BUN and other uremic products can result in dialysis disequilibrium, particularly if the child begins hemodialysis with a high BUN (greater than 120–150 mg/dL). The pathogenesis of this syndrome is complex and multifactorial but may be related to the removal of urea from the blood while brain levels decline slower, such that disequilibrium occurs; symptoms include restlessness, fatigue, headache, nausea, vomiting, leading to confusion, seizures and coma (95,96). This severe complication of hemodialysis can be prevented by slowly lowering the BUN during hemodialysis and by the prophylactic infusion of mannitol (0.5–1 g/kg body weight) during hemodialysis to counteract the decline in the serum osmolality that occurs during hemodialysis.

Vascular access in newborns can be provided by umbilical vessels while older infants and children require catheterization of a large vessel to obtain blood flows adequate for hemodialysis. Catheters can be placed in the internal or external jugular veins or in the femoral vein. To avoid hypotension, the total volume of the dialysate circuit, including the dialyzer and tubing, should not exceed 10% of the neonates' blood volume. Blood flow rates to achieve clearances of 1.5–3.0 ml/kg/min are utilized depending upon the indications for dialysis, the initial BUN level and degree of azotemia, and the clinical status of the newborn. Again, depending upon the clinical status of the child and the degree of azotemia, clearances can be increased to 3–5 cc/kg/min in subsequent dialysis sessions. To maintain adequate control of azotemia and to allow for adequate nutrition during acute renal failure, frequent hemodialysis as often as daily may be needed, especially in the newborn.

Another important consideration in treating the child with hemodialysis for acute renal failure is the choice of a dialysis membrane. Several studies in adults have shown that cuprophane membranes are bio-incompatible and activate complement (98) and polymorphonuclear neutrophiles (PMNs) to degranulate, produce reactive oxygen molecules, and initiate the generation of proinflammatory cytokines (97–100). The generation of these toxic products results in additional systemic and renal injury, potentially prolonging the course of renal failure. In other studies, the use of high-flux polyacrylonitrile (AN 69) membranes in patients receiving angiotensin converting enzyme inhibitors was associated with anaphylactic reactions (101–103).

Hemofiltration

Over the past several years, renal replacement therapy with hemofiltration, including continuous venovenous hemofiltration (CVVH) or with the addition of a dialysis circuit to the hemofilter, continuous venovenous hemodiafiltration (CVVHD), has become increasingly popular in the treatment of acute renal failure during childhood (82, 104–106). Hemofiltration without dialysis (CVVH) follows the principle of removal of large quantities of ultrafiltrate from plasma with the replacement of an isosmotic electrolyte solution, while hemofiltration with dialysis (CVVHD) also results in solute removal via the added dialysis circuit. The advantages of hemofiltration (with or without a dialysis circuit) include that it can result in rapid fluid removal, does not require the patient to be hemodynamically stable and is continuous, avoiding rapid solute and fluid shifts as occurs in hemodialysis. The disadvantages include that hemofiltration may require constant heparinization and there is a potential for severe fluid and electrolyte abnormalities due to the large volume of fluid removed and subsequently replaced (106). Hemofiltration/hemodiafiltration was found to allow good control of fluid, electrolyte and acid-base balance and has been used in newborns with inborn errors of metabolism (106,107). The survival rate in children weighing up to 10 kg undergoing CVVH is similar to older children and adolescents (108). As in hemodialysis, vascular access in newborns can be provided by umbilical vessels while older infants and children require catheterization of a large vessel to obtain blood flows adequate for hemofiltration. Catheters can be placed in the internal or external jugular veins or in the femoral vein. Similar to hemodialysis, the total volume of the extracorporeal circuit, including the hemofilter and tubing, should not exceed 10% of the newborn's blood volume.

PROGNOSIS

In the neonate, the prognosis and recovery from acute renal failure is highly dependent upon the underlying etiology of the acute renal failure (9–14,50–52). Factors that are associated with mortality include multiorgan failure, hypotension, need for pressors, hemodynamic instability, and need for mechanical ventilation and dialysis (9–14,50–52). Overall, mortality in newborns with acute renal failure ranges from 10–61% and is highest in infants with multiorgan failure (9–14). In infants maintained by peritoneal dialysis for acute renal failure, mortality was 64% in oligo/anuric infants compared to 20% in infants with adequate urine output (12). Long term follow up of children with acute renal failure has shown that death and renal sequelae are common 3–5 years following acute renal failure in pediatric patients, suggesting that the detrimental effects of acute renal failure are long lasting (109).

It is well known that neonates with congenital disease, such as dysplasia with or without obstructive uropathy, cortical necrosis, or cystic kidney diseases, are at risk for later development of chronic kidney disease. In contrast, it has been thought that ischemic and nephrotoxic renal injury is reversible with renal function returning to normal. However, recent studies have shown that hypoxic ischemic and nephrotoxic insults can result in alterations that can lead to kidney disease at a later time (1,2,44–47). Thus, acute renal failure from any cause is a risk factor for subsequent renal disease. Acute renal failure in the full term neonate is associated with renal disease later in life (43). In one study of 6 older children with a history of acute renal failure not requiring dialysis in the neonate, only two were normal, three had chronic renal failure and one was on dialysis (43). While the number of children studied was small, this study raises concern about the long term renal outcome for such children. An inverse relationship between the development of hypertension and proteinuria during adulthood and birth weight has been reported (43,44,47).

The long term effect of acute renal failure in the neonate is potentially compounded when the insult occurs before the full complement of nephrons has developed in utero. Since nephrogenesis proceeds until 34 weeks' gestation, acute renal failure before this time may result in reduced nephron number. Indeed, it has been shown that preterm neonates with acute renal failure have a high incidence of a low glomerular filtration rate and increasing proteinuria several years later (45) and that morphologic studies have shown decreased nephron number and glomerulomegaly (46). Several studies in animal models and some human studies have documented that hyperfiltration of the remnant nephron may eventually lead to progressive glomerulosclerosis of the remaining nephrons. Typically, the late development of chronic renal failure first becomes apparent with the development of hypertension, proteinuria, and eventually an elevated BUN and creatinine.

When premature neonates were investigated during childhood (ages 6.1 to 12.4 years) defects in tubular reabsorption of phosphorus were evident and the TRP was significantly lower and the urinary excretion of phosphorus significantly higher compared to control children (110). Urinary calcium excretion was also higher in children born prematurely compared to control children. Others have found nearly identical findings and the investigators attributed these alterations to aminoglycoside nephrotoxicity (111,112) In view of these alterations in renal function, increasing proteinuria and tubular dysfunction, neonates with acute renal failure and nephrotoxic insults need lifelong monitoring of their renal function, blood pressure, and urinalysis.

REFERENCES

1. Basile DP, Donohoe D, Roethe K, et al. Renal ischemic injury results in permanent damage to peritubular capillaries and influences long-term outcome. Am J Physiol 281:F887–F889, 2001.
2. Basile D. Rarefaction of peritubular capillaries following ischemic acute renal failure: a potential factor predisposing progressive nephropathy. Curr Opin Nephrol Hypertens 13:1–13, 2004.
3. Pryde PG, Sedman AB, Nugents CE, Basrr M. Angiotensin converting enzyme inhibitor fetopathy. J Am Soc Nephrol 3:1575–1582, 1993.
4. Lip GYH, Churchill D, Beevers M, et al. Angiotensin converting enzyme inhibitors in early pregnancy. Lancet 350:1446–1447, 1997.
5. Martinovic J, Benachi A, Laurent N, et al. Fetal toxic effects and angiotensin-II-receptor antagonists. Lancet 358:241–242, 2001.
6. Cooper WO, Hernandez-Diaz S, Arbogast PG, et al. Major congenital malformations after first-trimester exposure to ACE inhibitors. N Eng J Med 354:2443–2451, 2006.
7. Benini D, Fanos V, Cuzzolin L, Tato L. In utero exposure to nonsteroidal anti-inflammatory drugs: Neonatal acute renal failure. Pediatr Nephrol 19:232–234, 2004.
8. Hui-Stickle S, Brewer ED, Goldstein SL. Pediatric ARF epidemiology at a tertiary care center from 1999 to 2001. Am J Kidney Dis 45:96–101, 2005.
9. Mathews DE, West KW, Rescorla FJ, Vane DW, Grosfeld JL, Wappner RS, Bergstein J, Andreoli SP. Peritoneal dialysis in the first 60 days of life. J Pediatr Surg 25:110–116, 1990.
10. Andreoli SP. Acute renal failure. Curr Opin Pediatr 17:713–717, 2002.
11. Mogal NE, Brocklebank JT, Meadow SR. A review of acute renal failure in children: incidence, etiology and outcome. Clin Nephrol 49:91–95, 1998.
12. Karlowivz MG, Adelman RD. Nonoliguric and oliguric acute renal failure. Pediatr Nephrol 9:718–722, 1995.
13. Andreoli SP: Renal failure in the newborn init. In Polin RA, Yoder MC, Berg FD, (eds) Workbook in Practical Neonatology (pp. 322–337). Philadelphia, PA: W.B. Saunders Co., 2000.
14. Gouyon JB, Guignard JP. Management of acute renal failure in newborns. Pediatr Nephrol 14:1037–1044, 2000.
15. Vanpee M, Blennow M, Linne T, Herin P, Aperia A. Renal function in very low birth weight infants: Normal maturity reached during childhood. J Pediatr 121:784–788, 1992.

16. Drukker A, Guignard JP. Renal aspects of the term and preterm infant: a selective update. Current Opinion in Pediatrics 14:175–182, 2002.

17. Goldstein SL. Pediatric acute kidney injury: it's time for real progress. Pediatr Nephrol 21:891–895, 2006.

18. Martin-Ancel A, Garcia-Alix A, Gaya F, et al. Multiple organ involvement in perinatal asphyxia. J Pediatr 127:786–793, 1995.

19. Cataldi L, Leone R, Moretti U, et al. Potential risk factors for the development of acute renal failure in preterm newborn infants: A case controlled study. Arch Dis Child Fetal Neonatal Ed 90:514–519, 2005.

20. Aggarwal A, Kumar P, Chowkhary G, et al. Evaluation of renal function in asphyxiated newborns. J Trop Pediatr 51:295–299, 2005.

21. Cuzzolin L, Fanos V, Pinna B, et al. Postnatal renal function in preterm newborns: a role of diseases, drugs and therapeutic interventions. Pediatr Nephrol 21:931–938, 2006.

22. Airede A, Bello M, Werasingher HD. Acute renal failure in the newborn: Incidence and outcome. J Paediatr Child Health 33:246–249, 1997.

23. Nobilis A, Kocsis I, Toth-Heyn P, et al. Variance of ACE and AT1 receptor genotype does not influence the risk of neonatal acute renal failure. Pediatr Nephrol 16:1063–1066, 2001.

24. Vasarhelyi B, Toth-Heyn P, Treszl A, Tulassay T. Genetic polymorphism and risk for acute renal failure in preterm infants. Pediatr Nephrol 20:132–135, 2005.

25. Treszl A, Toth-Heyn P, Koscic I. Interleukin genetic variants and the risk of renal failure in infants with infection. Pediatr Nephrol 17:713–717, 2002.

26. Fekkete A, Treszl A, Toht-Heyn P, et al. Association between heat shock protein 72 gene polymorphism and acute renal failure in neonates. Pediatr Res 54:452–455, 2003.

27. Kelly KJ, Baird NR, Greene AL. Induction of stress response proteins and experimental renal ischemia/reperfusion. Kidney Int 59:1798–1802, 2001.

28. Toth-Heyn P, Dukker A, Guignard JP. The stressed neonatal kidney: from pathophysiology to clinical management of neonatal vasomotor nephropathy. Pediatr Nephrol 14:227–239, 2000.

29. Andreoli SP. Acute renal failure in the newborn. Seminars in Perinatology 28:112–123, 2004.

30. Badr KF, Ichikawa I. Prerenal failure: a deleterious shift from renal compensation to decompensation. N Engl J Med 319:623–628, 1988.

31. van Bel F, Guit GL, Schipper J, van de Bor M, Baan J. Indomethacin-induced changes in renal blood flow velocity waveform in premature infants investigated with color Doppler imaging. J Pediatr 118:621–626, 1991.

32. Cifuentes RF, Olley PR, Balfe JW, Radde IC, Soldin SJ. Indomethacin and renal function in premature infants with persistent patent ductus arteriosus. J Pediatr 95:583–587, 1979.

33. Allegaert K, Vanhole C, de Hoon J, et al. Nonselective cyclo-oxygensae inhibitors and glomerular filtration rate in preterm infants. Pediatr Nephrol 20:1557–1561, 2005.

34. Zanardo V, Vedovato S, Lago P, et al. Urinary ET-1, AVP and sodium in premature infants treated with indomethacin and ibuprofen for patent ductus arteriosus. Pediatr Nephrol 20:1552–1556, 2005.

35. Gersony WM, Peckham GJ, Ellison RC, Miettienen OS, Nadas AS. Effects of indomethacin in premature infants with patent ductus arteriosus: results of a national collaborative stud. J Pediatr 102:895–906, 1983.

36. Itabashi K, Ohno T, Nishda H. Indomethacin responsiveness of patent ductus arteriosus and renal abnormalities in preterm infants treated with indomethacin. J Pediatr 143:203–207, 2003.

37. Brater DC. Effects of nonsteroidial anti-inflammatory drugs on renal function: Focus on cyclooxygenase-2-selective inhibitors. Am J Med 107:65S–71S, 1999.

38. Perazella MA, Eras J. Are selective COX-2 inhibitors nephrotoxic? Am J Kidney 35:937–940, 2000.

39. Tack ED, Perlman JM. Renal failure in sick hypertensive premature infants receiving captopril therapy. J Pediatr 112:805–810, 1988.

40. Wood EG, Bunchman TE, Lynch RE. Captopril-induced reversible acute renal failure in an infant with coarctation of the aorta. Pediatrics 88:816–818, 1991.

41. Dutta S, Narnag A. Enalapril induced acute renal failure in a newborn infant. Pediatr Nephrol 18:570–572, 2003.

42. Hricik DE, Dunn MJ. Angiotensin converting enzyme inhibitor-induced acute renal failure: causes, consequences, and diagnostic uses. J Am Soc Nephrol 1:845–858, 1990.

43. Polito C, Papale MR, LaManna AL. Long-term prognosis of acute renal failure in the full term newborn. Clin Pediatr 37:381–386, 1998.

44. Tulassay T, Vasarheleyi B. Birth weight and renal function. Curr Opin Neph Hypertens 11:347–352, 2002.

45. Abitbol CL, Bauer CR, Montane B, et al. Long term follow-up of extremely low birth weight infants with neonatal renal failure. Pediatr Nephrol 18:887–893, 2003.

46. Rodriguez MM, Gomez A, Abitbol C, Chandar J, Montane B, Zilleruelo G. Comparative renal histomorphometry: A case study of oliogonephropathy of prematurity. Pediatr Nephrol 20:945–949, 2005.

47. Keijzer-Veen MG, et al. Microalbuminaria and lower glomerular filtration rate at young adult age in subjects born very prematurely and after intrauterine growth retardation. J Am Soc Nephrol 16:2762–2768, 2005.

48. Mathew OP, Jones AS, James E, Bland H, Groshong T. Neonatal renal failure: Usefulness of diagnostic indices. Pediatrics 65:57–60, 1980.

49. Ellis EN, Arnold WC. Use of urinary indexes in renal failure in the newborn. Am J Dis Child 136:615–617, 1982.
50. Perlman JM, Tack ED. Renal injury in the asphyxiated newborn infant: relationship to neurologic outcome. 113:875–879, 1988.
51. Stapleton FB, Jones DP, Green RS. Acute renal failure in neonates: incidence, etiology and outcome. Pediatr Nephrol 1:314–320, 1987.
52. Gallego N, Perez-Caballero C, Estepa R, Liano F, Ortuno J. Prognosis of patients with acute renal failure without cardiomyopathy. Arch Dis Childhood 84:258–260, 2001.
53. Humes HD. Aminoglycoside nephrotoxicity. Kidney Int 33:900–911, 1988.
54. Kasik JW, Leuschen MP, Bolam DL, Nelson RM. Rhabdomyolysis and myoglobinemia in neonates. Pediatrics 76:255–258, 1985.
55. Watanabe T. Rhabdomyolysis and acute renal failure in children. Pediatr Nephrol 16:1072–1075, 2001.
56. Andreoli SP. Reactive oxygen molecules, oxidant injury and renal disease. Pediatr Nephrol 5:733–742, 1991.
57. Payne RM, Martin TC, Bower RJ, Canter CE. Management and follow-up of arterial thrombosis in the neonatal period. J Pediatr 114:853–858, 1989.
58. Ellis D, Kaye RD, Bontempo FA. Aortic and renal artery thrombosis in a neonate: Recovery with thrombolytic therapy. Pediatr Nephrol 11:641–644, 1997.
59. Chevalier RL. What treatment do you advise for bilateral or unilateral renal thrombosis in the newborn, with or without thrombosis of the inferior vena cava? Pediatr Nephrol 5:679, 1991.
60. Mocan H, Beattie TJ, Murphy AV. Renal venous thrombosis in infancy: long-term follow-up. Pediatr Nephrol 5:45–49, 1991.
61. Christensen AM, Daouk GH, Norling LL, Catlin EA, Ingelfinger JR. Postnatal transient renal insufficiency in the feto-fetal transfusion syndrome. Pediatr Nephrol 13:117–120, 1999.
62. Cincotta RB, Gray PH, Phythian G, et al. Long term outcome of twin-twin transfusion syndrome. Arch Dis Child Fetal Med 83:F171–F176, 2000.
63. Beck M, Graf C, Ellenrieder B, et al. Long-term outcome of kidney function after twin-twin transfusion syndrome treated by intrauterine laser coagulation. Pediatr Nephrol 20:1657–1659, 2005.
64. Anand SK, Northway JD, Smith JA. Neonatal renal papillary and cortical necrosis. Am J Dis Child 131:773–777, 1977.
65. Kellum JA. Use of diuretics in the acute care setting. Kidney Int 53:67–70, 1998.
66. Denton MD, Chertow GM, Brady HR. 'Renal-dose' dopamine for the treatment of acute renal failure: Scientific rationale, experimental studies and clinical trials. Kidney Int 49:4–14, 1996.
67. Chertow GM, Sayegh MH, Allgren RL, Lazarus JM. Is the administration of dopamine associated with adverse or favorable outcomes in acute renal failure? Am J Med 101:498–553, 1996.
68. Australian and New Zealand Intensive Care Society Clinical Trials Group. Low dose dopamine in patients with early renal dysfunction: a placebo controlled trial. Lancet 356:2139–2143, 2000.
69. Kellum JA, Decker JM. Use of dopamine in acute renal failure: A meta-analysis. Crit Care Med 29:1526–1531, 2001.
70. Galley HF. Renal dose dopamine: will the message get through? Lancet 356:2112–2113, 2000.
71. Lauschke A, Teichgraber UKM, Frei U, Eckardt KU. 'Low-dose' dopamine worsens renal perfusion in patients with acute renal failure. Kidney Int 69:1669–1674, 2006.
72. Jenik AG, et al. A randomized, double blind, placebo-controlled trail of the effects of prophylactic theophylline on renal function in term neonates with perinatal asphyxia. Pediatrics 105:E45, 2000.
73. Bhat M, Shah ZA, Makidoomi MS, Mufti MH. Theophylline for renal function in term neonates with perinatal asphyxia: a randomized, placebo controlled trial. J Pediatrics 149:180–184, 2006.
74. Bark AF, et al. Prophylactic theophylline to prevent renal dysfunction in newborns exposed to perinatal asphyxia—a study in a developing country. Pediatr Nephrol 20:1249–1252, 2005.
75. Lemley KV. Can theophylline prevent the development of renal dysfunction in neonates with severe asphyxia? Nature Clinical Practice Nephrology 2:196–197, 2006.
76. Rodriguez-Soriano J. Potassium homeostasis and its disturbances in children. Pediatr Nephrol 9:364–374, 1995.
77. Malone TA. Glucose and insulin versus cation-exchange resin for the treatment of hyperkalemia in very low birth weight infants. J Pediatr 118:121–123, 1991.
78. Singh BS, Sadiq HF, Noguchi A, Keenan WJ. Efficacy of albuterol inhalation in treatment of hyperkalemia in premature neonates. J Pediatr 121:16–20, 2002.
79. Bunchman TE, Wood EG, Schenck MH, Weaver KA, Klein BL, Lynch RE. Pretreatment of formula with sodium polystyrene sulfonate to reduce dietary potassium intake. Pediatr Nephrol 5:29–32, 1991.
80. Gerstman BB, Kirkman R, Platt R. Intestinal necrosis associated with postoperative orally administered sodium polystyrene sulfonate in sorbitol. Am J Kid Dis 20:159–161, 1992.
81. Andreoli SP, Dunson JW, Bergstein JM. Calcium carbonate is an effective phosphorus binder in children with chronic renal failure. Am J Kidney Dis 9:206–210, 1987.
82. Belsha CW, Kohaut EC, Warady BA. Dialytic management of childhood acute renal failure: a survey of North American pediatric nephrologists. Pediatr Nephrol 9:361–363, 1995.
83. Steele BT, Vigneux A, Blatz D, Flavin M, Paes B. Acute peritoneal dialysis in infants weighing <1500 g. J Pediatr 110:126–129, 1987.
84. Rainey KE, DiGeronimo R, Pascual-Baralt J. Successful long term peritoneal dialysis in a very low birth weight infant with renal failure secondary to feto-fetal transfusion syndrome. Pediatrics 106:849–852, 2000.

85. Golej J, Kitzmueller E, Herman M, Boigner H, Burda G, Trittenwein G. Low-volume peritoneal dialysis in 116 neonatal and paediatic critical care patients. Eur J Pediatr 161:385–389, 2002.

86. Vaziri ND, Ness R, Wellikson L, Barton C, Greep N. Bicarbonate-buffered peritoneal dialysis. An effective adjunct in the treatment of lactic acidosis. Am J Med 67:392–396, 1979.

87. McNiece KL, Ellis EE, Drummond-Webb JJ, Fontenot EE, et al. Adequacy of peritoneal dialysis in children following cardiopulmonary bypass surgery. Pediatr Nephrol 20:972–976, 2005.

88. Ledermann SE, Scanes ME, Fernando ON, et al. Long-term outcome of peritoneal dialysis in infants. J Pediatr 136:24–29, 2000.

89. Ellis EN, Pearson D, Champion B, Wood EG. Outcome of infants on chronic peritoneal dialysis. Adv Perit Dial 11:266–269, 1995.

90. Donckerwolcke RA, Bunchman TE. Hemodialysis in infants and small children. Pediatr Nephrol 8:103–106, 1994.

91. Sadowski RH, Harmon WE, Jabs K. Acute hemodialysis of infants weighing less than five kilograms. Kidney Int 45:903–906, 1994.

92. Wigand C, Thompson T, Bock GH, Mathis RK, Kjellstrand CM, Mauer SM. The management of life-threatening hyperammonemia. J Pediatr 116:125–128, 1980.

93. Pinnick RV, Wiegmann TB, Diederich DA: Regional citrate anticoagulation for hemodialysis in the patient at high risk for bleeding. N Eng J Med 258–261, 1983.

94. Conger JF.. Does hemodialysis delay recovery form acute renal failure? Semin Dialy 3:146–147, 1990.

95. Arieff AI. Dialysis disequilibrium syndrome: Current concepts on pathogenesis and prevention. Kidney Int 45:629–635, 1994.

96. Silver SM, Sterns RH, Halperin ML. Brain swelling after dialysis: Old urea or new osmoles? Am J Kidney Dis 28:1–13, 1996.

97. Schulman G, Fogo A, Gung A, Badr K, Hakim R. Complement activation retards resolution of acute ischemic renal failure in the rat. Kidney Int 40:1069–1074, 1991.

98. Cheung AK, Parker CJ, Wilcox L, Janatova J. Activation of the alternative pathway of complement by cellulosic hemodialysis membranes. Kidney Int 36:257–265, 1989.

99. Himmelfarb J, Lazarus M, Hakim R. Reactive oxygen species production by monocytes and polymorphonuclear leukocytes during dialysis. Am J Kidney Dis 17:271–276, 1991.

100. Lazarus JM, Owen WF. Role of bio-incompatibility in dialysis morbidity and mortality. Am J Kidney Dis 24:1019–1032, 1994.

101. Verresen L, Waer M, Vanrenterghem Y, Michielsen P. Angiotensin-converting-enzyme inhibitors and anaphylactoid reactions to high-flux membrane dialysis. Lancet 336:1360–1362, 1990.

102. Brunet PH, Jaber K, Berland Y, Baz M. Anaphylactoid reactions during hemodialysis and hemofiltration: Role of associating AN69 membrane and angiotensin I-converting enzyme inhibitors. Am J Kidney Dis XIX:444–447, 1992.

103. Parnes EL, Shapiro WB. Anaphylactoid reactions in hemodialysis patients treated with AN69 dialyzer. Kidney Int 40:1148–1152, 1991.

104. Forni LG, Hilton PJ. Continuous hemofiltration in the treatment of acute renal failure. N Engl J Med 336:1303–1309, 1997.

105. Ronco C, Brendolan A, Bragantini L, Chiaramonte S, Feriani M, Fabris A, et al. Treatment of acute renal failure in newborns by continuous arterio-venous hemofiltration. Kidney Int 29:908–915, 1986.

106. Zobel G, Rod S, Urlesberger B, et al. Continuous renal replacement therapy in critically ill neonates. Kidney Int 53:S169–S173, 1998.

107. Falk MC, Knight JF, Roy LP, Wilcken B, Schell DN, O'Connell AJ, et al. Continuous venovenous hemofiltration in the acute treatment of inborn errors of metabolism. Pediatr Nephrol 8:330–333, 1994.

108. Symons JM, Brophy PD, Gregory MJ, et al. Continuous renal replacement therapy in children up to 10 kg. Am J Kid Dis 984:989, 2003.

109. Askenazi DJ, Feig DI, Graham NM, et al. 3–5 year longitudinal follow up of pediatric patients with acute renal failure. Kidney Int 69:184–189, 2006.

110. Rodriguez-Soriano J, Aguirre M, Oliveros R, Vallo A. Long-term follow-up of extremely low birth weight infants. Pediatr Nephrol 20:579–584, 2005.

111. Jones CA, Bowden LS, Watling R, et al. Hypercalcuria in ex-preterm children aged 7–8 years. Pediatr Nephrol 16:665–671, 2001.

112. Jones C, Judd B. Long term follow-up of extremely low birth weight infants. Pediatr Nephrol 21:299, 2006.

Chapter 14

Obstructive Uropathy: Assessment of Renal Function in the Fetus

Robert L. Chevalier, MD

Obstructive uropathy comprises the greatest identifiable cause of renal insufficiency and renal failure in infants and children (1). This group of disorders creates significant diagnostic and therapeutic challenges for the obstetrician, perinatologist, neonatologist, pediatric nephrologist and pediatric urologist. The hallmark of obstructive uropathy is hydronephrosis, which is most often first detected by fetal ultrasonography. The etiology of the lesions responsible for congenital urinary tract obstruction remains undetermined in most cases, although mutations in certain genes have been implicated in a variety of urinary tract malformations (2,3), and malformation syndromes (4). The natural history of obstructive uropathy remains poorly defined, and an improved understanding of pathophysiology will be necessary to advance diagnosis and management.

While the focus of this review is the assessment of renal function in the fetus, the rationale for measuring fetal renal function is as important as the evaluation itself. Moreover, renal function is inextricably linked to renal growth, development, and adaptation to injury (such as obstruction of the urinary tract). The physician caring for the fetus with obstructive uropathy must be aware of not only the fetal and neonatal outcome, but also the potential function of the kidneys and urinary tract throughout life (Fig. 14-1). The consequences of

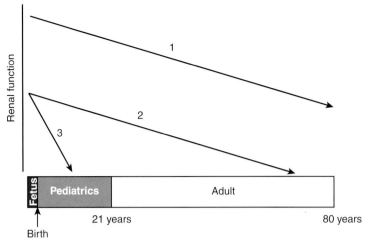

Figure 14-1 Scheme showing long-term impact of congenital obstructive uropathy. The urinary tract abnormality develops in embryonic and fetal life, but if mild (1), the consequences of the condition may become apparent only later in adulthood, if at all. If moderate (2), progression of renal insufficiency may develop earlier in adulthood. If severe (3), renal failure develops in infancy or childhood. Fetal intervention should take into account not only the health and welfare of fetus and mother, but the long-term implications of perinatal management.

urinary tract maldevelopment include not only the challenges of dialysis and transplantation, but also those of recurrent urinary tract infections and urinary incontinence. Any fetal intervention must therefore take into account its potential impact on the patient's expected quality of life through adulthood. For these reasons, the determination of renal function in the fetus is considered in the broad context of congenital obstructive uropathy.

PATHOGENESIS OF CONGENITAL OBSTRUCTIVE UROPATHY

The relative contribution of primary renal maldevelopment and altered renal development secondary to obstruction to urine flow remains unclear. Studies in animals have shown that experimentally induced fetal ureteral or urethral obstruction can result in dysplastic renal changes (generally following obstruction early in gestation), or hydronephrosis with varying degrees of impairment of renal growth and function (following obstruction later in gestation) (5,6). Experimental urinary tract obstruction in the fetal sheep results in a spectrum of renal responses that are remarkably similar to those in the human fetus with obstructive uropathy (7). Hydronephrotic kidneys most often result from bladder outlet obstruction or ureteral obstruction with spontaneous urinary decompression (Fig. 14-2). In contrast, cystic kidneys have grossly visible cysts with effacement of the medulla, while 'dysgenetic' kidneys are small, with decreased numbers of glomeruli and immature tubules surrounded by mesenchymal collars (Fig. 14-2) (7). The consequences of obstruction to urine flow during renal development are highly complex, involving tubular dilatation and altered epithelial–mesenchymal interaction, apoptosis, and cyst formation (Fig. 14-3) (8). If initiated early in fetal life, urinary tract obstruction alters branching morphogenesis, leading to altered induction of glomeruli, podocyte apoptosis, and glomerular cysts (Fig. 14-3). The result of these events is a decrease in nephron number. The severity of obstructive uropathy depends on the severity and timing of obstruction, as well as the site and duration of obstruction (9).

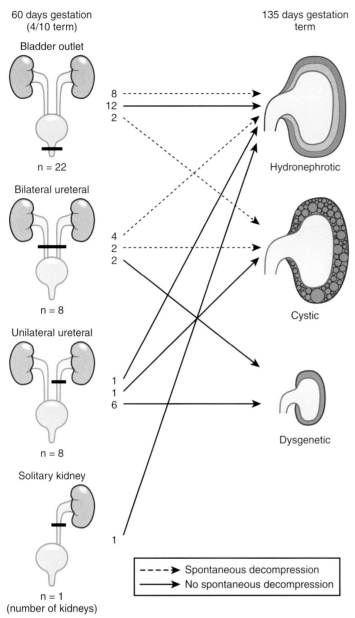

Figure 14-2 Effects of various types of experimental urinary tract obstruction in the fetal sheep. Bladder outlet obstruction most often leads to hydronephrosis (with or without spontaneous decompression), and preservation of corticomedullary differentiation. Bilateral ureteral obstruction with spontaneous decompression leads to hydronephrotic or cystic kidneys, but to dysgenetic kidneys if decompression does not occur. Unilateral ureteral obstruction most often leads to dysgenetic kidneys, but can result in hydronephrotic or cystic kidneys if spontaneous decompression occurs. Cystic kidneys all have spontaneous decompression, and have distortion of the renal architecture by cysts, with preservation of normal intervening structures. Dysgenetic kidneys are small, without visible cysts, without corticomedullary delineation, and with a reduced number of glomeruli, which are abnormal. (From Peters CA, Carr MC, Lais A et al: The response of the fetal kidney to obstruction. J Urol 148:503, 1992, with permission.)

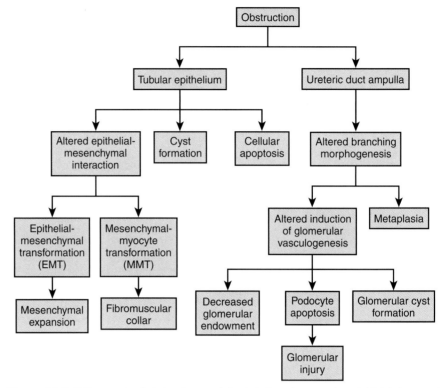

Figure 14-3 Pathogenesis of obstructive renal dysplasia based on experimental fetal sheep and monkey studies. The effects of obstruction involve a combination of renal maldevelopment and injury: first, there is abnormal branching morphogenesis leading directly to a reduction in glomerular development. Second, there is podocyte apoptosis, tubular apoptosis and epithelial-mesenchymal transformation, and interstitial cell transformation to myofibroblasts, which contribute to ongoing nephron loss. (From Matsell DG, Tarantal AF: Experimental models of fetal obstructive nephropathy. Pediatr Nephrol 17:470, 2002, with permission.)

DIFFERENTIAL DIAGNOSIS OF FETAL HYDRONEPHROSIS: INTRODUCTION TO THE CONTROVERSIES

Even the definition of clinically significant urinary tract obstruction is subject to debate. Peters has offered the following: 'obstruction is a condition of impaired urinary drainage, which, if uncorrected, will limit the ultimate functional potential of a developing kidney' (10). While this definition accounts for the relationship between renal function and renal development, it does not provide a useful clinical guide to determine a critical degree of urinary tract obstruction in the fetus or infant. In the fetus or infant with hydronephrosis, urinary tract obstruction must be distinguished from vesicoureteral reflux (VUR) and from physiologic renal pelvic dilatation (9). Additional nonobstructive causes of hydronephrosis include congenital extrarenal pelvis and nonrefluxing nonobstructed megaureter (Table 14-1) (11).

Ureteropelvic junction obstruction (UPJO) is the most common lesion resulting in congenital obstructive uropathy. Although it is most often unilateral, the contralateral kidney may be subject to other abnormalities, such as VUR (9). The major controversy surrounding the evaluation of UPJO is the selection of patients for surgical pyeloplasty (as well as the timing of the procedure), with the objective of maximizing long-term renal function. Ureterovesical obstruction and ureterocoele with ectopic ureter are additional sites for a congenital obstructive lesion, and must also be distinguished from uncomplicated VUR. Less commonly encountered,

Table 14-1   **Causes of Antenatal Hydronephrosis**
Anomalous ureteropelvic junction (UPJ)/UPJ obstruction
Multicystic kidney
Retrocaval ureter
Primary obstructive megaureter
Nonrefluxing nonobstructed megaureter
Vesicoureteral reflux
Midureteral stricture
Ectopic ureterocele
Ectopic ureter
Posterior urethral valves
Prune belly syndrome
Urethral atresia
Hydrocolpos
Pelvic tumor
Cloacal abnormality

From Elder JS: Antenatal hydronephrosis—Fetal and neonatal management. Pediatr Clin North Am 44:1299, 1997.

retrocaval ureter, primary obstructive megaureter, or midureteral stricture can also result in fetal hydronephrosis (Table 14-1). Multicystic dysplastic kidney can be confused sonographically with UPJO, and is thought to result from ureteral atresia and severe obstructive uropathy in early fetal development (12). These kidneys are nonfunctional, and generally involute either before or after parturition, and can be followed by serial ultrasonography. Other cystic kidney disorders, such as solitary cysts and polycystic kidney disease, are generally easier to differentiate from obstructive uropathy.

Although less common, bladder outlet obstruction constitutes a more serious cause of obstructive uropathy because both kidneys are compromised. The differential diagnosis of obstructive lesions in this site includes posterior urethral valves (PUV), prune belly syndrome, and urethral atresia (Table 14-1). The major controversy in the management of these lower tract lesions also relates to patient selection and the timing of surgical intervention, including fetal urinary diversion (discussed below) (13). Finally, hydrocolpos, neoplasms (such as sacrococcygeal tumors), or cloacal abnormalities rarely account for congenital urinary tract obstruction (Table 14-1).

FETAL RENAL DEVELOPMENT AND PHYSIOLOGY

To understand the assessment of renal function in the fetus with potential obstructive uropathy, it is first necessary to review normal fetal renal physiology. Since function follows morphology, it is useful to examine human fetal renal development (Fig. 14-4) (14). Following the initial appearance and disappearance of the pronephros and mesonephros in early embryonic life, the metanephros begins development at the end of the first trimester (Fig. 14-4). Nephrogenesis undergoes most rapid growth during the second trimester, with completion by 34 weeks' gestation, while renal mass increases exponentially throughout the second and third trimesters (Fig. 14-4). Fetal urine production normally increases dramatically in the third trimester, reaching rates of approximately 50 mL/h at term (Fig. 14-5) (15). For a 2.5 kg infant, this amounts to a urine flow rate of 20 mL/kg/h that would translate to a high rate of diuresis in the neonate. As described below, the high fetal urine flow rate contributes significantly to amniotic fluid volume (Fig. 14-6) (16), which becomes compromised in severe bilateral fetal obstructive uropathy.

Fetal renal blood flow increases linearly throughout the second half of pregnancy, from less than 20 mL/min at 20 weeks to 40–100 mL/min at

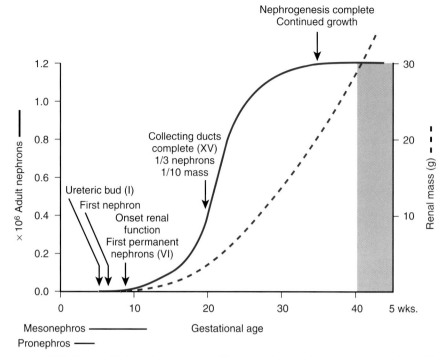

Figure 14-4 Human fetal renal development. The pronephros and mesonephros are formed in the first weeks of embryonic life and are replaced by the metanephros, which begins to produce urine at about the 10th week of gestation. The most rapid period of nephrogenesis is in the midtrimester, with nephrogenesis being complete by the 34th week. Renal mass follows an exponential increase throughout the second and third trimesters. (From Harrison MR, Golbus MS, Filly RA et al: Management of the fetus with congenital hydronephrosis. J Pediatr Surg 17:728, 1982, with permission.)

40 weeks (Fig. 14-7) (17). Fetal glomerular filtration rate (GFR) also increases progressively during the second half of gestation, and has been calculated from data obtained from a clinical fetal research center (18,19). Estimated fetal creatinine clearance increases from <1 mL/min below 25 weeks to >4 mL/min at term (Fig. 14-8a) (20). Urine concentrating capacity is reduced in the fetus due to anatomic immaturity of the renal medulla, decreased medullary concentration of sodium

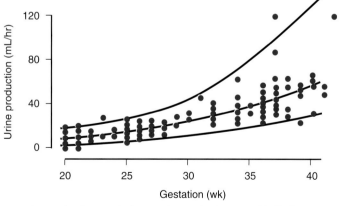

Figure 14-5 Urine production rate in human fetuses in the second half of gestation (individual patient data points [n = 85 fetuses], with lines showing mean and 95% confidence intervals). Data were obtained from serial measurements of fetal bladder volume using real-time ultrasonography at 2- to 5-min intervals. (From Rabinowitz R, Peters MT, Vyas S et al: Measurement of fetal urine production in normal pregnancy by real-time ultrasonography. Am J Obstet Gynecol 161:1264, 1989, with permission.)

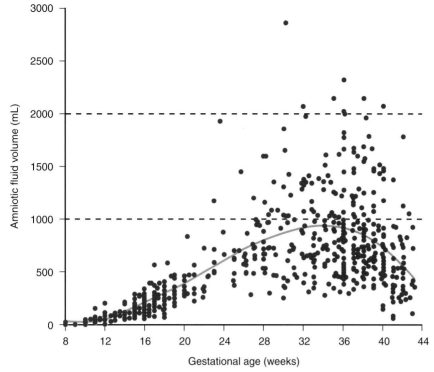

Figure 14-6 Amniotic fluid volume in human pregnancies in the second and third trimesters (individual data points [n = 705 pregnancies]). Solid line is polynomial regression. (From Brace RA, Wolf EJ: Normal amniotic fluid volume changes throughout pregnancy. Am J Obstet Gynecol 161:382, 1989, with permission.)

chloride and urea, and diminished responsiveness of collecting ducts to vasopressin (21). Recent studies show that this is due in part to a reduced density of aquaporins in the fetus (22,23), as well as to increased renal prostaglandin production, which counteracts the action of vasopressin (24). Fractional excretion of sodium decreases progressively throughout the second half of gestation, but remains at 5–20% of the filtered load (Fig. 14-8b) (20). This is due to progressive maturation of the proximal tubular sodium transporters (Na/H exchanger, chloride/formate exchanger and Na-K ATPase) in the fetus (25–27). In addition, sodium channels in the collecting duct also mature progressively (28). These changes lead to a progressive decrease in

Figure 14-7 Renal blood flow in human fetuses in the second half of gestation measured by color-pulsed Doppler evaluation of the renal artery (individual data points [n = 22 fetuses each studied three times], with lines showing mean and 95% confidence intervals). From Veille JC, Hanson RA, Tatum K et al: Quantitative assessment of human fetal renal blood flow. Am J Obstet Gynecol 169:1399, 1993, with permission.)

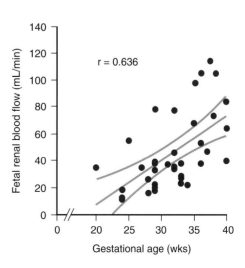

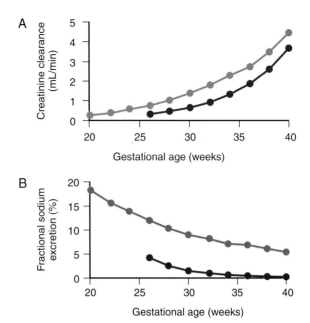

Figure 14-8 Renal function in the human fetus (●-● circles) and neonate (●-● circles) in the second half of gestation. A, Estimated creatinine clearance; B, Calculated fractional sodium excretion. Fetal values were calculated from several groups of data from a single human fetal research center (15,18,19), and postnatal values were previously reported (30). (From Haycock GB: Development of glomerular filtration and tubular sodium reabsorption in the human fetus and newborn. Br J Urol 81 (Suppl. 2):33, 1998, with permission.)

fetal urine sodium concentration from 16 to 36 weeks' gestation (Fig. 14-9) (29). Renal adaptation to parturition is revealed by a marked reduction in fractional excretion of sodium in neonates compared to fetuses of similar gestational age (Fig. 14-8b) (30). The fetal kidney is capable of proton excretion, and >80% of filtered bicarbonate is reabsorbed in the third trimester (31,32).

EVALUATION OF THE FETAL URINARY TRACT

The assessment of a fetus with hydronephrosis should first involve a detailed evaluation of the sonogram of the kidneys and urinary tract. The severity of fetal renal

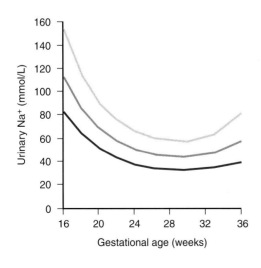

Figure 14-9 Fetal urinary sodium concentration based on data from 26 human fetuses 16–36 weeks' gestation with normal urinary tracts (mean and 95% confidence intervals). (From Nicolini U, Fisk NM, Rodeck CH et al: Fetal urine biochemistry: An index of renal maturation and dysfunction. Br J Obstet Gynaecol 99:46, 1992, with permission.)

Table 14-2 **Renal Pelvic Diameters on Antenatal and Postnatal Sonograms for Unobstructed, Possibly Obstructed, and Definitely Obstructed Kidneys**

Age	Unobstructed renal pelvis (mm) mean (range, SD)	Possibly obstructed renal pelvis (mm) mean (range, SD)	Obstructed renal pelvis (mm) mean (range, SD)
16–23 weeks' gestation	3 (0–11, 2)	4 (0–9, 3)	4 (0–10, 4)
24–30 weeks' gestation	5 (0–16, 3)	6 (0–11, 3)	11 (6–19, 4)
31–40 weeks' gestation	5 (0–17, 3)	8 (0–17, 4)	20 (7–56, 13)
6 days postnatal	6 (0–10, 2)	6 (0–11, 3)	18 (5–54, 11)
6 weeks postnatal	6 (3–10, 2)	10 (6–20, 4)	22 (11–60, 13)

From Clautice-Engle T, Anderson NG, Allan RB et al: Diagnosis of obstructive hydronephrosis in infants: Comparison sonograms performed 6 days and 6 weeks after birth. Am J Roentgenol 164:963, 1995.

pelvic dilatation does not always correlate well with renal functional outcome (33), but anteroposterior renal pelvic diameter exceeding 7 mm in the third trimester appears to be predictive of obstructive uropathy, with a 69–92% positive predictive value (34,35). Of note, variability in the measurement of fetal renal pelvic diameter averages 4 mm, such that 70% of fetuses had both 'normal' and 'abnormal' values during a 2-h study period (36). Comparison of renal pelvic diameters measured by antenatal ultrasonography and grouped by ultimate outcome shows a broad range for each gestational age (Table 14-2) (37). Discrimination clearly improves with gestational and postnatal age. Increased renal echogenicity or effacement of the corticomedullary junction in the fetal ultrasound has been associated with dysplastic changes in the kidney, and therefore an unfavorable prognosis (38). Although a correlation between gross renal anatomy (revealed by ultrasonography) and renal function (measured by postnatal diuretic renography) would be expected, this is often not the case. In fact, studies have shown that the relationship between renal histology and renal function in children with UPJO is very poor (39,40). There is evidence that fetal renal artery Doppler examination can distinguish nonfunctioning cystic kidneys from normal (41), but no studies document a reliable estimate of renal blood flow in fetal obstructive uropathy. Even postnatal measurement of the intrarenal resistive index has not proved reliable for the evaluation of obstructive uropathy (42).

Fetal ultrasonography also permits the examination of the lower urinary tract, paying particular attention to dilatation and thickening of the bladder, both of which are increased with significant bladder outlet obstruction, which occurs with PUV. In addition, ultrasonography provides an estimation of amniotic fluid volume, which is decreased in the second and third trimesters in any condition associated with decreased fetal urine production. This includes bilateral renal agenesis, renal hypoplasia, dysplasia, polycystic kidney disease, or obstructive uropathy. Severe oligohydramnios is associated with pulmonary hypoplasia, which becomes a major cause of neonatal mortality in fetal obstructive uropathy (43). In fact, when associated with severe urethral obstruction, mortality associated with second trimester oligohydramnios has been reported to be as high as 95% (44). This is important, as the prevention of pulmonary hypoplasia (rather than the prevention of renal insufficiency, as described below) constitutes the major justification for the clinical measurement of renal function in the human fetus.

Once detected by maternal ultrasonography, the mother of a fetus with urinary tract anomalies and oligohydramnios should receive consultation by appropriate specialists, including the perinatologist, genetic counselor, pediatric urologist, and pediatric nephrologist. Delivery of these infants should optimally be planned for a tertiary care center with the necessary experience and multidisciplinary team.

EVALUATION OF FETAL RENAL FUNCTION

The clinical evaluation of fetal renal function is challenging, and must be measured indirectly. As described above, fetal urine flow can be determined from timing fetal bladder filling and emptying (15), and amniotic fluid volume provides an estimate of fetal urine production in the second and third trimesters (16). Fetal urine sampling provides information regarding fetal renal function (Table 14-3). As stated above, however, the rationale for measuring fetal renal function is to confirm which fetuses with severe oligohydramnios have salvageable renal function, and therefore require intervention to permit pulmonary maturation (45).

Fetal serum β_2-microglobulin, normally less than 5.6 mg/L (Table 14-3), serves as a measure of glomerular function, and does not change with gestational age (46,47). This parameter can also be a useful predictor of renal injury in the fetus with obstructive uropathy (Fig. 14-10) (47). Although sampling of fetal serum β_2-microglobulin is more difficult than sampling urine, sensitivity and specificity are 80% and 99%, respectively (48), and it allows serial tracking of fetal renal function before and after surgical intervention. In contrast, fetal urinary β_2-microglobulin is increased as a consequence of tubular dysfunction, with values exceeding

Table 14-3 Concentrations of Biomarkers of Fetal Renal Function Associated with Favorable Renal Prognosis

Fetal serum markers	β_2-microglobulin (mg/L) (Nicolini & Spelzini 2001, Dommergues et al 2000, Berry et al 1995)	<5.6
Fetal urine markers	Sodium (mmol/L) (Nicolini & Spelzini 2001)	<100
	Chloride (mmol/L) (Johnson et al 1994)	<90
	Calcium (mmol/L) (Nicolini et al 1992)	<1.2
	Osmolality mOsm/L (Johnson et al 1994)	<200
	β_2-microglobulin (mg/L) (Muller et al 1993)	<2
	Total protein (mg/dL) (Johnson et al 1994)	<20
	N-acetyl-β-D-glucosaminidase (nmol/mL/h) (Tassis et al 1996)	<100
	Cystatin-C (mg/L) (Muller et al 1999)	<1
Amniotic fluid markers	Cystatin-C (mg/L) (Mussap et al 2002)	<1

Berry SM, Lecolier B, Smith RS et al: Predictive value of fetal serum beta 2-microglobulin for neonatal renal function. Lancet 345:1277, 1995.

Dommergues M, Muller F, Ngo S et al: Fetal serum β_2-microglobulin predicts postnatal renal function in bilateral uropathies. Kidney Int 58:312, 2000.

Johnson MP, Bukowski TP, Reitleman C et al: In utero surgical treatment of fetal obstructive uropathy: A new comprehensive approach to identify appropriate candidates for vesicoamniotic shunt therapy. Am J Obstet Gynecol 170:1770, 1994.

Muller F, Dommergues M, Mandelbrot L et al: Fetal urinary biochemistry predicts postnatal renal function in children with bilateral obstructive uropathies. Obstet Gynecol 82:813, 1993.

Muller F, Bernard MA, Benkirane A et al: Fetal urine cystatin C as a predictor of postnatal renal function in bilateral uropathies. Clin Chem 45:2292, 1999.

Mussap M, Fanos V, Pizzini C et al: Predictive value of amniotic fluid cystatin C levels for the early identification of fetuses with obstructive uropathies. Intl J Obstet Gynaec 109:778, 2002.

Nicolini U, Spelzini F: Invasive assessment of fetal renal abnormalities: urinalysis, fetal blood sampling and biopsy. Prenat Diagn 21:964, 2001.

Nicolini U, Fisk NM, Rodeck CH et al: Fetal urine biochemistry: An index of renal maturation and dysfunction. Br J Obstet Gynaecol 99:46, 1992.

Tassis BMG, Trespidi L, Tirelli AS et al: In fetuses with isolated hydronephrosis, urinary Beta2- microglobulin and N-acetyl-Beta-D-glucosaminidase (NAG) have a limited role in the prediction of postnatal renal function. Prenat Diagn 16:1087, 1996.

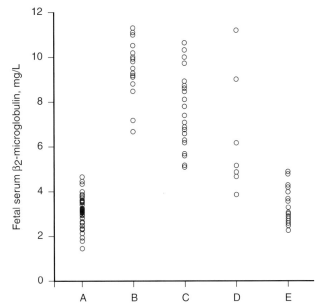

Figure 14-10 Fetal serum β2-microglobulin concentration. A, controls (n = 67); B, bilateral renal agenesis (n = 18); C, termination of pregnancy due to bilateral renal dysplasia (n = 26); D, infants with postnatal serum creatinine >50 μmol/L (n = 6); E, infants with postnatal serum creatinine <50 μmol/L (n = 28). (From Dommergues M, Muller F, Ngo S et al: Fetal serum β2-microglobulin predicts postnatal renal function in bilateral uropathies. Kidney Int 58:312, 2000, with permission.)

2 mg/L, suggesting a poor renal outcome (Table 14-3) (49). Similarly, fetal urinary N-acetyl-β-D-glucosaminidase (NAG) concentration is elevated in severe obstructive uropathy (>100 nmol/mL/h) (Table 14-3), although neither β_2-microglobulin nor NAG can be used independently to discriminate between fetuses with renal damage and those with normal function (50).

Urinary calcium concentration exceeding 1.2 mmol/L has also been reported to correlate with poor renal outcome (Table 14-3) (29). Following the beginning of metanephric function at the end of the first trimester (Fig. 14-4), tubular function matures throughout gestation, and urine becomes progressively hypotonic, with decreasing urinary sodium concentration from 16 to 30 weeks' gestation (Fig. 14-9) (29). It should be noted that in the early second trimester, fetal urine sodium concentration is normally similar to plasma, so that the effects of obstructive uropathy would not be detectable at 16 weeks (Fig. 14-9). However, because urine sodium concentration decreases throughout the second and third trimesters, values above 100 mEq/L beyond 20 weeks' gestation should be considered abnormal (Table 14-3) (46). In addition to urine sodium, urine chloride concentration has also been shown to be a useful marker of fetal renal dysfunction, with values above 90 mEq/L being abnormal (Table 14-3) (51). Similarly, urine osmolality exceeding 200 mOsm/L and total protein exceeding 20 mg/dL were found to be associated with significant fetal renal dysfunction (Table 14-3), with superior sensitivity and specificity to β_2-microglobulin or urine sodium concentration (51).

While fetal urine sodium and calcium concentration can discriminate severe renal dysfunction secondary to obstructive uropathy, these markers are less helpful in predicting moderate renal dysfunction (52). Although requiring sophisticated analytical equipment, proton nuclear magnetic resonance spectroscopy can provide superior resolution of potential biomarkers in 0.5 mL of fetal urine from patients, subsequently followed for at least 1 year with either normal GFR, decreased GFR, or severe renal dysplasia associated with fetal or neonatal death (53). Two-dimensional representation of fetal urine β_2-microglobulin and sodium concentration

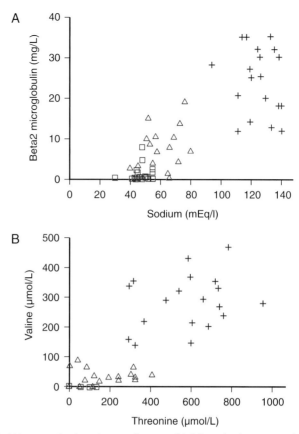

Figure 14-11 Urine samples from human fetuses with bilateral urinary tract obstruction examined by proton nuclear magnetic resonance. Group 1 (n = 21, squares) consisted of survivors for >1 year with serum creatinine <50 μmol/l; group 2 (n = 17, triangles) of survivors with serum creatinine >50 μmol/l; group 3 (n = 18, crosses) of those with histologic dysplasia associated with fetal (termination of pregnancy) or neonatal death. A, Relation between fetal urinary concentration of β2-microglobulin and sodium concentration. B, Relation between fetal urinary valine and threonine concentration. (From Eugene M, Muller F, Dommergues M et al: Evaluation of postnatal renal function in fetuses with bilateral obstructive uropathies by proton nuclear magnetic resonance spectroscopy. Am J Obstet Gynecol 170:595, 1994, with permission.)

discriminates between those with normal and decreased GFR (but survival) with 76% sensitivity, 81% specificity, and 81% negative predictive value (Fig. 14-11a) (53). Fetal urine valine-threonine concentration discriminates with 88% sensitivity, 86% specificity, and 90% negative predictive value (Fig. 14-11b) (53).

Recently, cystatin C has been investigated as a promising marker of fetal renal function. Cystatin C is a low molecular weight protein (13.3 kDa) that is produced by all nucleated human cells, does not cross the placenta, and is filtered by the glomerulus and completely reabsorbed by the tubule (54). Fetal *urine* cystatin C has a similar sensitivity and specificity to urinary sodium and β2-microglobulin in distinguishing severe renal dysfunction, but has the advantage of not varying with gestational age (Fig. 14-12a) (54). In contrast, studies have shown that *amniotic fluid* cystatin C concentration normally decreases with gestational age from 22 weeks to 36 weeks (Fig. 14-12b), but that concentrations of cystatin C in amniotic fluid from pregnancies with fetal uropathies are significantly higher (1.1–1.8 mg/L) than normal (0.5–0.8 mg/L) (Table 14-3) (55).

An enhancement of sensitivity in discrimination by urinary biomarkers has been achieved by sequential sampling of three fetal bladder aspirations, each 48 h apart (56). The rationale for this is as follows: the first urine sample represents

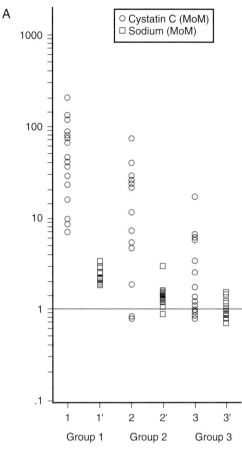

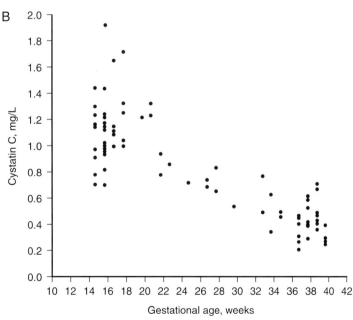

Figure 14-12 Fetal urine and amniotic fluid cystatin C concentration. A, Fetal urine cystatin C and sodium concentration expressed as multiples of the median (MoM) on a logarithmic scale. Group 1 (n = 19), termination of pregnancy or neonatal death due to bilateral renal dysplasia; group 2 (n = 19), infants with postnatal serum creatinine >50 μmol/L; group 3 (n = 33), infants with postnatal creatinine <50 μmol/L. B, Amniotic fluid cystatin C in the second and third trimesters for normal fetuses (n = 96). Values for 22–36 week fetuses with obstructive uropathy ranged from 1.08 to 1.75 mg/L. (From Muller F., Bernard MA, Benkirane A et al: Fetal urine cystatin C as a predictor of postnatal renal function in bilateral uropathies. Clin Chem 45:2292, 1999; Mussap M, Fanos V, Pizzini C et al: Predictive value of amniotic fluid cystatin C levels for the early identification of fetuses with obstructive uropathies. Intl J Obstet Gynaec 109:778, 2002, with permission.)

'bladder' urine, while the second represents urine that was flushed into the bladder from the dilated upper urinary tracts, and the third represents newly produced urine that drained into the bladder following temporary relief of obstruction by the bladder aspirations (Fig. 14-13) (51,56). It should be recalled that with bladder outlet obstruction, renal function is often impaired asymmetrically. Thus, bladder

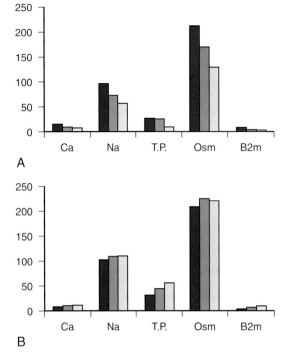

Figure 14-13 Sequential urinary electrolyte and protein concentration in representative fetuses with obstructive uropathy. A, Fetus demonstrates sequential improvement in all parameters, a pattern associated with the absence of underlying renal dysplasia and good predicted postnatal outcome after shunt placement. B, Fetus demonstrates sequential worsening in parameters associated with significant irreversible underlying renal fibrosis and dysplasia and poor postnatal outcome. Ca, calcium; Na, sodium; T.P., total protein; Osm, osmolality; B2m, β2-microglobulin. (From Johnson MP, Bukowski TP, Reitleman C et al: In utero surgical treatment of fetal obstructive uropathy: A new comprehensive approach to identify appropriate candidates for vesicoamniotic shunt therapy. Am J Obstet Gynecol 170:1770, 1994, with permission.)

urine indices will reflect function of the more severely affected kidney, and may underestimate the recoverability of the less damaged kidney. For this reason, if there is a marked difference in hydronephrosis between kidneys, aspiration of the renal pelves can be performed (45).

Three variables have been identified as independent predictors of adverse outcome in fetal hydronephrosis: oligohydramnios, postnatal GFR <20 mL/min, and prematurity (57). The nadir plasma creatinine concentration is a useful marker of prognosis: fetuses with a nadir of >1.0 mg/dL all progressed to renal failure, whereas 75% of those with a nadir serum creatinine of <0.8 mg/dL maintained normal GFR for over 4 years (45). While oligohydramnios and reduced GFR are directly linked to functioning renal mass, the role of prematurity is less obvious. The fetus with significant bladder outlet obstruction is more likely to be born before term (58). Of greater concern is the recent discovery that nephrogenesis may not progress postnatally in very low birth weight infants, such that the ultimate number of nephrons may remain permanently decreased (59,60). Since severe congenital bladder outlet obstruction can itself significantly reduce the number of nephrons in the human fetus (61), the added complication of prematurity becomes an important variable.

FETAL SURGICAL INTERVENTION FOR OBSTRUCTIVE UROPATHY

In the setting of oligohydramnios with bladder distension and bilateral hydronephrosis, after other serious anomalies have been ruled out by fetal ultrasonography (with amnioinfusion if necessary), fetal karyotype should be obtained from chorionic villus sampling or amniotic fluid (Fig. 14-14) (62). A minimum of three serial fetal urine samples should then be obtained at 48–72 h intervals as described above, and fetuses are characterized as good prognosis (Table 14-3), borderline prognosis (maximum of 2 abnormal values), or poor prognosis (maximum of 3 abnormal values). Parents are then offered the option of prenatal

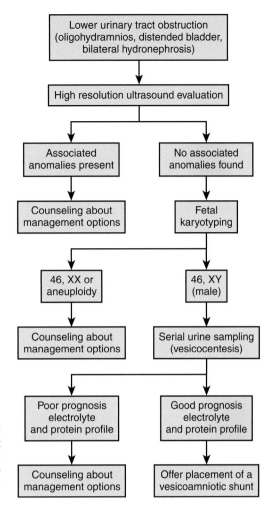

Figure 14-14 Algorithm for the prenatal evaluation and management of fetuses with suspected lower urinary tract obstruction. (From Biard JM, Johnson MP, Carr MC et al: Long-term outcomes in children treated by prenatal vesicoamniotic shunting for lower urinary tract obstruction. Obstet Gynecol 106:503, 2005, with permission.)

intervention if the karyotype is normal male with isolated lower urinary tract obstruction and good or borderline urine markers (62). Vesicoamniotic shunting is a temporary percutaneous intervention that provides diversion of fetal urine to the amniotic space, and has been described in detail (13). As discussed below, the ultimate outcome of patients undergoing fetal intervention for obstructive uropathy is variable, with survival largely dependent on the specific underlying diagnosis and the criteria for patient selection (62–64). In the absence of a large prospective study, the impact of vesicoamniotic shunting on even pulmonary maturation remains to be established conclusively.

HISTOLOGY OF THE FETAL KIDNEY IN OBSTRUCTIVE UROPATHY

Kidneys from human fetuses with severe bladder outlet obstruction showed both dysplastic and cystic changes, with increased apoptosis of mesenchymal and tubular cells (65). Examination of kidneys from human fetuses with severe bladder outlet obstruction or multicystic dysplasia with ureteral atresia showed expansion of glomerular and tubular cysts with retention of the macula densa and primitive loop structure, suggesting that the abnormalities developed after initial nephron differentiation (66). In another study of human fetuses of 14–37 weeks' gestation with severe bilateral hydronephrosis, histologic findings revealed a range of dysplastic changes, including cessation of nephrogenesis, disappearance or myofibroblastic differentiation of metanephric blastema, and increased expression of α-smooth muscle actin by mesenchymal cells (67). These changes are clearly irreversible, and correlate with oligohydramnios, ultrasound evidence of renal dysplasia (loss of corticomedullary differentiation, renal hyperechogenicity, and presence of renal cortical cysts), and abnormal fetal urine sodium and/or β$_2$-microglobulin concentration (67).

Attempts to perform renal biopsies in fetuses with obstructive uropathy have been of marginal usefulness. In the largest series reported to date, a successful renal specimen was obtained by percutaneous needle aspiration in 50% of 10 biopsies performed in fetuses with bilateral obstructive uropathy (68). Normal fetal renal histology was found in four of these cases, with renal dysplasia being found in the remaining patient, who went on to develop renal failure despite a fetal urine sodium concentration of 60 mEq/L (68). The authors conclude that, while the technique is feasible and safe, it is limited by the difficulties in obtaining an adequate sample and the concern that needle biopsy does not provide representative samples of the entire kidney (68).

POSTNATAL FOLLOW UP

Bilateral Hydronephrosis

The infant with antenatal diagnosis of bilateral hydronephrosis should have prompt postnatal abdominal ultrasonography, voiding cystourethrography, and nuclide renography to determine whether there is evidence for bilateral upper tract obstruction or VUR, or bladder outlet obstruction. In such patients, continuous bladder drainage through an indwelling catheter is necessary to determine the renal functional potential before deciding on definitive surgical intervention (9). During the transition from fetal to extrauterine life, infants with severe obstructive uropathy (especially after relief of obstruction) may manifest an exaggeration of the normal postnatal diuresis and natriuresis (69,70). This is due to the altered expression of renal sodium transporters and aquaporins in bilateral obstructive uropathy (71,72), and mediated by upregulation of cyclooxygenase 2 in the renal medulla (73).

Unilateral Hydronephrosis

Ultrasonography of the kidneys and urinary tract should be performed after birth in all infants with suspected antenatal hydronephrosis (Fig. 14-15). In the immediate postnatal period, infants with renal pelvic diameter less than 15 mm were found not to have significant renal abnormalities, while of those with greater pelvic dilatation, 79% had urinary tract obstruction or VUR (74). Although there is concern that physiologic volume contraction in the early postnatal period could underestimate hydronephrosis if neonatal ultrasonography is performed within the first two days of life, there is no significant difference in ultimate outcome gained by waiting until 7–10 days of life (75). However, to enhance the reliability of the neonatal study, most practitioners suggest a delay (75). Follow up of fetuses with persistent postnatal hydronephrosis should include voiding cystourethrography to rule out VUR, and diuretic renography (76) to determine the severity of functional obstruction (Fig. 14-15) (77). A progressive increase in the severity of hydronephrosis by ultrasonography may be a more reliable index of severity of obstruction than the pattern of diuretic renography (77,78). Calyceal dilatation on ultrasound examination may be a better index of progression than the measured pelvic diameter, although all infants with pelvic diameter exceeding 50 mm should have pyeloplasty, regardless of calyceal dilatation (79).

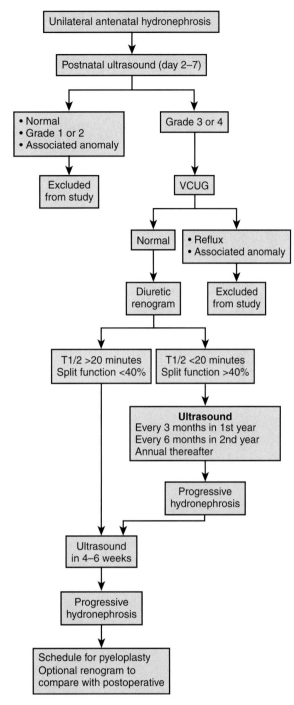

Figure 14-15 Algorithm for the postnatal evaluation and management of infants with unilateral hydronephrosis determined by antenatal ultrasonography. Ultrasound grading of hydronephrosis is by the Society for Fetal Urology (77). VCUG, voiding cystourethrogram; T1/2, nuclide clearance half time. (From Hafez AT, McLorie G, Bägli D et al: Analysis of trends on serial ultrasound for high grade neonatal hydronephrosis. J Urol 168:1518, 2002, with permission.)

A significant controversy has developed regarding the indications for pyeloplasty in infants with a diagnosed UPJO. Koff and his associates argue that close monitoring by renal ultrasonography and diuretic renography can avert surgical intervention in all but approximately 25% of patients with unilateral UPJO (80), and 35% of bilateral UPJO (81). There are several concerns with this "conservative" approach, which has been termed "aggressive observation" by DiSandro and Kogan (82). There is substantial experimental and clinical evidence indicating that the severity of renal injury from UPJO can be related to the duration of obstruction (9,82). Retrospective studies of patients with UPJO detected prenatally had better outcome than those diagnosed postnatally (83–85) and, in one study, pyeloplasty resulted in improved function only in the group diagnosed prenatally (85). Therefore, waiting for measurable functional deterioration may lead to irreversible nephron loss. Of particular concern is the failure of patients to adhere to a schedule of follow up studies, which may contribute to an even greater incidence of renal deterioration in patients for whom pyeloplasty is deferred (86).

LONG-TERM IMPLICATIONS OF CONGENITAL OBSTRUCTIVE UROPATHY

The management of obstructive uropathy in the fetus and neonate should be governed by the expected long-term outcomes for these patients. While patients with unilateral disease and a normal contralateral kidney should enjoy normal long-term renal function, there may be an increased prevalence of abnormalities of the contralateral kidney that may not be detected (9). Even after pyeloplasty, patients with either unilateral or bilateral hydronephrosis may manifest ongoing tubular dysfunction, such as renal tubular acidosis or a renal concentrating defect (87,88). In patients with PUV and normal renal function, distal renal tubular acidosis can persist long after ablation of the valves (89).

While ongoing postnatal renal maturation of children with bilateral severe obstructive uropathy can permit a period of years of life with conservative medical management, the needs of continued growth often lead to renal failure and the need for renal replacement therapy (90). Thus, relentless progression of renal insufficiency characterizes many cases of PUV, with the onset of renal failure by the second decade (90). In a recent report, the long-term outcome among patients with antenatal diagnosis of PUV was not different from those detected postnatally (91). Although prenatal surgical intervention for fetal obstructive uropathy was developed in San Francisco 25 years ago to avoid this outcome, the experience has been variable. In a retrospective review of the San Francisco program from 1981 to 1999, 14 fetuses with PUV and "favorable" urinary electrolytes underwent surgery; of these six died, with five of the survivors developing chronic renal insufficiency (63). The investigators concluded that favorable urinary electrolytes and surgical intervention may not change the outcome (63). The experience for prenatal intervention for lower urinary tract obstruction at Detroit, another major center, was similar: 38% died and 50% lived beyond 2 years of age, with 57% of these developing chronic renal insufficiency or renal failure (64). Disturbingly, height was below the 5th percentile in 50%, although "acceptable continence" was achieved in 50% (64). A long-term additional complication of survivors includes chronic respiratory disorders (45). In the most recent report from the Children's Hospital of Philadelphia (a third major center for fetal intervention in obstructive uropathy), 1-year survival was 91%, with 18 surviving candidates yielding fetal urinary prognostic indices that were good in 13 cases and borderline or poor in 5 cases (62). Six of the 18 children developed renal failure, 8 had persistent respiratory problems, 9 had musculoskeletal problems, and 9 had frequent urinary tract infections (62). Neurological development was normal in all but three patients, and the patients and their families reported that their life is worthwhile, with a "quality of life" score not different from that of the healthy population (62). This last outcome measure is perhaps more meaningful than any of the other statistical analysis that we can apply to our patients.

THE FUTURE

The current state of the art allows us to visualize the fetal urinary tract as well as to evaluate renal function in the fetus throughout the second half of gestation.

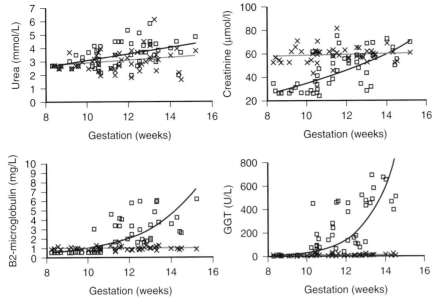

Figure 14-16 Biochemical indices of fetal renal maturation in early pregnancy. Urea, creatinine, β2-microglobulin and γ-glutamyltransferase were measured in paired samples of amniotic fluid (squares) and maternal serum (crosses) collected at the time of pregnancy termination between 8 and 14 weeks, and in women undergoing early transabdominal amniocentesis between 11 and 16 weeks' gestation. The increase in creatinine, β2-microglobulin and γ-glutamyltransferase amniotic fluid concentrations after 10 weeks' gestation reflects the maturation of fetal GFR at a time when tubular reabsorption remains immature. (From Gulbis B, Jauniaux E, Jurkovic D et al: Biochemical investigation of fetal renal maturation in early pregnancy. Pediatr Res 39:731, 1996, with permission.)

Unfortunately, for severe forms of obstructive uropathy, much of the damage sustained by the kidneys as a result of obstruction occurs between the 8th and 16th weeks. Analysis of amniotic fluid creatinine, gamma-glutamyltransferase, and β2-microglobulin concentration during this interval shows an abrupt increase after 10 weeks' gestation (Fig. 14-16) (92) that likely reflects the onset of glomerular filtration by the newly formed metanephros (Fig. 14-4). Unfortunately, fetal kidneys are difficult to visualize during the first trimester, and because of nephron immaturity, fetal urine or amniotic fluid indices cannot reflect significant renal maldevelopment at this point (Figs 14-4, 14-6 and 14-9).

There are many factors that converge to impact the delicate process of renal morphogenesis in the fetus. In addition to the genome of the fetus that may contain mutations in genes expressed by the developing metanephros, maternal and uterine environmental factors can alter gene activity (Fig. 14-17) (93). There is considerable experimental data to support a major role for fetal urinary flow impairment as another factor that significantly alters gene activity (Fig. 14-17).

Advances in imaging and the discovery of new biomarkers of fetal renal function and injury should lead to new diagnostic and therapeutic approaches to congenital urinary tract obstruction. Three-dimensional ultrasonography can provide improved resolution of fetal gross anatomy (94), and may enhance prenatal evaluation of obstructive uropathy. There is also increasing appreciation of the complex alterations in renal gene expression and cellular responses to congenital urinary tract obstruction (9). Microarray analysis of renal gene expression in mice or rats with experimental or spontaneous ureteral obstruction has revealed significant upregulation or downregulation of many molecules (95–97). Preliminary microarray analysis of human fetal and infant kidneys with congenital urinary tract

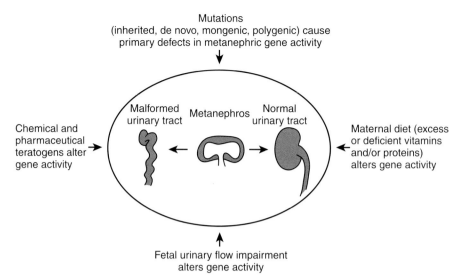

Figure 14-17 Influences on gene expression during development of the urinary tract: mutations, teratogens, alterations in the maternal diet, and obstruction to urine flow in the fetus. (From Woolf AS: A molecular and genetic view of human renal and urinary tract malformations. Kidney Int 58:500, 2000, with permission.)

obstruction is consistent with patterns found in the animal models (Fig. 14-18) (98). Further study of such changes can lead to the development of new biomarkers of obstructive uropathy (99).

Candidate markers that are upregulated in the kidney of experimental animals with ureteral obstruction include transforming growth factor-β1, tumor necrosis factor-α, and monocyte chemoattractant protein-1, while epidermal growth factor is downregulated (100–102). The urinary excretion of these molecules is altered in children with unilateral UPJO, and may therefore prove useful also in fetal urine assays (103–105). Over the past five years, the renal expression of dozens of molecules has been shown to be altered by urinary tract obstruction (95–97), and experimental manipulation of some pathways can attenuate the renal lesions (106). Some of the salutary effects in experimental models have been achieved by gene therapy (106). Because much of the renal injury resulting from congenital obstructive uropathy takes place in the prenatal or early perinatal period, fetal gene therapy is theoretically an attractive option (107). Moreover, the fetus has larger populations of less differentiated cells (such as stem cells) that may be more responsive to such an approach. Moreover, the fetus is also immunologically naïve and therefore susceptible to induction of tolerance (107).

Finally, there are human gene polymorphisms of the renin-angiotensin system that predict the development and progression of congenital uropathies. Mutations in the angiotensin type 2 receptor gene are associated with an increased incidence of congenital anomalies of the kidney and urinary tract in several populations (108,109). Italian children with congenital uropathies and renal parenchymal lesions have a higher prevalence of the D/D genotype of angiotensin converting enzyme (ACE) than patients without parenchymal lesions (109). European children with chronic renal failure due to renal malformations and the D/D genotype have a more rapid rate of loss of GFR than those with I/D or I/I genotype (Fig. 14-19) (110). Similarly, Indian children with congenital uropathies (including PUV) and D allele also have an adverse prognosis (111). Fetal testing for such polymorphisms may lead to improved long-term management of patients with congenital obstructive uropathy.

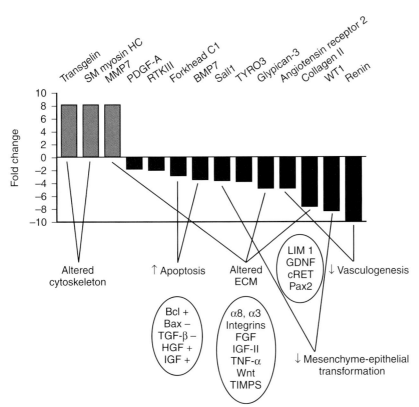

Figure 14-18 Microarray analysis was performed on kidneys from patients with congenital obstructive uropathy (n = 6), ranging from fetuses of 18 weeks' gestation to children 1 year of age, as well as on kidneys from age-matched controls (n = 6). Differential expression of selected candidate genes (from 8400 screened) were sorted based on at least a 5-fold difference in expression. Genes given a − value are decreased, and upregulated genes are to the left of the graph. Most of the genes are downregulated. Genes involved in vasculogenesis in humans and mesenchymal-epithelial transformation are downregulated. Genes in ovals are candidate genes suggested from animal studies, with potential synergistic effect, but not represented in this set of GeneChip data. Extracellular matrix (ECM) genes are increased or decreased. Decreased forkhead C1 and BMP7 may contribute to increased apoptosis, and additional apoptosis-related genes are implicated as well. Increased smooth muscle actin and transgelin represent altered cytoskeletal genes. (From Liapis H: Biology of congenital obstructive nephropathy. Exp Nephrol 93:87, 2003, with permission.)

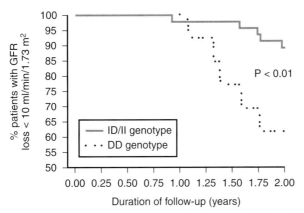

Figure 14-19 Renal "survival" analysis in children with chronic renal failure due to renal malformations (n = 59). During 2 years of follow-up, loss of GFR >10 mL/min per 1.73 m2 was observed in 39% of patients with ACE D/D genotype, compared to only 11% in those with I/D or I/I genotype. (From Hohenfellner K, Wingen A-M, Nauroth O et al: Impact of ACE I/D gene polymorphism on congenital renal malformations. Pediatr Nephrol 16:356, 2001, with permission.)

SUMMARY AND CONCLUSIONS

Assessment of renal function in the fetus with obstructive uropathy is a complex and multidisciplinary process that requires an understanding of fetal renal development and physiology, as well as of the causes and consequences of maldevelopment of the urinary tract. This review addresses a number of major questions relating to the evaluation and management of congenital obstructive uropathy, and provides arguments for the following conclusions:

1. What is the natural history of obstructive uropathy? Based on animal models, as well as the follow up of infants born with urinary tract obstruction, the evolution of this group of disorders is extremely heterogeneous and dependent on many variables. These include the timing and location of the obstructive lesion, the severity of obstruction, and the gestational age at birth.

2. What is the relative contribution of primary renal maldevelopment versus altered renal development secondary to obstructive injury? The patient's genome, as well as the fetal-maternal environment, are shared determinants of the renal functional outcome. A better understanding of mutations accounting for altered renal morphogenesis, as well as polymorphisms modulating the progression of secondary renal injury, will lead to better preventive measures. Advances in understanding the cellular and molecular mechanisms responsible for both abnormal renal development and the secondary adaptive responses will lead to improved therapies.

3. What constitutes a definition of significant urinary tract obstruction? Significant obstruction 'is a condition of impaired urinary drainage, which, if uncorrected, will limit the ultimate functional potential of a developing kidney' (10). This definition emphasizes the importance of long-term outcome in any evaluation or intervention of the affected fetus.

4. What is the correlation of fetal renal pelvic dilatation with functional outcome? Unfortunately, with the exception of extreme hydronephrosis, the lack of precision in the measurement of fetal renal pelvic dilation results in a poor correlation between this parameter and renal functional outcome. Improved imaging techniques as well as standardization of procedures are needed.

5. What is the correlation of fetal renal histologic changes with functional outcome? Attempts to correlate fetal histologic changes with renal prognosis have been disappointing. Even postnatal renal histology in children with unilateral ureteropelvic junction obstruction shows poor correlation with relative renal function. Refined approaches, such as immunohistochemistry or laser capture microscopy, are needed.

6. Which patients should undergo pyeloplasty for ureteropelvic junction obstruction, and what should be the criteria? The fetus with unilateral hydronephrosis and normal amniotic fluid volume should not undergo measurement of renal function or intervention before birth. The infant with high grade progressive hydronephrosis should undergo early postnatal pyeloplasty, regardless of relative renal function.

7. Which patients should undergo fetal intervention for obstructive nephropathy, and what should be the criteria? Selected fetuses with bilateral hydronephrosis, distended bladder, and oligohydramnios may undergo serial ultrasonography, karyotyping, and urine sampling. Those with favorable sonographic and urine biomarker profiles should be considered for placement of a vesicoamniotic shunt by an experienced team of specialists in an established center. At the present time, fetal intervention cannot be

mandated in any individual patient, in view of the lack of rigorous prospective controlled studies.

8. What is the impact of fetal intervention on the long-term prognosis? In properly selected patients, the prevention of pulmonary hypoplasia is the most important outcome of successful fetal intervention for severe obstructive uropathy, and survival can be 90% at one year. Optimization of renal function is difficult to document, and 30–60% of survivors develop chronic renal insufficiency or renal failure.

9. What will the future bring? Advances in imaging and the discovery of new biomarkers of renal development and injury (proteomics) will allow evaluation in the first trimester. Progress in genomics should permit the identification of mutations or polymorphisms predictive of renal malformations or risk of progression of the renal lesions of obstructive uropathy. Gene therapy is also theoretically more likely to be effective in the fetus than postnatally.

REFERENCES

1. Seikaly MG, Ho PL, Emmett L, et al. Chronic renal insufficiency in children: The 2001 annual report of the NAPRTCS. Pediatr Nephrol 18:796, 2003.
2. Woolf AS, Winyard PJ. Molecular mechanisms of human embryogenesis: developmental pathogenesis of renal tract malformations. Pediatric & Developmental Pathology 5:108, 2002.
3. Woolf AS, Thiruchelvam N. Congenital obstructive uropathy: its origin and contribution to end-stage renal disease in children. Adv Ren Replace Ther 8:157, 2001.
4. Woolf AS. Emerging roles of obstruction and mutations in renal malformations. Pediatr Nephrol 12:690, 1998.
5. Peters CA. Obstruction of the fetal urinary tract. J Am Soc Nephrol 8:653, 1997.
6. Peters CA. Animal models of fetal renal disease. Prenat Diagn 21:917, 2001.
7. Peters CA, Carr MC, Lais A, et al. The response of the fetal kidney to obstruction. J Urol 148:503, 1992.
8. Matsell DG, Tarantal AF. Experimental models of fetal obstructive nephropathy. Pediatr Nephrol 17:470, 2002.
9. Chevalier RL, Roth JA. Obstructive uropathy. In Avner ED, Harmon WE, Niaudet P, (eds): Pediatric Nephrology, 5th edn (pp 1049–1076). Philadelphia, PA: Lippincott Williams and Wilkins, 2004.
10. Peters CA. Urinary tract obstruction in children. J Urol 154:1874, 1995.
11. Elder JS. Antenatal hydronephrosis—Fetal and neonatal management. Pediatr Clin North Am 44:1299, 1997.
12. Woolf AS. Unilateral multicystic dysplastic kidney. Kidney Int 69:190, 2006.
13. Johnson MP. Fetal obstructive uropathy. In Harrison MR, Evans MI, Adzick NS, Holzgreve W, (eds): The Unborn Patient, 3rd edn (pp 259–286). Philadelphia, PA: W.B. Saunders Co., 2001.
14. Harrison MR, Golbus MS, Filly RA, et al. Management of the fetus with congenital hydronephrosis. J Pediatr Surg 17:728, 1982.
15. Rabinowitz R, Peters MT, Vyas S, et al. Measurement of fetal urine production in normal pregnancy by real-time ultrasonography. Am J Obstet Gynecol 161:1264, 1989.
16. Brace RA, Wolf EJ. Normal amniotic fluid volume changes throughout pregnancy. Am J Obstet Gynecol 161:382, 1989.
17. Veille JC, Hanson RA, Tatum K, et al. Quantitative assessment of human fetal renal blood flow. Am J Obstet Gynecol 169:1399, 1993.
18. Nicolaides KH, Cheng HH, Snijders RJM, et al. Fetal urine biochemistry in the assessment of obstructive uropathy. Am J Obstet Gynecol 166:932, 1992.
19. Moniz CF, Nicolaides KH, Bamforth FJ, et al. Normal reference ranges for biochemical substances relating to renal, hepatic, and bone function in fetal and maternal plasma during pregnancy. J Clin Pathol 38:468, 1985.
20. Haycock GB. Development of glomerular filtration and tubular sodium reabsorption in the human fetus and newborn. Br J Urol 81(Suppl. 2):33, 1998.
21. Stanier MW. Development of intra-renal solute gradients in foetal and postnatal life. Pfluegers Arch 336:263, 1972.
22. Devuyst O, Burrow CR, Smith BL, et al. Expression of aquaporins-1 and -2 during nephrogenesis and in autosomal dominant polycystic kidney disease. Am J Physiol 271:F169–F183, 1996.
23. Wintour EM, Earnest L, Alcorn D, et al. Ovine AQP1: cDNA cloning, ontogeny, and control of renal gene expression. Pediatr Nephrol 12:545, 1998.
24. Melendez E, Reyes JL, Escalante BA, et al. Development of the receptors to prostaglandin E2 in the rat kidney and neonatal renal functions. Dev Pharmacol Ther 14:125, 1990.

25. Guillery EN, Karniski LP, Mathews MS, et al. Maturation of proximal tubule Na/H antiporter activity in sheep during the transition from fetus to newborn. Am J Physiol 267:F537–F545, 1994.

26. Guillery EN, Huss DJ. Developmental regulation of chloride/formate exchange in the guinea pig proximal tubule. Am J Physiol 269:F686–F695, 1995.

27. Guillery EN, Huss DJ, McDonough AA, et al. Posttranscriptional upregulation of Na+-K+-ATPase activity in newborn guinea pig renal cortex. Am J Physiol Renal Physiol 273:F254–F263, 1997.

28. Watanabe S, Matsushita K, McCray PBJ, et al. Developmental expression of the epithelial Na+ channel in kidney and uroepithelia. Am J Physiol Renal Physiol 276:F304–F314, 1999.

29. Nicolini U, Fisk NM, Rodeck CH, et al. Fetal urine biochemistry: An index of renal maturation and dysfunction. Br J Obstet Gynaecol 99:46, 1992.

30. Al-Dahhan J, Haycock GB, Chantler C. Sodium homeostasis in term and preterm neonates. Arch Dis Child 58:335, 1983.

31. Kesby GJ, Lumbers ER. Factors affecting renal handling of sodium, hydrogen ions, and bicarbonate by the fetus. Am J Physiol 251:F226–F231, 1986.

32. Kesby GJ, Lumbers ER. The effects of metabolic acidosis on renal function of fetal sheep. J Physiol 396:65, 1988.

33. Hanna MK. Antenatal hydronephrosis and ureteropelvic junction obstruction: The case for early intervention. Urology 55:612, 2000.

34. Ismaili K, Hall M, Donner C, et al. Results of systematic screening for minor degrees of fetal renal pelvis dilatation in an unselected population. Am J Obstet Gynecol 188:242, 2003.

35. Kent A, Cox D, Downey P, et al. A study of mild fetal pyelectasia—outcome and proposed strategy of management. Prenat Diagn 20:206, 2000.

36. Persutte WH, Hussey M, Chyu J, et al. Striking findings concerning the variability in the measurement of the fetal renal collecting system. Ultrasound Obst Gynec 15:186, 2000.

37. Clautice-Engle T, Anderson NG, Allan RB, et al. Diagnosis of obstructive hydronephrosis in infants: Comparison sonograms performed 6 days and 6 weeks after birth. Am J Roentgenol 164:963, 1995.

38. Mouriquand PDE, Troisfontaines E, Wilcox DT. Antenatal and perinatal uro-nephrology: current questions and dilemmas. Pediatr Nephrol 13:938, 1999.

39. Elder JS, Stansbrey R, Dahms BB, et al. Renal histological changes secondary to ureteropelvic junction obstruction. J Urol 154:719, 1995.

40. Zhang PL, Peters CA, Rosen S. Ureteropelvic junction obstruction: morphological and clinical studies. Pediatr Nephrol 14:820, 2000.

41. Gill B, Bennett RT, Barnhard Y, et al. Can fetal renal artery Doppler studies predict postnatal renal function in morphologically abnormal kidneys? A preliminary report. J Urol 156:190, 1996.

42. Rawashdeh YF, Djurhuus JC, Mortensen J, et al. The intrarenal resistive index as a pathophysiological marker of obstructive uropathy. J Urol 165:1397, 2001.

43. Nakayama DK, Harrison MR, de Lorimier AA. Prognosis of posterior urethral valves presenting at birth. J Ped Surg 21:43, 1986.

44. Mahony BS, Callen PW, Filly RA. Fetal urethral obstruction. Ultrasound evaluation. Radiology 157:221, 1985.

45. Freedman AL, Johnson MP, Gonzalez R. Fetal therapy for obstructive uropathy: past, present..... future? Pediatr Nephrol 14:167, 2000.

46. Nicolini U, Spelzini F. Invasive assessment of fetal renal abnormalities: urinalysis, fetal blood sampling and biopsy. Prenat Diagn 21:964, 2001.

47. Dommergues M, Muller F, Ngo S, et al. Fetal serum β_2-microglobulin predicts postnatal renal function in bilateral uropathies. Kidney Int 58:312, 2000.

48. Berry SM, Lecolier B, Smith RS, et al. Predictive value of fetal serum beta 2-microglobulin for neonatal renal function. Lancet 345:1277, 1995.

49. Muller F, Dommergues M, Mandelbrot L, et al. Fetal urinary biochemistry predicts postnatal renal function in children with bilateral obstructive uropathies. Obstet Gynecol 82:813, 1993.

50. Tassis BMG, Trespidi L, Tirelli AS, et al. In fetuses with isolated hydronephrosis, urinary Beta2-microglobulin and N-acetyl-Beta-D-glucosaminidase (NAG) have a limited role in the prediction of postnatal renal function. Prenat Diagn 16:1087, 1996.

51. Johnson MP, Bukowski TP, Reitleman C, et al. In utero surgical treatment of fetal obstructive uropathy: A new comprehensive approach to identify appropriate candidates for vesicoamniotic shunt therapy. Am J Obstet Gynecol 170:1770, 1994.

52. Guez S, Assael BM, Melzi ML, et al. Shortcomings in predicting postnatal renal function using prenatal urine biochemistry in fetuses with congenital hydronephrosis. J Pediatr Surg 31:1401, 1996.

53. Eugene M, Muller F, Dommergues M, et al. Evaluation of postnatal renal function in fetuses with bilateral obstructive uropathies by proton nuclear magnetic resonance spectroscopy. Am J Obstet Gynecol 170:595, 1994.

54. Muller F, Bernard MA, Benkirane A, et al. Fetal urine cystatin C as a predictor of postnatal renal function in bilateral uropathies. Clin Chem 45:2292, 1999.

55. Mussap M, Fanos V, Pizzini C, et al. Predictive value of amniotic fluid cystatin C levels for the early identification of fetuses with obstructive uropathies. Intl J Obstet Gynaec 109:778, 2002.

56. Johnson MP, Corsi P, Bradfield W, et al. Sequential urinalysis improves evaluation of fetal renal function in obstructive uropathy. Am J Obstet Gynecol 173:59, 1995.

57. Oliveira EA, Diniz JSS, Cabral ACV, et al. Prognostic factors in fetal hydronephrosis: a multivariate analysis. Pediatric Nephrology 13:859, 1999.

58. Hedrick HL, Flake AW, Crombleholme TM, et al. History of fetal diagnosis and therapy: Children's Hospital of Philadelphia experience. Fetal Diagn Ther 18:65, 2003.

59. Rodriguez MM, Gomez A, Abitbol C, et al. Comparative renal histomorphometry: a case study of oligonephropathy of prematurity. Pediatr Nephrol 20:945, 2005.

60. Rodriguez MM, Gomez AH, Abitbol CL, et al. Histomorphometric analysis of postnatal glomerulogenesis in extremely preterm infants. Pediatr Devel Pathol 7:17, 2004.

61. Gasser B, Mauss Y, Ghnassia JP, et al. A quantitative study of normal nephrogenesis in the human fetus: Its implication in the natural history of kidney changes due to low obstructive uropathies. Fetal Diagn Ther 8:371, 1993.

62. Biard JM, Johnson MP, Carr MC, et al. Long-term outcomes in children treated by prenatal vesicoamniotic shunting for lower urinary tract obstruction. Obstet Gynecol 106:503, 2005.

63. Holmes N, Harrison MR, Baskin LS. Fetal surgery for posterior urethral valves: Long-term postnatal outcomes. Pediatrics 108:36, 2001.

64. Freedman AL, Johnson MP, Smith CA, et al. Long-term outcome in children after antenatal intervention for obstructive uropathies. Lancet 354:374, 1999.

65. Poucell-Hatton S, Huang M, Bannykh S, et al. Fetal obstructive uropathy: Patterns of renal pathology. Pediatr Devel Pathol 3:223, 2000.

66. Shibata S, Shigeta M, Shu Y, et al. Initial pathological events in renal dysplasia with urinary tract obstruction in utero. Virchows Arch Int J Pathol 439:560, 2001.

67. Daiekha-Dahmane F, Dommergues M, Muller F, et al. Development of human fetal kidney in obstructive uropathy: Correlations with ultrasonography and urine biochemistry. Kidney Int 52:21, 1997.

68. Bunduki V, Saldanha LB, Sadek L, et al. Fetal renal biopsies in obstructive uropathy: Feasibility and clinical correlations – Preliminary results. Prenat Diagn 18:101, 199.

69. Lorenz JM, Kleinman LI, Ahmed G, et al. Phases of fluid and electrolyte homeostasis in the extremely low birth weight infant. Pediatrics 96:484, 1995.

70. Terzi F, Assael BM, Claris Appiani A, et al. Increased sodium requirement following early postnatal surgical correction of congenital uropathies in infants. Pediatr Nephrol 4:581, 1990.

71. Li CL, Wang WD, Kwon TH, et al. Altered expression of major renal Na transporters in rats with bilateral ureteral obstruction and release of obstruction. Am J Physiol Renal Physiol 285:F889–F901, 2003.

72. Li C, Wang W, Kwon TH, et al. Downregulation of AQP1, -2, and -3 after ureteral obstruction is associated with a long-term urine-concentrating defect. Am J Physiol 281:F163–F171, 2001.

73. Norregard R, Jensen BL, Li C, et al. COX-2 inhibition prevents downregulation of key renal water and sodium transport proteins in response to bilateral ureteral obstruction. Am J Physiol 289:F322–F333, 2005.

74. Johnson CE, Elder JS, Judge NE, et al. The accuracy of antenatal ultrasonography in identifying renal abnormalities. Am J Dis Child 146:1181, 1992.

75. Wiener JS, O'Hara SM. Optimal timing of initial postnatal ultrasonography in newborns with prenatal hydronephrosis. J Urol 168:1826, 2002.

76. Conway JJ, Maizels M. The "well tempered" diuretic renogram: A standard method to examine the asymptomatic neonate with hydronephrosis or hydroureteronephrosis. J Nucl Med 33:2047, 1992.

77. Hafez AT, McLorie G, Bägli D, et al. Analysis of trends on serial ultrasound for high grade neonatal hydronephrosis. J Urol 168:1518, 2002.

78. Fernbach SK, Maizels M, Conway JJ. Ultrasound grading of hydronephrosis: Introduction to the system used by the Society for Fetal Urology. Pediatr Radiol 23:478, 1993.

79. Dhillon HK. Prenatally diagnosed hydronephrosis: The Great Ormond Street experience. Br J Urol 81:39, 1998.

80. Ulman I, Jayanthi VR, Koff SA. The long-term followup of newborns with severe unilateral hydronephrosis initially treated nonoperatively. J Urol 164:1101, 2000.

81. Onen A, Jayanthi VR, Koff SA. Long-term followup of prenatally detected severe bilateral newborn hydronephrosis initially managed nonoperatively. J Urol 168:1118, 2002.

82. DiSandro MJ, Kogan BA. Ureteropelvic junction obstruction. Urol Clin North Am 25:187, 1998.

83. McAleer IM, Kaplan GW. Renal function before and after pyeloplasty: Does it improve? J Urol 162:1041, 1999.

84. Capolicchio G, Leonard MP, Wong C, et al. Prenatal diagnosis of hydronephrosis: Impact on renal function and its recovery after pyeloplasty. J Urol 162:1029, 1999.

85. Chertin B, Fridmans A, Knizhnik M, et al. Does early detection of ureteropelvic junction obstruction improve surgical outcome in terms of renal function? J Urol 162:1037, 1999.

86. Eskild-Jensen A, Jorgensen TM, Olsen LH, et al. Renal function may not be restored when using decreasing differential function as the criterion for surgery in unilateral hydronephrosis. BJU Int 92:779, 2003.

87. Chandar J, Abitbol C, Zilleruelo G, et al. Renal tubular abnormalities in infants with hydronephrosis. J Urol 155:660, 1996.

88. Marra G, Goj V, Appiani AC, et al. Persistent tubular resistance to aldosterone in infants with congenital hydronephrosis corrected neonatally. J Pediatr 110:868, 1987.

89. Sharma RK, Sharma AP, Kapoor R, et al. Prognostic factors for persistent distal renal tubular acidosis after surgery for posterior urethral valve. Am J Kid Dis 38:488, 2001.

90. Roth KS, Carter WH Jr, Chan JCM. Obstructive nephropathy in children: Long-term progression after relief of posterior urethral valve. Pediatrics 107:1004, 2001.

91. Ylinen E, Ala-Houhala M, Wikstrom S. Prognostic factors of posterior urethral valves and the role of antenatal detection. Pediatr Nephrol 19:874, 2004.

92. Gulbis B, Jauniaux E, Jurkovic D, et al. Biochemical investigation of fetal renal maturation in early pregnancy. Pediatr Res 39:731, 1996.

93. Woolf AS. A molecular and genetic view of human renal and urinary tract malformations. Kidney Int 58:500, 2000.

94. Hsieh YY, Chang CC, Lee CC, et al. Fetal renal volume assessment by three-dimensional ultrasonography. Am J Obstet Gynecol 182:377, 2000.

95. Higgins DF, Lappin DWP, Kieran NE, et al. DNA oligonucleotide microarray technology identifies fisp-12 among other potential fibrogenic genes following murine unilateral ureteral obstruction (UUO): Modulation during epithelial-mesenchymal transition. Kidney Int 64:2079, 2003.

96. Silverstein DM, Travis BR, Thornhill BA, et al. Altered expression of immune modulator and structural genes in neonatal unilateral ureteral obstruction. Kidney Int 64:25, 2003.

97. Seseke F, Thelen P, Ringert RH. Characterization of an animal model of spontaneous congenital unilateral obstructive uropathy by cDNA microarray analysis. Eur Urol 45:374, 2004.

98. Liapis H. Biology of congenital obstructive nephropathy. Exp Nephrol 93:87, 2003.

99. Chevalier RL. Biomarkers of congenital obstructive nephropathy: Past, present and future. J Urol 172:852, 2004.

100. Chung KH, Chevalier RL. Arrested development of the neonatal kidney following chronic ureteral obstruction. J Urol 155:1139, 1996.

101. Misseri R, Meldrum DR, Dinarello CA, et al. TNF-alpha mediates obstruction-induced renal tubular cell apoptosis and proapoptotic signaling. Am J Physiol 288:F406–F411, 2004.

102. Stephan M, Conrad S, Eggert T, et al. Urinary concentration and tissue messenger RNA expression of monocyte chemoattractant protein-1 as an indicator of the degree of hydronephrotic atrophy in partial ureteral obstruction. J Urol 167:1497, 2002.

103. El Sherbiny MT, Mousa M, Shokeir AA, et al. Role of urinary transforming growth factor-β1 concentration in the diagnosis of upper urinary tract obstruction in children. J Urol 168:1798, 2002.

104. Valles P, Pascual L, Manucha W, et al. Role of endogenous nitric oxide in unilateral ureteropelvic junction obstruction in children. Kidney Int 63:1104, 2003.

105. Grandaliano G, Gesualdo L, Bartoli F, et al. MCP-1 and EGF renal expression and urine excretion in human congenital obstructive nephropathy. Kidney Int 58:182, 2000.

106. Chevalier RL. Obstructive nephropathy: Towards biomarker discovery and gene therapy. Nat Clin Prac Nephrol 2:157, 2006.

107. Yang EY, Flake AW, Adzick NS. Prospects for fetal gene therapy. Sem Perinatol 23:524, 1999.

108. Pope JC, Brock JW III, Adams MC, et al. Congenital anomalies of the kidney and urinary tract—Role of the loss of function mutation in the pluripotent angiotensin type 2 receptor gene. J Urol 165:196, 2001.

109. Rigoli L, Chimenz R, di Bella C, et al. Angiotensin-converting enzyme and angiotensin type 2 receptor gene genotype distributions in Italian children with congenital uropathies. Pediatr Res 56:988, 2004.

110. Hohenfellner K, Wingen A-M, Nauroth O, et al. Impact of ACE I/D gene polymorphism on congenital renal malformations. Pediatr Nephrol 16:356, 2001.

111. Bajpai M, Pratap A, Somitesh C, et al. Angiotensin converting enzyme gene polymorphism in Asian Indian children with congenital uropathies. J Urol 171:838, 2004.

Index

A

acid-base balance
  fetal kidneys and, 67
  normal growth and, 72, 73
  sodium homeostasis and, 47, 48
  See also acidosis
acid load
  elimination
    fetoplacental, 67, 68
    postnatal, 68–70
  See also acid-base balance; acid load; acidosis: metabolic;
    alkalosis
acidosis
  metabolic
    fetal, 67–70
    maternal renal compensation of, 68
    in premature infants, 73
    renal compensation of, 69
  respiratory, 67
  See also acid-base balance; acid load; alkalosis
acute tubular necrosis (ATN), 212, 213
adenosine
  glomerular filtration rate and, 81
  tubuloglomerular feedback and, 118
adenosine triphosphate (ATP), 118
ADH-escape, 131. *See also* antidiuretic hormone
adrenocortical hormones
  fetal programming and, 46, 47
  receptors, 108, 109
aldosterone
  -mediated distal reabsorption, 35
  plasma concentration, 45
  potassium secretion and, 58, 59
  relative insensitivity to, 70
alkalosis
  metabolic, 69, 71
  respiratory, 70, 71
  See also acid-base balance; acidosis
amiloride-sensitive epithelial sodium channel (ENaC),
  37, 38
amniotic fluid
  arginine vasopressin and, 132
  composition, 5
  developmental changes in, 44, 45
  dynamics, 26, 27
  nitrogenous waste products in, 5
  sodium metabolism in, 27
  sources, 6
  volume, 5, 6
    developmental changes in, 155, 231
    intrauterine growth restriction and, 155
    metabolism, 27
    regulation, 8, 26, 27
angiotensin
  I (Ang I), 107, 108, 120
  II (Ang II)
    action, 108, 111–113
    glomerular filtration and, 81
    heteromeric G-proteins and, 110
    metabolites, 108, 109

angiotensin *(Continued)*
  production, 107–109, 111
  receptors, 114, 115
    AT_1, 109, 111, 114, 119, 120
    AT_2, 109, 111
    AT_3, 110
    AT_4, 110
    gene targeting of, 110
  -related genes, 113
  See also angiotensin converting enzyme; renin-
    angiotensin-aldosterone system
angiotensin converting enzyme
  action, 107, 108
  expression, 108
  fetal growth and development and, 113, 114, 208, 209
  See also angiotensin; angiotensin converting enzyme
    inhibitor
angiotensin converting enzyme inhibitor (ACEI), 91,
  113, 114
angiotensinogen, 107–109, 114
angiotensin receptor blocker (ARB), 113, 114, 208, 209
angiotensin II receptor antagonists (ARA), 91
antidiuretic hormone (ADH), 131, 134
anuria, 113, 114, 209, 210, 215
aquaglyceroporins, 13
aquaporins
  arginine vasopressin and, 130, 131
  brain-specific (AQP4), 25, 26
  characteristics, 13, 14
  density, 229–232
  expression, 15, 131, 201
  forms of, 14
  function, 13, 14, 107
  mechanism of action, 8
  membrane, 14, 15
  placental, 14, 15,
arginine vasopressin
  action, 130, 131
    modulation of, 131
    in neonatal kidney, 132
    placental, 131, 132
  in amniotic fluid, 132
  aquaporins and, 130, 131 (*see also* aquaporins)
  characteristics, 129
  in fetus, 132
  genes, 129
  modulation of water excretion by, 129, 131
  in newborn, 132, 133
  receptors, 130–132
  secretion, 129, 130
  synthesis, 129
AT_1 receptor-associated protein (ATRAP), 110. *See also*
  angiotensin: receptors
AT_2 receptor-interacting protein (ATIP1), 110
atrial natriuretic peptide (ANP)
  actions, 135, 136
    in cardiovascular disease, 140
    in circulatory transition at birth, 30, 138, 139
    in kidney, 138
    modulation of, 136